The Clinical Practice of Chinese Medicine:

Pelvic Inflammatory Disease & Miscarriage

by **Huang Jian-ling & Liang Xue-fang**

Translated by **Jiang Qian, Mei Li & Song Qi**

Editied by **Mei Li**

CBS Publishers & Distributors Pvt Ltd

New Delhi • Bengaluru • Chennai • Kochi • Kolkata • Mumbai
Bhubaneswar • Hyderabad • Jharkhand • Nagpur • Patna • Pune • Uttarakhand

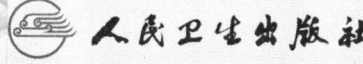

PMPH   PEOPLE'S MEDICAL PUBLISHING HOUSE

The Clinical Practice of Chinese Medicine:
Pelvic Inflammatory Disease & Miscarriage
中医临床实用系列：盆腔炎与流产

ISBN: 978-93-86827-74-6

CBS Edition: 2019

This edition has been published by CBS Publishers & Distributors under arrangement with People's Medical Publishing House

First published: 2006

PMPH ISBN: 7-117-08060-4/R · 8061

Not for sale outside India, Pakistan, Nepal, Bhutan and Sri Lanka.

Library of Congress Cataloguing in Publication Data:
A catalog record for this book is available from the Library of Congress

Published by Satish Kumar Jain and produced by Varun Jain for

CBS Publishers & Distributors Pvt Ltd
4819/XI Prahlad Street, 24 Ansari Road, Daryaganj, New Delhi 110 002, India.
Ph: 23289259, 23266861, 23266867   Website: www.cbspd.com
Fax: 011-23243014   e-mail: delhi@cbspd.com; cbspubs@airtelmail.in.

Corporate Office: 204 FIE, Industrial Area, Patparganj, Delhi 110 092
Ph: 4934 4934   Fax: 4934 4935   e-mail: publishing@cbspd.com; publicity@cbspd.com

Branches

- **Bengaluru:** Seema House 2975, 17th Cross, K.R. Road, Banasankari 2nd Stage, Bengaluru 560 070, Karnataka, India
  Ph: +91-80-26771678/79   Fax: +91-80-26771680   e-mail: bangalore@cbspd.com

- **Chennai:** 7, Subbaraya Street, Shenoy Nagar, Chennai 600 030, Tamil Nadu, India.
  Ph: +91-44-26680620, 26681266   Fax: +91-44-42032115   e-mail: chennai@cbspd.com

- **Kochi:** 42/1325, 1326, Power House Road, Opposite KSEB Power House, Ernakulam 682 018, Kochi, Kerala, India.
  Ph: +91-484-4059061-65   Fax: +91-484-4059065   e-mail: kochi@cbspd.com

- **Kolkata:** 6/B, Ground Floor, Rameswar Shaw Road, Kolkata-700 014, West Bengal, India
  Ph: +91-33-22891126, 22891127, 22891128   e-mail: kolkata@cbspd.com

- **Mumbai:** 83-C, Dr E Moses Road, Worli, Mumbai-400018, Maharashtra, India
  Ph: +91-22-24902340/41   Fax: +91-22-24902342   e-mail: mumbai@cbspd.com

Representatives
- **Bhubaneswar** 0-9911037372   • **Hyderabad** 0-9885175004   • **Jharkhand** 0-9811541605   • **Nagpur** 0-9021734563
- **Patna** 0-9334159340   • **Pune** 0-9623451994   • **Uttarakhand** 0-9716462459

Printed at Nutech Print Services - India

About the Authors

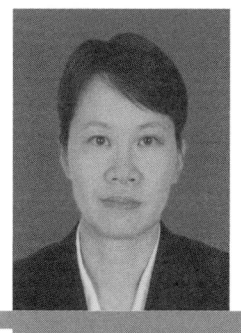

梁雪芳　教授

Professor **Liang Xue-fang** serves as an associate professor and state-approved Master's level advisor at the Second Clinical Medical College of Guangzhou University of Chinese Medicine (also known as Traditional Chinese Medicine Hospital of Guangdong Province). She has worked in the Chinese medical clinical department of gynecology for 17 years, and specializes in treating diseases such as endometriosis, pelvic inflammatory masses, infertility, benign and malignant tumors, and other gynecological diseases. Due to her solid foundation in Chinese medical theory and her rich clinical experience, her expertise is the treatment of obstinate gynecological disease. In 2004, she was appointed by the State Hospital of Hong Kong to develop clinical and scientific research in the field of Chinese medicine.

Professor Liang participated in the editing and publication of *Integration of Chinese and Western Medicine in Gynecology and Obstetrics* and *Integration of Chinese and Western Medicine in the Treatment of Endometriosis*. She managed the "Preclinical Research on *E Leng* Capsules 莪棱胶囊", a study funded by the State Administration of Traditional Chinese Medicine. She also managed the exploratory development of teaching methods using "Case Introduction Form" in the gynecology & obstetrics department of the seven-year integrative medicine program at Guangzhou TCM University. The clinical research on the usage of E Leng Capsules to treat endometriosis was awarded the "Second Prize of Science & Improvement" in 1999 by the Traditional Chinese Medicine Administration of Guangdong Province.

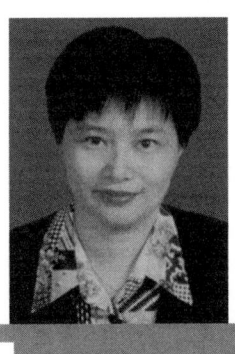

黄健玲　教授

Professor **Huang Jian-ling** was born on April, 1956. She is a professor, chief physician, and state-approved Doctoral advisor at the Second Clinical Medicine College of Guangzhou University of Chinese Medicine (also known as Chinese Medicine Hospital of Guangdong Province). She is also the Director of the Genealogy Department at this hospital. She was chosen to be a successor of a famous senior physician in the national Master and Apprentice Education Program. In addition, she is a standing member of the Family Planning Board under the Guangdong Branch of the Chinese Medicine Association, as well as a member of the Obstetrics and Gynecology Board of the Guangdong Provincial Medicine Association.

Professor Huang is fond of of clinical practice and scientific research, and advocates treatment based on pattern differentiation of signs and symptoms. She specializes in using classical formulas to treat gynecological emergencies and intractable diseases. She is particularly masterful at treating urgent & chronic PID, pelvic inflammation, infertility associated with salpingemphraxis and endometriosis using an integration of traditional Chinese medical and Western medical approaches. She has acquired many Master's and Doctoral level students, and has helped to foster a large group of experts in the field of Chinese medical gynecology.

Professor Huang has 24 years of clinical experience in gynecology, and a strong teaching and research background in the integration of traditional Chinese medicine & Western medicine. She has hosted & participated in 13 topics of scientific research on national, provincial and bureau levels, and has published 30 research papers in several magazines, as well as 6 monographs. She has won 8 clinical and teaching achievement awards.

Foreword

Chinese medicine is a broad and profound art of healing. It is a well-established and comprehensive system of medicine with an ancient origin and a long rich history. Throughout the ages, it has made a significant contribution to the prosperity of the Chinese civilization. The system of pattern differentiation and treatment fully reflects the Chinese medical view of health and disease as a holistic concept, the emphasis on the body's ability to regulate itself and adapt to the environment, and the need for individualized treatment. The integration of diseases and syndromes is the consummation of treatment based on pattern differentiation; it fully displays the superior characteristic of this discipline, and has an extensive influence on the development of the art of Chinese medicine.

The intention of this series of books is to introduce accurate Chinese medical diagnosis and treatment of various diseases to overseas readers.

The Chinese edition of *The Clinical Practice of Chinese Medicine* was edited by the Traditional Chinese Medicine Hospital of Guangdong Province (also known as the Second Affiliated Hospital of Guangzhou Chinese Medical University), and published by People's Medical Publishing House. When the series was published in 2000, it was widely accepted in clinical practice due to its originality, distinguishing features, richness in content, completeness, accuracy, and outstanding emphases. This series has become a trademark of standard in the eyes of Chinese and integrative medical practitioners. During the second printing of this series of books, Professor Deng Tie-tao praised, "For a series to be printed a multiple number of times, shows that it is highly regarded and has received excellent reviews." In order to keep up with the constant development of medical science, this series was revised and re-published in 2004 by People's Medical Publishing House. Due to its popularity, it has been reprinted numerous times since.

The English edition of this series of books includes 17 volumes:
- ✧ *COPD & Asthma*
- ✧ *Stroke & Parkinson's Disease*
- ✧ *Coronary Artery Disease & Hyperlipidemia*
- ✧ *Chronic Gastritis & Irritable Bowel Syndrome*
- ✧ *Diabetes & Obesity*
- ✧ *Gout & Rheumatoid Arthritis*
- ✧ *Menstrual Disorders I: Dysfunctional Uterine Bleeding & Amenorrhea*
- ✧ *Menstrual Disorders 2: Premenstrual Syndrome, Dysmenorrhea & Perimenopause*
- ✧ *Endometriosis & Uterine Fibroids*
- ✧ *Pelvic Inflammatory Disease & Miscarriage*
- ✧ *Insufficient Lactation & Fibrocystic Breast Disease*
- ✧ *Male & Female Infertility*
- ✧ *Eczema, Urticaria & Atopic Dermatitis*
- ✧ *Connective Tissue Diseases of the Skin*
- ✧ *Diseases of the Accessory Organs ot the Skin*
- ✧ *Fungal Infections & Pigmentary Disorders of the Skin*
- ✧ *Psoriasis, Cutaneous Pruritis & Herpes Zoster*

Clinical application varies by individual and by location; when this is combined with the rapid development of medical science, the treatment methods and medicinal dosages may also vary accordingly. When using these books as a reference guide, overseas readers should confirm the formulas and dosages of medicinals according to the individual health condition of the patient, as well as take into account the origin of the Chinese medicinals.

The quotes in these books were taken from various medical literature during the compilation process. We have deleted some of the contents of the original texts for the purpose of uniformity and ease in readability. We ask for the reader's forgiveness and express our respect and gratitude toward the original authors.

Due to the complicated nature of the diagnoses and treatments covered in these books, and the wide range of topics they touches upon, it is inevitable that one may encounter errors while reading through them. We respectively welcome constructive criticism and corrections from our readers.

The clinical practice of medicine changes with the constant development of medical science. The books in this series will be revised regularly to continuously adapt to the development of traditional Chinese medicine.

Editorial Board of the English edition of
The Clinical Practice of Chinese Medicine series
September, 2006

Editor's Preface

People's Medical Publishing House has invested much time into researching the Chinese medical education and practice overseas. The knowledge we have gathered from our investigation has given us a better understanding of what is needed to help further the development of Chinese medicine outside of China. The publication of the English edition of *The Clinical Practice of Chinese Medicine* series is the outcome of this arduous effort to improve the skill level of practitioners. We sincerely believe that this series of books will assist students of Chinese medicine in honing their ability to diagnose and treat a wide range of common clinical diseases.

In these books, readers shall find a very organized and thorough presentation of each disease, including its brief overview, etiology, pathomechanism, Chinese medical treatment using various treatment modalities, integrative treatment approaches, quotes from classical texts, comments of famous physicians, case studies, and modern research. We believe that these books will prove useful and valuable to all those involved in the field of Chinese medicine, which includes practitioners, students, teachers, patients and anyone who may be seeking answers to their questions about the efficacy of Chinese medicine.

Due to the nature of clinical medicine, we apologize for any out-dated or incorrect information that may appear in these books, and hope that readers will not hesitate to offer their comments and suggestions on how to improve the content of this material.

Mei Li, editor

September, 2006

Contents

Miscarriage ······· 149

盆腔炎

Pelvic Inflammatory Disease
by Huang Jian-ling, He Cheng-qun & Shen Bi-qiong

- ✦ OVERVIEW
- ✦ CHINESE MEDICAL ETIOLOGY AND PATHOMECHANISM
- ✦ CHINESE MEDICAL TREATMENT
- ✦ PROGNOSIS
- ✦ PREVENTIVE HEALTHCARE
- ✦ CLINICAL EXPERIENCE OF RENOWNED PHYSICIANS
- ✦ PERSPECTIVES OF INTEGRATIVE MEDICINE
- ✦ SELECTED QUOTES FROM CLASSICAL TEXTS
- ✦ MODERN RESEARCH
- ✦ REFERENCES

OVERVIEW

Pelvic inflammatory disease (PID) refers to the inflammation of the female internal genital organs (including the uterus, the fallopian tube and the ovaries), the surrounding connective tissue and pelvic peritoneum. The inflammation may be confined to one location or occur simultaneously in several locations. Depending on the onset of the disease, the clinical manifestations can be divided into two categories – acute pelvic inflammatory disease (acute PID) and chronic pelvic inflammatory disease (chronic PID). The chief symptoms of acute PID are aversion to cold, fever and chills (high fever and shivering if severe), lower abdominal pain that refuses pressure, and profuse thick, yellow, foul-smelling vaginal discharge. When the disease is active during menstruation, there may be profuse menstrual bleeding and prolonged menstruation. If there is peritonitis, it may be accompanied by symptoms of the digestive tract, such as nausea, vomiting, abdominal distention and diarrhea. If the urethra is affected, there may be difficult, frequent and painful urination. Involvement of the rectum may manifest as tenesmus, diarrhea or constipation.

Patients often present with a sickly complexion, elevated body temperature, rapid heart rate, abdominal distention, muscular tension, tenderness and rebound tenderness in the lower abdomen, and decreased or an absence of bowel sounds. Gynecological examination will reveal an increase in purulent vaginal discharge, tenderness of the fornix (the upper part of the vagina surrounding the cervix), pronounced lifting pain of the cervix, slight enlargement of the uterine body with tenderness and limitation of motion, bilateral thickening of the uterus, or palpable masses with pronounced tenderness.

The main symptoms of chronic PID are heaviness, distention, and pain of the lower abdomen, aching pain in the lumbosacral portion that is always exacerbated by exertion and sexual intercourse, and intensified before and after menstruation. It may be accompanied by symptoms of low-grade fever, profuse menses, menstrual irregularities, excessive leukorrhea and infertility. Some patients may suffer from depression, discomfort of the entire body and insomnia. When the patient's natural resistance to disease is compromised, she will be susceptible to acute or subacute episodes. Gynecological examination will often reveal retroposition of the uterus with limited mobility, thickening of one or both sides of the uterus, or palpable masses with pronounced tenderness.

In biomedicine, it is believed that a woman's natural defense is damaged by labor, abortion, poor menstrual hygiene, and surgeries of the uterus and pelvic cavity. This allows the pathogens to invade the internal genitals, the surrounding connective tissues and the pelvic cavity, thus resulting in PID. The pathogens originate from two sources --the microbial population that lives inside the vagina, and pathogens that come from the external environment. The pathogens may be simple aerobes, simple anaerobes, or a combination of both, and may be accompanied by sexually transmitted disease. The diagnosis can be determined from the case history, signs and symptoms. Routine blood test, routine urinalysis, inspection of the secretions of the cervical canal and puncturing of the posterior fornix are required to confirm the diagnosis.

The treatment of acute PID is focused on the integration of Chinese medicine and biomedicine. Biomedical treatment is primarily to prescribe antibiotics of maximum dosage. If there is abscess formation, surgery is required. Chinese medical treatment with Chinese medicinals can, not only alleviate the side effects of antibiotics, but also assist the antibiotics to reinforce the anti-inflammatory effect, which can quickly control the patient's condition and speed recovery. For chronic PID, Chinese medical treatment has advantages over biomedicine. Using a combination of treatment modalities is stressed, including the internal administration of Chinese medicinals, external application of Chinese medicinals, herbal enemas, acupuncture and moxibustion, and physical therapy. In order to prevent and cure recurrent attacks of chronic PID, lifestyle modification should be emphasized as well. It is imperative that patients consume light food and beverages, regulate their emotions, and participate in physical exercise to strengthen their constitution.

In Chinese medicine, PID belongs to the categories of "leukorrhea", "abdominal pain", "heat entering the blood chamber", "postpartum fever", and "concretions and conglomerations (abdominal masses)."

CHINESE MEDICAL ETIOLOGY AND PATHOMECHANISM

Chinese medicine views acute PID as a disease that is commonly induced by factors such as childbirth, abortion, operations involving the uterine cavity, menstruation, and sexual intercourse. During these situations, the uterus and uterine vessels are empty and weak. The blood chamber (referring to the penetrating vessel or uterus) is open, normal qi and blood has been consumed, and static blood accumulation has not yet been exhausted. If the patient is improperly nursed back to health, or if there is incomplete sterilization of tools during surgery, dampness, heat and toxic evil would invade the body due to the insufficiency of right qi. They will combine with qi and blood, and accumulate in the uterus, uterine vessels, uterine collaterals, governing and conception vessels. This struggle between evil qi and right qi causes acute PID.

In Chinese medicine, chronic PID is related to the following factors:

a. Binding Constraint of Damp-heat and Blood Stasis

This is due internal accumulation of damp-heat pouring downward into the lower jiao, obstructing the flow of qi and blood, and causing the accumulation of blood stasis in the penetrating and conception vessels. Another possible cause is accumulated static blood lingering after menstruation or childbirth, leading to the contraction of damp-heat evil. The damp-heat combined with blood obstructs the penetrating vessel, the conception vessel and blood, resulting in this disease.

b. Qi Stagnation and Blood Stasis

Innate depressed disposition or excessive anger influences the free coursing of liver qi, obstructs qi dynamic, and causes qi stagnation and blood stasis, which obstructs the penetrating vessel, conception vessel and uterine vessels, and disturbs the blood, resulting in this disease.

c. Congealing Cold-damp

During menstruation or after childbirth, remnant blood still remains. Walking in the rain, wading, catching colds, cold drink, or living in a cold damp environment for a long period of time leads to cold-dampness injuring the uterine vessel. Blood is congealed by cold-dampness. It obstructs the penetrating and conception vessels and the blood, resulting in this disease.

d. Spleen Deficiency with Binding Constraint of Dampness and Blood Stasis

Innate spleen deficiency, improper diet, exhaustion and tiredness, or excessive thinking injures the function of the spleen. Spleen deficiency leads to a disturbance in transformation and transportation, causing interior turbid dampness which flows downward into the lower burner and combines with blood stasis. The combination of dampness and blood stasis injures the penetrating and conception vessels, resulting in this disease.

e. Kidney Yang Deficiency

Innate deficiency of kidney qi, excessive sexual intercourse, and waning of the life gate fire (*ming men* fire) all lead to a decline in kidney yang. Other factors include poor health habits and contracting wind-cold during menstruation, thus allowing cold evil to invade the interior of the body and harm kidney yang. This leads to the failure to warm the penetrating and conception vessels, and causes the deficient cold of the uterine vessel, resulting in this pattern.

Acute PID occurs mostly as an excess pattern and chronic PID occurs mostly as a combined pattern of excess and deficiency.

CHINESE MEDICAL TREATMENT

1. Pattern Differentiation and Treatment

Acute PID is mostly attributed to exuberant heat toxins or the binding constraint of damp-heat and blood stasis. Chronic PID is mainly attributed to qi stagnation and blood stasis, binding constraint of damp-heat and blood stasis, stagnation of congealing cold-damp, binding constraint of blood stasis, dampness due to spleen deficiency, and deficiency of kidney yang. Treatment should be determined according to the different stages and disease patterns.

a. Exuberant Heat Toxins

【Syndrome Characteristics】 High fever, shivering, lower abdominal pain that refuses pressure, copious thick, sticky, yellow, foul-smelling leukorrhea, dryness and bitter taste in the mouth, nausea, poor appetite, scanty yellow urine, constipation, red tongue with dry yellow or thick greasy coating, and slippery rapid pulse.

【Treatment Principle】 Clear heat, resolve toxins, and drain dampness.

【Commonly Used Medicinals】 Use *jīn yín huā* (Flos Lonicerae Japonicae), *pú gōng yīng* (Herba Taraxaci), *shé shé cǎo* (Herba Hedyotis), *bài jiàng cǎo* (Herba Patriniae) and *hǔ zhàng* (Rhizoma et Radix Polygoni Cuspidati) to clear heat and resolve toxins. Use *huáng bǎi* (Cortex Phellodendri Chinensis), *zé xiè* (Rhizoma Alismatis) and *chē qián zǐ* (Semen Plantaginis) to drain dampness. Use *dà huáng* (Radix et Rhizoma Rhei), *hòu pò* (Cortex Magnoliae Officinalis) and *zhǐ shí* (Fructus Aurantii Immaturus) to purge the bowels and move qi. Use *chì sháo* (Radix Paeoniae Rubra) and *mǔ dān pí* (Cortex Moutan) to invigorate blood and transform blood stasis.

【Representative Formula】 Modified combination of *Wu Wei Xiao Du Yin* 五味消毒饮 and *Xiao Cheng Qi Tang* 小承气汤

【Ingredients】

金银花	jīn yín huā	15g	Flos Lonicerae Japonicae
蒲公英	pú gōng yīng	20g	Herba Taraxaci
黄柏	huáng bǎi	12g	Cortex Phellodendri Chinensis
大黄	dà huáng	10g	Radix et Rhizoma Rhei
厚朴	hòu pò	15g	Cortex Magnoliae Officinalis
枳实	zhǐ shí	15g	Fructus Aurantii Immaturus
败酱草	bài jiàng cǎo	30g	Herba Patriniae
虎杖	hǔ zhàng	15g	Rhizoma et Radix Polygoni Cuspidati
赤芍	chì sháo	15g	Radix Paeoniae Rubra
牡丹皮	mǔ dān pí	15g	Cortex Moutan

Internal Use: Add *dà huáng* (Radix et Rhizoma Rhei) to the decoction in the last 5 to 10 minutes of cooking. The decoction is boiled until 200 ml of liquid remains. Take one half of the warm decoction each time, 2 times a day.

【Formula Analysis】 Use *jīn yín huā* (Flos Lonicerae Japonicae), *pú gōng yīng* (Herba Taraxaci), *huáng bǎi* (Cortex Phellodendri Chinensis), *bài jiàng cǎo* (Herba Patriniae) and *hǔ zhàng* (Rhizoma et Radix Polygoni Cuspidati) to clear heat, resolve toxins, drain dampness and promote discharge of pus. Use *chì sháo* (Radix Paeoniae Rubra) and *mǔ dān pí* (Cortex Moutan) to clear heat and cool the blood. Use *dà huáng* (Radix et Rhizoma Rhei), *hòu pò* (Cortex Magnoliae Officinalis) and *zhǐ shí* (Fructus Aurantii Immaturus) to eliminate heat by purging the bowels.

【Modifications】 For exuberant heat presenting with high fever, add *huáng qín* (Radix Scutellariae) 12g and *lián qiào* (Fructus Forsythiae) 15g to reinforce the effect of clearing heat and resolving toxins.

For dampness presenting with profuse leukorrhea, add *yì yǐ rén* (Semen Coicis) 30g, *zé xiè* (Rhizoma Alismatis) 15g and *chē qián zǐ* (Semen Plantaginis) 15g to drain dampness.

For severe lower abdominal pain, add *xiāng fù* (Rhizoma Cyperi) 12g, *mù xiāng* (Radix Aucklandiae) 9g and *yán hú suǒ* (Rhizoma Corydalis) 12g to regulate qi and alleviate pain.

b. Binding Constraint of Damp-heat and Blood Stasis

【Syndrome Characteristics】 Lower abdominal pain, aching pain in the lumbosacral portion, profuse thick, yellow or white leukorrhea, possibly accompanied by low-grade fever, dryness and bitter taste in the mouth, chest oppression, poor appetite, scanty dark-colored urine, constipation, dusky red tongue with stasis spots, stasis maculae and yellow greasy coating, and wiry rapid or soggy rapid pulse.

【Treatment Principle】 Clear heat and drain dampness; invigorate blood and transform stasis.

【Commonly Used Medicinals】 Use *bài jiàng cǎo* (Herba Patriniae), *Yín huā téng* (Caulis Lonicerae Japonica), *yú xīng cǎo* (Herba Houttuyniae), *chē qián zǐ* (Semen Plantaginis) and *zé xiè* (Rhizoma Alismatis) to clear heat and drain dampness. Use *chì sháo* (Radix Paeoniae Rubra), *mǔ dān pí* (Cortex Moutan) and *dān shēn* (Radix et Rhizoma Salviae Miltiorrhizae) to invigorate blood and transform stasis.

【Representative Formula】 Modified *Zhi Dai Fang* 止带方

【Ingredients】

赤芍	chì sháo	15g	Radix Paeoniae Rubra
牡丹皮	mǔ dān pí	15g	Cortex Moutan
丹参	dān shēn	15g	Radix et Rhizoma Salviae Miltiorrhizae
车前子	chē qián zǐ	15g	Semen Plantaginis
泽泻	zé xiè	15g	Rhizoma Alismatis
栀子	zhī zǐ	10g	Fructus Gardeniae
败酱草	bài jiàng cǎo	20g	Herba Patriniae
银花藤	yín huā téng	20g	Caulis Lonicerae Japonica
大黄	dà huáng	10g	Radix et Rhizoma Rhei
鱼腥草	yú xīng cǎo	20g	Herba Houttuyniae

Internal Use: Add *dà huáng* (Radix et Rhizoma Rhei) to the decoction in the last 5 to 10 minutes of cooking. The decoction is boiled until 100 ml of liquid remains. Take one half of the decoction warm, 2 times a day.

【Formula Analysis】 This formula uses *Yín huā téng* (Caulis Lonicerae Japonica), *bài jiàng cǎo* (Herba Patriniae), *yú xīng cǎo* (Herba Houttuyniae), *zhī zǐ* (Fructus Gardeniae), etc. to clear heat and drain dampness. Use *chì sháo* (Radix Paeoniae Rubra), *mǔ dān pí* (Cortex Moutan) and *dān shēn* (Radix et Rhizoma Salviae Miltiorrhizae), etc. to clear heat, cool blood, invigorate blood and transform blood stasis. Use *chē qián zǐ* (Semen Plantaginis) and *zé xiè* (Rhizoma Alismatis) to promote water flow and leach out dampness. Use *dà huáng* (Radix et Rhizoma Rhei) to eliminate heat by purging the bowels, invigorate blood and transform stasis.

【Modifications】 For exuberant heat with fever, dryness and bitter taste in the mouth, add *huáng qín* (Radix Scutellariae) 12g and *huáng bǎi* (Cortex Phellodendri Chinensis) 12g to clear heat.

For excessive dampness with profuse leukorrhea, add *chuān bì xiè* (Rhizoma Dioscoreae Septemlobae) 15g and *tǔ fú líng* (Rhizoma Smilacis Glabrae) 15g to clear heat, and drain dampness.

For severe lower abdominal pain, add *xiāng fù* (Rhizoma Cyperi) 12g and *yán hú suǒ* (Rhizoma Corydalis) 12g to regulate qi and alleviate pain.

For inflamed palpable masses, add *sān léng* (Rhizoma Sparganii) 10g and *é zhú* (Rhizoma Curcumae) 10g to invigorate blood and disperse concretions.

c. Qi Stagnation and Blood Stasis

【Syndrome Characteristics】 Lower abdominal pain, lower abdominal distention and heaviness, aching pain in the lumbosacral area, profuse thick, yellow or white leukorrhea, depression, belching, sighing, premenstrual breast distention and pain, dusky red tongue with stasis spots, stasis maculae and thin white coating, and wiry rough pulse.

【Treatment Principle】 Invigorate blood and transform stasis. Regulate qi and alleviate pain.

【Commonly Used Medicinals】 Use *dāng guī* (Radix Angelicae Sinensis), *chì sháo* (Radix Paeoniae Rubra), *dān shēn* (Radix et Rhizoma Salviae Miltiorrhizae) and *mǔ dān pí* (Cortex Moutan) to invigorate blood and transform stasis. Use *xiāng fù* (Rhizoma Cyperi), *mù xiāng* (Radix Aucklandiae) and *zhǐ qiào* (Fructus Aurantii) to regulate qi and move stagnation.

【Representative Formula】 Modified *Pen Yan Fang* 盆炎方
【Ingredients】

当归	dāng guī	12g	Radix Angelicae Sinensis
赤芍	chì sháo	15g	Radix Paeoniae Rubra
牡丹皮	mǔ dān pí	12g	Cortex Moutan
丹参	dān shēn	20g	Radix et Rhizoma Salviae Miltiorrhizae
香附	xiāng fù	12g	Rhizoma Cyperi
木香	mù xiāng	9g	Radix Aucklandiae
枳壳	zhǐ qiào	12g	Fructus Aurantii
车前子	chē qián zǐ	15g	Semen Plantaginis
败酱草	bài jiàng cǎo	15g	Herba Patriniae
毛冬青	máo dōng qīng	15g	Radix Ilicis Pubescentis

Internal Use: Add *mù xiāng* (Radix Aucklandiae) in the last 5 to 10 minutes of cooking. The decoction is boiled until 100 ml of liquid remains. Take one half of the warm decoction each time, 2 times a day.

【Formula Analysis】 In this formula, *chì sháo* (Radix Paeoniae Rubra), *mǔ dān pí* (Cortex Moutan) and *dān shēn* (Radix et Rhizoma Salviae Miltiorrhizae) are used to clear heat, cool blood, invigorate blood and transform stasis. *Dāng guī* (Radix Angelicae Sinensis) is used to nourish blood, invigorate blood and transform stasis. *Xiāng fù* (Rhizoma Cyperi), *mù xiāng* (Radix Aucklandiae) and *zhǐ qiào* (Fructus Aurantii) regulate qi and alleviate pain. *Chē qián zǐ* (Semen Plantaginis) and *bài jiàng cǎo* (Herba Patriniae) clear heat, resolve toxins and drain dampness. *Máo dōng qīng* (Radix Ilecis Pubescens) is used here to invigorate blood, transform blood stasis, clear heat and drain dampness.

【Modifications】 For pronounced severe lower abdominal pain, add *yán hú suǒ* (Rhizoma Corydalis) 12g and *wū yào* (Radix Linderae) 12g to regulate qi and alleviate pain.

For cold and blood stasis pattern presenting with lower abdominal coldness and pain, add *guì zhī* (Ramulus Cinnamomi) 10g and *xiǎo huí xiāng* (Fructus Foeniculi) 6g to warm the channels and disperse cold.

For exuberant dampness pattern with profuse leukorrhea, add *chuān bì xiè* (Rhizoma Dioscoreae Septemlobae) 15g, *yì yǐ rén* (Semen Coicis) 30g and *zé xiè* (Rhizoma Alismatis) 15g to clear heat and drain dampness.

d. Congealing Cold-damp

【Syndrome Characteristics】 Lower abdominal pain with coldness and limitation of motion that is alleviated by warmth, aching pain in the lumbosacral area, profuse thin white leukorrhea, physical cold and cold limbs, greenish white complexion, pale dusky tongue, white greasy coating and deep tight pulse.

【Treatment Principle】 Disperse cold and eliminate dampness; invigorate blood and transform stasis.

【Commonly Used Medicinals】 Use *guì zhī* (Ramulus Cinnamomi) and *xiǎo huí xiāng* (Fructus Foeniculi) to warm the channels and dispel cold-damp. Use *dāng guī* (Radix Angelicae Sinensis), *dān shēn* (Radix et Rhizoma Salviae Miltiorrhizae), *chì sháo* (Radix Paeoniae Rubra) and *chuān xiōng* (Rhizoma Chuanxiong) to invigorate blood and transform stasis. Use *yán hú suǒ* (Rhizoma Corydalis) and *tái wū yào* (Radix Linderae) to regulate qi and alleviate pain.

【Representative Formula】 Modified *Shao Fu Zhu Yu Tang* 少腹逐瘀汤

【Ingredients】

桂枝	guì zhī	10g	Ramulus Cinnamomi
小茴香	xiǎo huí xiāng	6g	Fructus Foeniculi
当归	dāng guī	15g	Radix Angelicae Sinensis
川芎	chuān xiōng	10g	Rhizoma Chuanxiong
赤芍	chì sháo	12g	Radix Paeoniae Rubra
丹参	dān shēn	15g	Radix et Rhizoma Salviae Miltiorrhizae
茯苓	fú líng	20g	Poria
白木	bái zhú	15g	Rhizoma Atractylodis Macrocephalae
台乌药	tái wū yào	12g	Radix Linderae
延胡索	yán hú suǒ	12g	Rhizoma Corydalis

Internal Use: The decoction is boiled until 100 ml of liquid remains. Take one half of the decoction warm, 2 times a day.

【Formula Analysis】 In this formula, use *guì zhī* (Ramulus Cinnamomi) and *xiǎo huí xiāng* (Fructus Foeniculi) to warm the channels, disperse cold and alleviate pain. Use *dāng guī* (Radix Angelicae Sinensis), *chuān xiōng* (Rhizoma Chuanxiong) and *chì sháo* (Radix Paeoniae Rubra) to invigorate blood and transform stasis. Use *tái wū yào* (Radix Linderae) and *yán hú suǒ* (Rhizoma Corydalis) to regulate qi and alleviate pain. Use *fú ling* (Poria) and *bái zhú* (Rhizoma Atractylodis Macrocephalae) to warm the middle jiao and strengthen the spleen.

【Modifications】 For predominant dampness pattern with profuse leukorrhea, add *chuān bì xiè* (Rhizoma Dioscoreae Septemlobae) 15g and *yì yǐ rén* (Semen Coicis) 20g to drain dampness.

For cases accompanied by spleen deficiency with the symptoms of lassitude and weakness, add *dǎng shēn* (Radix Codonopsis) 15g and *huáng qí* (Radix Astragali) 15g to strengthen the spleen and benefit qi.

For cases accompanied by kidney deficiency with the symptom of aching pain in the lumbosacral area, add *chuān xù duàn* (Radix Dipsaci) 15g and *sāng jì shēng* (Herba Taxilli) 15g to warm and invigorate kidney qi.

For severe lower abdominal pain, add *bài jiàng cǎo* (Herba Patriniae) 15g and *máo dōng qīng* (Radix Ilicis Pubescentis) 20g to clear heat, drain dampness, invigorate blood and transform stasis.

e. Spleen Deficiency with Binding Constraint of Dampness and Blood Stasis

【**Syndrome Characteristics**】 Dull pain in the lower abdomen, lower abdominal distention and heaviness, aching pain in the lumbosacral area that is worse on exertion, slightly increased quantity of thin white leukorrhea without foul odor, lassitude and weakness, poor appetite, loose stool, pale dusky tongue with stasis spots, stasis maculae, white or greasy coating, and moderate weak pulse.

【**Treatment Principle**】 Strengthen the spleen and transform dampness; invigorate blood and transform stasis.

【**Commonly Used Medicinals**】 Use *dǎng shēn* (Radix Codonopsis), *bái zhú* (Rhizoma Atractylodis Macrocephalae), *cāng zhú* (Rhizoma Atractylodis) and *fú líng* (Poria) to strengthen the spleen and drain dampness. Use *dāng guī* (Radix Angelicae Sinensis), *chì sháo* (Radix Paeoniae Rubra), *dān shēn* (Radix et Rhizoma Salviae Miltiorrhizae), *yù jīn* (Radix Curcumae) and *xiāng fù* (Rhizoma Cyperi) to invigorate blood and transform stasis.

【**Representative Formula**】 Modified combination of *Wan Dai Tang* 完带汤 and *Pen Yan Fang* 盆炎方

【Ingredients】

丹参	dān shēn	15g	Radix et Rhizoma Salviae Miltiorrhizae
赤芍	chì sháo	12g	Radix Paeoniae Rubra
当归	dāng guī	12g	Radix Angelicae Sinensis
茯苓	fú líng	20g	Poria
白术	bái zhú	12g	Rhizoma Atractylodis Macrocephalae
党参	dǎng shēn	15g	Radix Codonopsis
郁金	yù jīn	15g	Radix Curcumae
香附	xiāng fù	12g	Rhizoma Cyperi
车前子	chē qián zǐ	15g	Semen Plantaginis
苍术	cāng zhú	10g	Rhizoma Atractylodis
炙甘草	zhì gān cǎo	6g	Radix et Rhizoma Glycyrrhizae Praeparata cum Melle

Internal Use: Take 1 bag a day. The decoction is boiled to 100 ml. Take one half of the decoction after warming every time, 2 times a day.

【Formula Analysis】 In this formula, use *bái zhú* (Rhizoma Atractylodis Macrocephalae), *shān yào* (Rhizoma Dioscoreae) and *fú líng* (Poria) to strengthen the spleen and transform dampness. Use *dǎng shēn* (Radix Codonopsis) to tonify middle qi. Use *cāng zhú* (Rhizoma Atractylodis) to dry dampness and move the spleen so as to reinforce the functions of dispelling dampness and transforming turbidity. Use *dān shēn* (Radix et Rhizoma Salviae Miltiorrhizae), *chì sháo* (Radix Paeoniae Rubra), *dāng guī* (Radix Angelicae Sinensis), *xiāng fù* (Rhizoma Cyperi) and *yù jīn* (Radix Curcumae) to invigorate blood and transform stasis. Use *chē qián zǐ* (Semen Plantaginis) to clear heat and drain dampness.

【Modifications】 For pronounced constitutional deficiency, add *huáng qí* (Radix Astragali) 15g to reinforce tonifying qi and strengthening the spleen.

For especially severe lower abdominal pain, add *yán hú suǒ* (Rhizoma Corydalis) 12g and *bài jiàng cǎo* (Herba Patriniae) 20g to regulate qi, drain dampness and alleviate pain.

For exuberant dampness, add *yì yǐ rén* (Semen Coicis) 30g and *chuān bì xiè* (Rhizoma Dioscoreae Septemlobae) 15g to enhance the function of draining dampness.

f. Kidney Yang Deficiency

【**Syndrome Characteristics**】 Profuse thin watery leukorrhea, fear of cold, cold limbs, dizziness, tinnitus, a sore lower back (as if sprained), cold sensation of the lower abdomen, lesser abdominal pain with heaviness, urine, frequent clear copious urination, increased nocturia, loose stools, pale tongue with thin white coating, and deep slow pulse.

【**Treatment Principle**】 Warm the kidney and nourish original qi; check leukorrhea by securing and astricting.

【**Commonly Used Medicinals**】 Use *shú fù zǐ* (Radix Aconiti Lateralis Praeparata), *ròu guì* (Cortex Cinnamomi), *bǔ gǔ zhī* (Fructus Psoraleae) and *yín yáng huò* (Herba Epimedii) to warm the kidney and nourish original qi. Use *huáng qí* (Radix Astragali), *bái zhú* (Rhizoma Atractylodis Macrocephalae), *fú líng* (Poria) and *dǎng shēn* (Radix Codonopsis), to warm and tonify spleen yang. Use *sāng piāo xiāo* (Oötheca Mantidis) and *jīn yīng zǐ* (Fructus Rosae Laevigatae) to stop leukorrhea by securing and astricting.

【**Representative Formula**】 Modified *Nèi Bǔ Wán* 内补丸

【**Ingredients**】

熟附子	shú fù zǐ	9g	Radix Aconiti Lateralis Praeparata
肉桂	ròu guì	1.5g	Cortex Cinnamomi
补骨脂	bǔ gǔ zhī	15g	Fructus Psoraleae
淫羊藿	yín yáng huò	12g	Herba Epimedii
菟丝子	tù sī zǐ	15g	Semen Cuscutae
黄芪	huáng qí	20g	Radix Astragali
白术	bái zhú	15g	Rhizoma Atractylodis Macrocephalae
茯苓	fú líng	20g	Poria
当归	dāng guī	15g	Radix Angelicae Sinensis
桑螵蛸	sāng piāo xiāo	9g	Oötheca Mantidis

Internal Use: Steam *ròu guì* (Cortex Cinnamomi) for internal use and put the other medicinals in water to decoct. The decoction is boiled until 100 ml of liquid remains. Take one half of the decoction warm each time, 2 times a day.

【Formula Analysis】 In this formula, *shú fù zǐ* (Radix Aconiti Lateralis Praeparata), *ròu guì* (Cortex Cinnamomi), *bǔ gǔ zhī* (Fructus Psoraleae) and *yín yáng huò* (Herba Epimedii) to warm and invigorate kidney yang, tonify kidney and nourish original qi. Use *huáng qí* (Radix Astragali) to replenish the middle jiao and tonify qi. Use *bái zhú* (Rhizoma Atractylodis Macrocephalae), *fú líng* (Poria) and *dāng guī* (Radix Angelicae Sinensis) to warm the middle jiao, strengthen the spleen and alleviate pain. Use *sāng piāo xiāo* (Oötheca Mantidis) to arrest spontaneous emission and leukorrhea.

【Modifications】 For blood stasis pattern with severe lesser abdominal pain, add *chì sháo* (Radix Paeoniae Rubra) 15g and *dān shēn* (Radix et Rhizoma Salviae Miltiorrhizae) 20g to invigorate blood and transform stasis.

For cases accompanied by spleen deficiency, add *dǎng shēn* (Radix Codonopsis) 15g and *chǎo biǎn dòu* (Semen Lablab Album) 20g to strengthen the spleen.

For cases accompanied by dampness, add *yì yǐ rén* (Semen Coicis) 30g and *cāng zhú* (Rhizoma Atractylodis) 15g to dry dampness.

2. Additional Treatment Modalities

a. Chinese Patent Medicine

a) *Fu Yan Kang* 妇炎康:
Function: Clear heat and drain dampness. Replenish qi and transform stasis.

Application: Use to treat chronic PID of the qi deficiency and damp-heat pouring downward pattern .

Dose: Take 4 to 6 pills, 3 times a day.

b) *Hua Hong Pian* 花红片:

Function: Clear heat, drain dampness and transform stasis.

Application: Use to treat the pattern of binding constraint of damp-heat and blood stasis of PID.

Dose: Take 4 to 5 pills, 3 times a day.

c) *Fu Ke Qian Jin Pian* 妇科千金片:

Function: Strengthen the spleen, drain dampness and transform blood stasis.

Application: Use to treat the pattern of spleen deficiency and damp-heat of PID.

Dose: Take 6 pills, 3 times a day.

d) *Jin Ji Jiao Nang* 金鸡胶囊:

Function: Clear heat and drain dampness.

Application: Use to treat PID of the damp-heat pouring downward pattern.

Dose: Take 4 pills, 3 times a day.

e) *Jin Gang Teng Jiao Nang* 金刚藤胶囊:

Function: Clear heat and drain dampness. Transform blood stasis and alleviate pain.

Application: Use to treat PID of the binding constraint of damp-heat and blood stasis pattern.

Dose: Take 4 pills, 3 times a day.

f) *Tai Nuo Qing Fu Ke Bai Dai Pian* 太诺清妇科白带片:

Function: Strengthen the spleen, drain dampness and transform blood stasis.

Application: Use to treat PID of the spleen deficiency and excessive dampness type.

Dose: Take 4 to 5 pills, 3 times a day.

g) *Shao Fu Zhu Yu Wan* 少腹逐瘀丸:

Function: Warm the channels, disperse cold and alleviate pain.

Application: Use to treat PID of the congealing cold-damp pattern.

Dose: Take 1 pill, 2 times a day.

b. Acupuncture and Moxibustion

a) Acupuncture Using Filiform Needle

【Indications】 Chronic PID

【Point Selection】

RN 3	zhōng jí	中极
ST 25	tiān shū	天枢
ST 29	guī laí	归来
SP 6	sān yīn jiāo	三阴交
SP 9	yīn líng quán	阴陵泉
BL 26	guān yuán shū	关元俞

【Point Modification】 For lower abdominal masses, add *ashi* points.

【Manipulation】 All the points are punctured with even method.

b) Auricular Acupuncture

【Indications】 Chronic PID

【Point Selection】

AH 8	fù bù	腹部
TF 2	nèi shēng zhí qū	内生殖区
CO 18	nèi fēn mì	内分泌
CO 17	sān jiāo	三焦
TG 2p	shèn shàng xiàn	肾上腺
CO 12	gān	肝

【Manipulation】 Apply needle embedding, or seed embedding. Treatment is carried out 2 or 3 times a week.

c) Electro-Acupuncture

【Indications】 Chronic PID

【Point Selection】

天枢	tiān shū	ST 25
血海	xuè hǎi	SP 10
中极	zhōng jí	RN 3
三阴交	sān yīn jiāo	SP 6

【Manipulation】 Select variable-density wave of medium intensity. Apply electric stimulation to the needles for 20 minutes. Treatment is carried out once every day or every other day.

c. External Application

a) *Si Huang Shui Mi* 四黄水蜜 : Take sufficient *Si Huang San* (Four Yellow Powder), which includes *dà huáng* (Radix et Rhizoma Rhei), *huáng qín* (Radix Scutellariae), *huáng bǎi* (Cortex Phellodendri Chinensis) and *huáng lián* (Rhizoma Coptidis). Add warm boiled water and mix them thoroughly to form a cake-like shape. Spread honey on its surface and wrap it with a cloth. Apply it externally on the lower abdomen. This treatment is carried out 1 to 2 times a day, and 10 sessions constitute one treatment course. The treatment may be carried out continuously, but suspended during menstruation.

Application: Use to treat acute and chronic PID.

b) *Shuang Bai Shui Mi* 双柏水蜜 : Take sufficient *Shuang Bai San* (Two White Powder), which includes *cè bǎi yè* (Cacumen Platycladi), *dà huáng* (Radix et Rhizoma Rhei), *huáng bǎi* (Cortex Phellodendri Chinensis), *zé lán* (Herba Lycopi) and *bò hé* (Herba Menthae). Add warm boiled water and mix them thoroughly to form a cake-like shape. Spread honey on its surface and wrap it with a cloth. Apply it externally on the lower abdomen. This treatment is carried out 1 to 2 times a day, and 10 sessions constitute one treatment course. The treatment is suspended during menstruation.

Application: Use to treat acute and chronic PID.

c) *Fu Yan San* 妇炎散 : Select *dà huáng* (Radix et Rhizoma Rhei), *jiāng huáng* (Rhizoma Curcumae Longae), *bài jiàng cǎo* (Herba Patriniae), *dān shēn* (Radix et Rhizoma Salviae Miltiorrhizae), *chì sháo* (Radix Paeoniae Rubra), *rǔ xiāng* (Olibanum), *yán hú suǒ* (Rhizoma Corydalis), *qiāng huó* (Rhizoma et Radix Notopterygii), *dú huó* (Radix Angelicae Pubescentis), *qiān nián jiàn* (Rhizoma Homalomenae) and *tòu gǔ cǎo* (Caulis Impatientis). Cut into thin slices or grind into powder, add warm water and wine and then mix them into paste. Apply the paste externally on the lower abdomen. This treatment is carried out 1 to 2 times a day, and 10 sessions constitute one treatment course. The treatment may be carried out continuously, but suspended during menstruation.

Application: Use to treat acute and chronic PID.

d. Herbal Enema

a) 复方毛冬青灌肠液 *Fu Fang Mao Dong Qing Guan Chang Ye*: It is physic liquor of 100 ml for retention enema, which includes *máo dōng qīng* (Radix Ilicis Pubescentis), *dà huáng* (Radix et Rhizoma Rhei), *huáng qí* (Radix Astragali) and *é zhú* (Rhizoma Curcumae). The treatment is carried out once a day. The treatment is suspended during menstruation.

Application: Use to treat acute and chronic PID.

b) *Kang Ning Tang* 康宁汤: Contains *zǐ huā dì dīng* (Herba Violae), *pú gōng yīng* (Herba Taraxaci), *bài jiàng cǎo* (Herba Patriniae), *bái huā shé shé cǎo* (Herba Hedyotis) *and kǔ shēn* (Radix Sophorae Flavescentis), which is cooked into 100 ml of thick decoction for retention enema. This treatment is carried out once a day, but suspended during menstruation.

Application: Use to treat acute and chronic PID.

e. Simple Prescriptions and Empirical Formulas

a) *Yin Qiao Hong Jiang Jie Du Tang* 银翘红酱解毒汤
【Ingredients】

金银花	jīn yín huā	30g	Flos Lonicerae Japonicae
连翘	lián qiào	30g	Fructus Forsythiae
红藤	hóng téng	30g	Caulis Sargentodoxae

败酱草	bài jiàng cǎo	30g	Herba Patriniae
薏苡仁	yì yǐ rén	12g	Semen Coicis
牡丹皮	mǔ dān pí	9g	Cortex Moutan
栀子	zhī zǐ	12g	Fructus Gardeniae
赤芍	chì sháo	12g	Radix Paeoniae Rubra
桃仁	táo rén	12g	Semen Persicae
延胡索	yán hú suǒ	9g	Rhizoma Corydalis
川楝子	chuān liàn zǐ	9g	Fructus Toosendan
乳香	rǔ xiāng	4.5g	Olibanum
没药	mò yào	4.5g	Myrrha

Internal Use: The decoction is divided into two or three portions. Take one portion every 6 hours, 1 decoction a day.

Application: Use to treat acute PID of the exuberant heat toxins type.

b) *Qing Gong Yin* 清宫饮
【Ingredients】

金银花	jīn yín huā	20g	Flos Lonicerae Japonicae
连翘	lián qiào	20g	Fructus Forsythiae
蒲公英	pú gōng yīng	20g	Herba Taraxaci
薏苡仁	yì yǐ rén	20g	Semen Coicis
甘草	gān cǎo	15g	Radix et Rhizoma Glycyrrhizae
黄柏	huáng bǎi	15g	Cortex Phellodendri Chinensis
滑石	huá shí	15g	Talcum
丹皮	dān pí	15g	Cortex Moutan
苍术	cāng zhú	15g	Rhizoma Atractylodis
茯苓	fú líng	15g	Poria
车前子	chē qián zǐ	15g	Semen Plantaginis
龙胆草	lóng dǎn cǎo	10g	Radix Gentianae

Internal Use: Take 1 bag a day. Decoct the medicinals with water for internal use.

Application: Use to treat acute PID of the exuberant heat toxins and the binding constraint of damp-heat and blood stasis patterns.

c) *Yue Ji Hua Gen Jian* 月季花根煎
【Ingredients】

月季花根	yuè jì huā gēn	15g	Rosa Chinensis Jacq.

Internal Use: It is the best to select fresh *yuè jì huā gēn* (Rosa Chinensis Jacq.). Wash and mince, then decoct it with water for internal intake. Take 1 bag a day.

Application: Use to treat chronic PID with leukorrhea due to dampness.

d) *Guo Yao Tang* 果药汤
【Ingredients】

煨白果	wēi bái guǒ	10g	Semen Ginkgo Praeparata
怀山药	huái shān yào	15g	Rhizoma Dioscoreae

Internal Use: Take 1 bag a day. Decoct the medicinals with water for internal use. Take one half of the decoction in the morning and the other in the evening.

Application: Use to treat spleen deficiency type PID.

e) *Lian Ou Ji Guan Hua Yin* 莲藕鸡冠花饮
【Ingredients】

鲜莲藕	xiān lián ǒu	100g	Nelumbinis Rhizome Recens
鸡冠花	jī guān huā	3 flowers	Flos Celosiae Cristatae

Internal Use: Wrap *xiān lián ǒu* (Nelumbinis Rhizome Recens) with a cloth and squeeze to obtain its juice. Then, put the juice and *jī guān huā* (Flos Celosiae Cristatae) together in water, and cook for 20 minutes. Finally, add sugar as desired. Take 50ml to 100ml every time, 2 times a day, or take as a tea throughout the day.

Application: Use to treat acute PID and chronic PID with profuse yellow vaginal discharge.

f) *Wu Mei Wu Zei San* 乌梅乌贼散

【Ingredients】

乌梅	wū méi	15g	Fructus Mume
乌贼骨	wū zéi gǔ	30g	Endoconcha Sepiae
红糖	hóng táng	20g	brown sugar

Internal Use: Char *wū méi* (Fructus Mume) and grind it into a powder. Calcine *wū zéi gǔ* (Endoconcha Sepiae) and grind it into a powder. Mix the two powders together and add brown sugar. Take the mixture with warm boiled water in the morning and in the evening.

Application: Use to treat chronic PID with red vaginal discharge.

g) *Yu Pu Yin Hua Yin* 鱼蒲银花饮

【Ingredients】

鱼腥草	yú xīng cǎo	30-60g	Herba Houttuyniae
蒲公英	pú gōng yīng	30g	Herba Taraxaci
银花藤	yín huā téng	30g	Caulis Lonicerae Japonicae

Internal Use: If fresh *yú xīng cǎo* (Herba Houttuyniae) is used, double the dosage. Decoct the medicinals in water for oral administration.

Application: Use to treat chronic PID with red vaginal discharge and lower abdominal pain.

h) *Yu Pen Yin* 愈盆饮

【Ingredients】

当归	dāng guī	9g	Radix Angelicae Sinensis
香附	xiāng fù	9g	Rhizoma Cyperi
益母草	yì mǔ cǎo	12g	Herba Leonuri

Internal Use: Decoct the medicinals with water for oral intake. Take 1 bag a day.

Application: Use to treat chronic PID of the qi stagnation and blood stasis syndrome.

i) *Da Huang Ji Dan Jian* 大黄鸡蛋煎
【Ingredients】

大黄	dà huáng	15g	Radix et Rhizoma Rhei
鸡蛋	jī dàn	5	eggs

Internal Use: Grind raw *dà huáng* (Radix et Rhizoma Rhei) into powder. The powder is then divided into 5 portions. Pierce a hole in the eggshell, remove the egg white and then put the powdered *dà huáng* (Radix et Rhizoma Rhei) 3g inside the egg. Cook the egg. After menstruation, take 1 egg every night before sleep. 5 continuous sessions constitute one treatment course.

Application: Use to treat PID of the blood stasis type.

j) *Hong Teng Tang* 红藤汤灌肠
【Ingredients】

红藤	hóng téng	30g	Caulis Sargentodoxae
败酱草	bài jiàng cǎo	30g	Herba Patriniae
蒲公英	pú gōng yīng	30g	Herba Taraxaci
鸭跖草	yā zhí cǎo	30g	Herba Commelinae
紫花地丁	zǐ huā dì dīng	30g	Herba Violae

Internal Use: Decoct the medicinals in water until 100 ml of liquid remains. Insert a no. 14 urethral catheter at least 15 centimeters into the anus. Administer enema for 30 minutes and then lay in bed for 30 minutes. Retention enema is given once a day, except during menstruation.

Application: Use to treat all types of PID.

k) *Pen Qiang Yan Gao* 盆腔炎膏外敷
【Ingredients】

当归	dāng guī	500g	Radix Angelicae Sinensis
白芍	bái sháo	500g	Radix Paeoniae Alba
红花	hóng huā	500g	Flos Carthami
生地黄	shēng dì huáng	240g	Radix Rehmanniae Recens

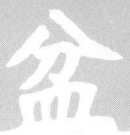

益母草	yì mǔ cǎo	240g	Herba Leonuri
川芎	chuān xiōng	120g	Rhizoma Chuanxiong
牛膝	niú xī	120g	Radix Achyranthis Bidentatae
牡丹皮	mǔ dān pí	120g	Cortex Moutan
桂枝	guì zhī	120g	Ramulus Cinnamomi
黄柏	huáng bǎi	120g	Cortex Phellodendri Chinensis
黄芩	huáng qín	120g	Radix Scutellariae
刘寄奴	liú jì nú	120g	Artemisiae Anomale
蒲黄	pú huáng	120g	Pollen Typhae
桃仁	táo rén	120g	Semen Persicae
郁金	yù jīn	90g	Radix Curcumae
艾叶	ài yè	90g	Folium Artemisiae Argyi
乳香	rǔ xiāng	90g	Olibanum
没药	mò yào	90g	Myrrha
血竭	xuè jié	90g	Sanguis Draconis
香油	xiāng yóu	5000g	Oleum Sesami (sesame oil)
广丹	guǎng dān	3500g	Plumbum Rubrum

External Use: Soak all the medicinals except *rǔ xiāng* (Olibanum), *mò yào* (Myrrha), *xuè jié* (Sanguis Draconis), *bīng piàn* (Borneolum Syntheticum) and *guǎng dān* (Plumbum Rubrum) in sesame oil for 2 hours, then decoct and deep-fry. After filtering the decoction and putting aside the medicinals, dissolve *rǔ xiāng* (Olibanum), *mò yào* (Myrrha) *xuè jié* (Sanguis Draconis) and *bīng piàn* (Borneolum Syntheticum) in the decoction. Repeat filtering and decoct the medicinals again. When the decoction can drip like beads, add *guǎng dān* (Plumbum Rubrum) to form a paste. Ask the patient to lie down. Clean the lower abdominal area with warm water. (Warm and melt the medicinal paste.) First, apply the sesame oil and then apply the warm medicinal paste, making sure the temperature is not too hot that it would scald the skin. When the paste gets cold, apply another warm paste. Repeat the treatment 4 times (which takes about 1 hour). After warm application, affix one medicinal paste to the lower abdomen. Apply once a day. 10 sessions constitute one treatment course.

Application: Use to treat all patterns of chronic PID.

PROGNOSIS

Generally, through timely and effective treatment, physical signs and symptoms of pelvic inflammatory disease will completely disappear, leading to a full recovery. Acute pelvic inflammatory disease may be complicated by septicemia and pyemia due to the powerful toxicity of pathogens, weak resistance of patients and improper treatment. Chronic pelvic inflammatory disease may lead to salpingemphraxis (obstruction of the fallopian tubes), which can cause infertility and influence the physical and mental health of patients. Therefore, the importance of the treatment of pelvic inflammatory disease should be highly stressed.

PREVENTIVE HEALTHCARE

1. Lifestyle Modification

Pay attention to personal hygiene and well-being during menstruation, during pregnancy, and after childbirth. Keep personal sanitary supplies clean and avoid the use of contaminated substitutions. Avoid excessive or unclean intercourse. Medical staff should strictly adhere to the guidelines of cleanliness when inducing abortion, inserting intrauterine devices, uterine and pelvic surgeries, and during childbirth. Patients of chronic pelvic inflammatory disease should balance work and rest, avoid overexertion, and actively participate in physical exercise. This will help strengthen the constitution and increase the body's resistance to disease.

2. Dietary Recommendation

Consume light food and drink, and avoid sweet or spicy foods of high fat and protein content (such as shrimp and crab) in order to avoid producing internal damp-heat and exacerbating the disease. During acute episodes, patients may choose easy-to-digest food that is abundant in nutrients and vitamins, and make sure they get drink plenty of liquids.

a) *Pu Gong Ying Di Ding Dang Gui Tang* 蒲公英地丁当归汤
【Ingredients】

蒲公英	pú gōng yīng	15g	Herba Taraxaci
紫花地丁	zǐ huā dì dīng	15g	Herba Violae
当归	dāng guī	6g	Radix Angelicae Sinensis
红糖	hóng táng		brown sugar

Internal Use: Put the 3 medicinals together in a pot. Decoct and filter out the dregs to obtain the liquid. Add brown sugar as desired. Take one half of the decoction each time, 2 times a day, not exceeding 1 decoction a day. 5 to 7sessions constitute one treatment course.

Application: This formula can clear heat, resolve toxins, invigorate blood and eliminate inflammation. Use to treat PID of the binding constraint of damp-heat and blood stasis type.

b) *Yi Yi Ren Bai Zhu Zhou* 薏苡仁白术粥
【Ingredients】

生薏苡仁	shēng yì yǐ rén	30g	Semen Coicis
白术	bái zhú	10g	Rhizoma Atractylodis Macrocephalae
大米	dà mǐ	50g	rice
白糖	bái táng		white sugar

Internal Use: Wrap *bái zhú* (Rhizoma Atractylodis Macrocephalae) with a clean gauze. Put all the medicinals in a pot, add water and cook to make a porridge. Remove the wrapped herb from the cooked porridge, add the desired amount of sugar and serve. Take this formula once every other day. 5 to 7 sessions constitute one treatment course.

Application: This formula can strengthen the spleen and drain dampness. Use to treat spleen deficiency pattern.

c) *Dang Gui Chuan Xiong Di Yu Jian* 当归川芎地榆煎
【Ingredients】

当归	dāng guī	12g	Radix Angelicae Sinensis
川芎	chuān xiōng	12g	Rhizoma Chuanxiong
生地榆	shēng dì yú	10g	Radix Sanguisorbae Recens
红糖	hóng táng	20g	brown sugar

Internal Use: Put 3 medicinals in a pot to cook for 20 minutes and filter out the dregs to obtain the liquid. Add brown sugar and bring to a boil. The decoction is divided into two or three portions. Take one portion each time, 2 or 3 times a day. Take 1 decoction a day. 5 to 7 continuous sessions constitute one treatment course.

Application: This formula can invigorate and cool blood. Use to treat these two patterns of chronic PID -- qi stagnation and blood stasis type, and stasis and heat obstruction type.

d) *Cang Zhu Niu Xi Chen Pi Zhou* 苍术牛膝陈皮粥
【Ingredients】

苍术	cāng zhú	10g	Rhizoma Atractylodis
牛膝	niú xī	10g	Radix Achyranthis Bidentatae
陈皮	chén pí	6g	Pericarpium Citri Reticulatae
大米	dà mǐ	100g	rice

Internal Use: Decoct the 3 herbs with water. Drain the decoction, discard the dregs and save the liquid. Add rice to the liquid and cook to make porridge. The porridge is divided into two portions. Take one portion each time, 2 times a day. Take 1 decoction a day. 5 to 7 continuous sessions constitute one treatment course.

Application: This formula can eliminate dampness, transform phlegm, regulate qi and unblock the channels. Use to treat stagnation of phlegm and dampness type of chronic PID.

e) *Dan Cao Huang Qin Yin Hua Tang* 胆草黄芩银花汤
【Ingredients】

龙胆草	lóng dǎn cǎo	15g	Radix Gentianae
黄芩	huáng qín	6g	Radix Scutellariae
银花	yín huā	20g	Flos Lonicerae Japonicae
冰糖	bīng táng		rock sugar

Internal Use: Put the 3 medicinals in a pot to cook and then filter out the dregs to obtain the liquid. Add rock sugar to taste. The soup is divided into two or three portions. Take one portion each time, 2 or 3 times a day. Drinking this decoction continuously for 2 to 5 days constitutes one treatment course.

Application: This formula can clear heat. Use to treat damp-heat pattern of acute and chronic PID.

f) *Bai Guo Yi Yi Ren Zhu Xiao Du Tang* 白果薏苡仁猪小肚汤
【Ingredients】

白果	bái guǒ	20 seeds	Semen Ginkgo
生薏苡仁	shēng yì yǐ rén	30g	Semen Coicis Recens
猪小肚	zhū xiǎo dù	2	pig bladders

Internal Use: Peel off *bái guǒ* (Semen Ginkgo) and separate the impurities from *shēng yì yǐ rén* (Semen Coicis Recens). Wash the medicinals and pig bladders, and put them all in an earthenware pot. Add 5 bowls of clean water. Cook them over strong flame. After the soup boils, stew them on low flame until two small bowls of liquid remains. Add some common salt for flavor. Drink the soup and its contents.

Application: Strengthens the spleen and transforms dampness. Use to treat spleen deficiency pattern of chronic PID.

g) *Ma Chi Xian Zhi Dun Ji Dan* 马齿苋汁炖鸡蛋
【Ingredients】

鲜马齿苋	xiān mǎ chǐ xiàn	200g	Herba Portulacae Recens
鸡蛋	jī dàn	1	egg
白糖	bái táng		white sugar

Internal Use: Clean *xiān mǎ chǐ xiàn* (Herba Portulacae Recens) and cut off the roots. Soak and wash them in cool boiled water for a while, and then stir and squeeze them to get the juice. Break open an egg and add some sugar and fresh juice of purslane herb. Mix and stir all the ingredients, and then put them in a bowl which is placed in a big pot of water. Steam and serve.

Application: Clears heat, drains dampness and stops leukorrhea. Use to treat chronic PID of the damp-heat pouring downward pattern.

h) *Ji Guan Hua Shou Rou Tang* 鸡冠花瘦肉汤
【Ingredients】

鸡冠花	jī guān huā	30g	Flos Celosiae Cristatae
猪瘦肉	zhū shòu ròu	100g	lean pork

Internal Use: Wash *jī guān huā* (Flos Celosiae Cristatae) and the lean pork. Cut the pork into thick pieces. Put them all in an earthenware pot and add 4 small bowls of clean water. Cook them on slow fire until one small bowl of soup remains. Then, add some common salt for flavor. Drink the soup and eat the meat.

Application: Clear heat and drain dampness. Use to treat damp-heat pattern of acute PID and chronic PID.

i) *Xian Ying Zhu Ti Tang* 仙樱猪蹄汤
【Ingredients】

仙茅	xiān máo	15g	Rhizoma Curculiginis
金樱子	jīn yīng zǐ	20g	Fructus Rosae Laevigatae
猪蹄	zhū tí	1 foot	pig foot

Internal Use: Remove the fur from the pig foot. Cut it into small pieces. Wash all the ingredients and put them together in an earthenware pot. Then, add 6 bowls of water. Cook over strong flame. After the soup boils, simmer on low flame until two bowls of soup remains. Add common salt for flavor. Drink the soup and eat pig foot.

Application: Strengthens the kidney to arrest leukorrhea. Use to treat kidney yang deficiency pattern of chronic PID.

3. Regulation of Emotional and Mental Health

PID patients should avoid mental stimuli, keep an optimistic attitude and have confidence that the disease can be cured.

CLINICAL EXPERIENCE OF RENOWNED PHYSICIANS

1. Empirical Formulas

a) *Xiao Zheng Yin* 消癥饮 used to treat chronic PID
【Prescription】

当归	dāng guī	12g	Radix Angelicae Sinensis
丹参	dān shēn	12g	Radix et Rhizoma Salviae Miltiorrhizae
海藻	hái zǎo	15g	Sargassum
茯苓	fú líng	6g	Poria
薏苡仁	yì yǐ rén	30g	Semen Coicis
炮山甲	páo shān jiǎ	12g	Squama Manis Praeparata
川芎	chuān xiōng	6g	Rhizoma Chuanxiong
银花	yín huā	9g	Flos Lonicerae Japonicae
连翘	lián qiào	10g	Fructus Forsythiae
橘核	jú hé	12g	Semen Citri Reticulatae
青皮	qīng pí	6g	Pericarpium Citri Reticulatae Viride
延胡索	yán hú suǒ	9g	Rhizoma Corydalis

Internal Use: Take 1 bag a day. Decoct the medicinals with water.

【Indications】 Chronic PID

【Formula Analysis】 In this formula, *dāng guī* (Radix Angelicae Sinensis), *dāng shēn* (Radix et Rhizoma Salviae Miltiorrhizae) and *chuān xiōng* (Rhizoma Chuanxiong) are used to invigorate blood and transform blood stasis. *Páo shān jiǎ* (Squama Manis Praeparata) is used to transform blood stasis, dissipate nodules, disperse swelling and expel pus. *Fú líng* (Poria) and *yì yǐ rén* (Semen Coicis) drains dampness, strengthens the spleen and leaches out dampness. In addition, *yì yǐ rén* (Semen Coicis) has the effect of expelling pus and dispersing abscesses as well. *Qīng pí* (Pericarpium Citri Reticulatae Viride) courses the liver and breaks qi, and is often paired with *jú hé* (Semen Citri Reticulatae) to regulate qi, dissipate nodules and alleviate pain. *Hái zǎo* (Sargassum) disperses phlegm, softens hard masses and dissipates nodules. *Yín huā* (Flos Lonicerae Japonicae) and *lián qiào* (Fructus Forsythiae) clear heat and resolve toxins, disperse swelling and alleviate pain. These two medicinals are often combined with *hái zǎo* (Sargassum) and *jú hé* (Semen Citri Reticulatae) to treat abdominal masses (concretions and conglomerations). This entire formula is used to treat salpingo-oophoritis, and is especially effective for the chronic PID.

【Modifications】 For the thickening of the adnexa and lingering adnexal cysts, add *sān léng* (Rhizoma Sparganii), *é zhú* (Rhizoma Curcumae), *kūn bù* (Thallus Laminariae; Thallus Eckloniae) and *mǔ lì* (Concha Ostreae). For qi deficiency pattern, add *dǎng shēn* (Radix Codonopsis) and *huáng qí* (Radix Astragali). For blood deficiency pattern, add *jī xuè téng* (Caulis Spatholobi) and *zǐ hé chē* (Placenta Hominis). For the pattern of spleen and stomach deficiency, add *bái zhú* (Rhizoma Atractylodis Macrocephalae), *dà zǎo* (Fructus Jujubae) and *zhì gān cǎo* (Radix et Rhizoma Glycyrrhizae Praeparata cum Melle). For spleen and kidney yin deficiency, add *gǒu qǐ zǐ* (Fructus Lycii), *huái shān yào* (Rhizoma Dioscoreae) and *shú dì huáng* (Radix Rehmanniae Praeparata). For the pattern of qi stagnation due to congealing cold, add *xiǎo huí xiāng* (Fructus Foeniculi) and *gān jiāng* (Rhizoma Zingiberis).

(Hu Ximing. *Compendium of Secret Chinese Medical Formulas* 中国中医秘方大全 . Shanghai: Wenhui Publishing House, 1989.142)

b) *Yin Jia Tang* 银甲汤 used to treat binding constraint of damp-heat
【**Prescription**】

金银花	jīn yín huā	15g	Flos Lonicerae Japonicae
连翘	lián qiào	15g	Fructus Forsythiae
升麻	shēng má	15g	Rhizoma Cimicifugae
红藤	hóng téng	24g	Caulis Sargentodoxae
蒲公英	pú gōng yīng	24g	Herba Taraxaci
生鳖甲	shēng biē jiǎ	24g	Carapax Trionycis Recens
紫花地丁	zǐ huā dì dīng	30g	Herba Violae
生蒲黄	shēng pú huáng	12g	Pollen Typhae Recens
椿根皮	chūn gēn pí	12g	Cortex Ailanthi
大青叶	dà qīng yè	12g	Folium Isatidis
琥珀末	hǔ pò mò	12g	Succinum
桔梗	jié gěng	12g	Radix Platycodonis
茵陈	yīn chén	13g	Herba Artemisiae Scopariae

Internal Use: Take 1 bag a day. Decoct the medicinals with water for internal use. Drink the decoction in intervals. Also, the medicinals can be ground into powder, then mixed with honey to form honey pills. Take 3 honey pills at a time, 3 times a day.

【**Indications**】 Leukorrhea due to the binding constraint of damp-heat with yellow or red vaginal discharge (it is equivalent to diseases of modern biomedicine such as PID, endometritis, and cervicitis).

【**Formula Analysis**】 This formula includes many medicinals for clearing heat and resolving toxins as the main herbs, such as *jīn yín huā* (Flos Lonicerae Japonicae), *lián qiào* (Fructus Forsythiae), *pú gōng yīng* (Herba Taraxaci), *zǐ huā dì dīng* (Herba Violae), *hóng téng* (Caulis Sargentodoxae), *dà qīng yè* (Folium Isatidis) and *shēng má* (Rhizoma

Cimicifugae). Use medicinals that clear heat and remove dampness, such as *yīn chén* (Herba Artemisiae Scopariae) and *chūn gēn pí* (Cortex Ailanthi) as the auxiliary herbs. Use *shēng biē jiǎ* (Carapax Trionycis Recens) *shēng pú huáng* (Pollen Typhae Recens) and *hǔ pò* (Succinum) as the assisting medicinals to invigorate blood, transform blood stasis, soften hard masses and dissipate nodules. Use *jié gěng* (Radix Platycodonis) to clear heat and expel filth. The combination of all the medicinals mentioned above enhances the effects of clearing heat, removing dampness, resolving toxins and dispelling evils.

(Chai Yuejian. *The Quintessence of Chinese Contemporary Famous Doctors* 中华当代名医妙方精华. Changchun: Changchun Publishing House, 1992.421)

c) *Hao Pu Jie Du Tang* 蒿蒲解毒汤 used to treat acute PID
【Prescription】

青蒿	qīng hāo	12g	Herba Artemisiae Annuae
牡丹皮	mǔ dān pí	12g	Cortex Moutan
黄柏	huáng bǎi	12g	Cortex Phellodendri Chinensis
蒲公英	pú gōng yīng	30g	Herba Taraxaci
白薇	bái wēi	20g	Radix et Rhizoma Cynanchi Atrati
丹参	dān shēn	20g	Radix et Rhizoma Salviae Miltiorrhizae
连翘	lián qiào	20g	Fructus Forsythiae
赤芍	chì sháo	15g	Radix Paeoniae Rubra
桃仁	táo rén	15g	Semen Persicae
青皮	qīng pí	10g	Pericarpium Citri Reticulatae Viride
川楝子	chuān liàn zǐ	10g	Fructus Toosendan

Internal Use: Add *qīng hāo* (Herba Artemisiae Annuae) in the last 5 to 10 minutes of cooking. Decoct the medicinals with water twice. Take the decoction in several intervals throughout the day. Take 1 or 2 doses a day.

【Indications】 Acute PID with symptoms of strong fever, aversion to cold, scorching hot sensation of the lower abdomen, abdominal pain, dark-colored urine, constipation, and profuse thick, yellow, foul-smelling leukorrhea.

【Formula Analysis】 In this formula, use *qīng hāo*'s (Herba Artemisiae Annuae) cold property and bitter flavor to clear heat, and its fragrant odor to penetrate and dissipate. Moreover, it excels in clearing and draining heat from the liver and gallbladder, as well as from the blood level. Use *pú gōng yīng* (Herba Taraxaci), *huáng bǎi* (Cortex Phellodendri Chinensis) and *lián qiào* (Fructus Forsythiae) to clear heat and resolve toxins. Use *bái wēi* (Radix et Rhizoma Cynanchi Atrati) and *mǔ dān pí* (Cortex Moutan) to clear heat and cool blood. Use *dān shēn* (Radix et Rhizoma Salviae Miltiorrhizae), *chì sháo* (Radix Paeoniae Rubra) and *táo rén* (Semen Persicae) to invigorate blood and transform blood stasis. Use *qīng pí* (Pericarpium Citri Reticulatae Viride) and *chuān liàn zǐ* (Fructus Toosendan) to regulate qi and resolve constraint. The combination of all the medicinals strengthens the effects of clearing heat, resolving toxins, moving qi and transforming blood stasis.

【Modifications】 For constipation, add *dà huáng* (Radix et Rhizoma Rhei) 12g. Be sure to add *dà huáng* (Radix et Rhizoma Rhei) in the last 5 to 10 minutes of decocting.

For nausea, vomiting and poor appetite, add fresh *zhú rú* (Caulis Bambusae in Taenia) 15g and *huò xiāng* (Herba Pogostemonis) 10g.

For stinging pain during urination, add *Liu Yi San* 20g.

【Comments】 Luo believes the principal treatment of PID is to move qi, invigorate blood and transform stasis. The selection of the medicinals for moving qi, activating blood and transforming blood stasis varies according to the individual and the presenting pattern. Generally speaking, for exuberant heat toxins, it is imperative to clear heat and resolve toxins. Therefore, one must select the appropriate medicinals for clearing heat and resolving toxins, such as *qīng hāo* (Herba Artemisiae Annuae), *huáng bǎi* (Cortex Phellodendri Chinensis) and *lián qiào* (Fructus

Forsythiae). And it is better to select *pú gōng yīng* (Herba Taraxaci) and *bài jiàng cǎo* (Herba Patriniae), which can not only resolve toxins, but also disperse carbuncles, reduce swelling, cool blood and transform blood stasis. The dosage for these medicinals should be a slightly higher than usual. This summarizes Dr. Luo's valuable clinical experience from his use of medicinals.

(Luo Yuankai. *Luo Yuankai's Treatise on Chinese Medical Treatment* 罗元恺论医集 . Beijing: People's Medical Publishing House, 1990.61)

d) *Qing Re Jie Du Tang* 清热解毒汤 used to treat damp toxins and exuberant heat
【**Prescription**】

金银花	jīn yín huā	15g	Flos Lonicerae Japonicae
连翘	lián qiào	15g	Fructus Forsythiae
蒲公英	pú gōng yīng	15g	Herba Taraxaci
紫花地丁	zǐ huā dì dīng	15g	Herba Violae
黄芩	huáng qín	9g	Radix Scutellariae
车前子	chē qián zǐ	9g	Semen Plantaginis
丹皮	dān pí	9g	Cortex Moutan
地骨皮	dì gǔ pí	9g	Cortex Lycii
瞿麦	qú mài	12g	Herba Dianthi
萹蓄	biǎn xù	12g	Herba Polygoni Avicularis
冬瓜子	dōng guā zǐ	30g	Semen Benincasae
赤芍	chì sháo	6g	Radix Paeoniae Rubra

Internal Use: Take 1 or 2 doses a day. Decoct the medicinals with water. Take the decoction at intervals.

【**Indications**】 Use to treat the pattern of excessive toxic dampness and heat of acute PID and chronic PID.

【**Formula Analysis**】 The formula is used to treat the pattern of damp toxins directly attacking the uterus. In this formula, *jīn yín huā* (Flos Lonicerae Japonicae), *lián qiào* (Fructus Forsythiae), *pú gōng yīng* (Herba Taraxaci), *zǐ huā dì dīng* (Herba Violae) and *huáng qín* (Radix Scutellariae) are used to clear heat and resolve toxins. *Chē qián zǐ* (Semen Plantaginis), *qú mài* (Herba Dianthi), *biǎn xù* (Herba Polygoni Avicularis) and *dōng guā zǐ* (Semen Benincasae) drain dampness. *Chì sháo* (Radix Paeoniae Rubra) and *dān pí* (Cortex Moutan) to invigorate blood and transform blood stasis. *Dì gǔ pí* (Cortex Lycii) cools blood and clears heat. The combination of all the medicinals strengthens the effects of clearing heat, resolving toxins, draining dampness, invigorating blood, dispersing swelling and alleviating pain.

【Comments】The pathogenic evil of damp toxins directly attacks the lower jiao, invading the vulva and uterus, which always causes foul-smelling yellow vaginal discharge. In the beginning, the pattern mostly resembles excess and heat. Therefore, the treatment centers on clearing heat and resolving toxins, assisted by draining dampness and expelling blood stasis. Liu excels at using medicinals for clearing heat, draining dampness and invigorating blood for the elimination of toxic heat, dampness evil, and static blood, thus allowing for recovery.

(Beijing Chinese Medical Hospital, Bejing Chinese Medical College. *Liu Fengwu Experience in Gynecology* 刘奉五妇科经验 . Beijing: People's Medical Publishing House, 1977.290)

e) *Qing Re Xiao Yu Guan Chang Fang* 清热消瘀灌肠方 used to treat PID
【Prescription】

红藤	hóng téng	15g	Caulis Sargentodoxae
败酱草	bài jiàng cǎo	15g	Herba Patriniae
鱼腥草	yú xīng cǎo	15g	Herba Houttuyniae
蒲公英	pú gōng yīng	15g	Herba Taraxaci
炙乳香	zhì rǔ xiāng	6g	Olibanum Praeparata
炙没药	zhì mò yào	6g	Myrrha Praeparata
三棱	sān léng	5g	Rhizoma Sparganii
莪术	é zhú	5g	Rhizoma Curcumae
丹皮	dān pí	3g	Cortex Moutan

External Use: Cook the medicinals mentioned above with water into 100 ml of thick decoction for retention enema, administered once a day.

【Indications】 Acute and chronic PID

【Formula Analysis】 In this formula, *hóng téng* (Caulis Sargentodoxae), *bài jiàng cǎo* (Herba Patriniae), *yú xīng cǎo* (Herba Houttuyniae) and *pú gōng yīng* (Herba Taraxaci) clear heat, resolve toxins, disperse swelling and alleviate pain. *Rǔ xiāng* (Olibanum), *mò yào* (Myrrha), *sān léng* (Rhizoma Sparganii) and *é zhú* (Rhizoma Curcumae) regulate qi, invigorate blood, transform stasis and alleviate pain. *Dān pí* (Cortex Moutan) clears heat and cools blood. This pattern can be treated effectively with a combination of medicinals for internal and external use.

(Hu Ximing: Editor-in-chief. *Compendium of Secret Chinese Medical Formulas* 中国中医秘方大全 . Shanghai: Wenhui Publishing House, 1989.137)

2. Selected Case Studies

(1) Pu Fuzhou's Case Studies: Puerperal Infection

Song, female, 37 years old, admitted to hospital.

History of Present Illness: The patient was 4.5 months pregnant when she fell while trying to sit down, and developed vaginal bleeding as a result of the accident. She was sent to the emergency room on August 22nd.

Examination revealed the following: The vulvae were normal; the external cervical os was dilated and the internal cervical os was closed; the fundus was one horizontally-placed finger distance below the umbilicus; fetal sounds were abnormal, and there was vaginal bleeding. Tocolysis (inhibition of uterine contractions) was administered. However, there was profuse menses-like vaginal bleeding the following day. Surgery to remove the contents of the uterus was performed immediately, and was a success. High fever occurred right after the operation, for which Tetracycline was administered orally. The high fever and shivering lasted for 4 days, at a temperature of 39.6℃ . There was also slight distention of the abdomen, decreased bowel sounds, tenderness below the xyphoid process radiating to the entire abdomen with muscular tension, rebound tenderness (+), shifting dullness (±), abdominal pain with groaning, and scanty vaginal bleeding. Chemical examination revealed the following -- Blood routine: HB 11.7g/100 ml, WBC 19,000/ mm³, N% 90%, M 2%, L 8%. Urine routine: Urinary protein: small volume, RBC 3-4/HP, WBC 7-8/ HP, blood pressure 120/80mmHg, pulse rate 18 beats per minute, blood culture (−). At the time, the diagnosis was advanced-stage infectious miscarriage and septicemia. The patient was then continuously given oxytetracycline, chlorotetracycline, streptomycin and a couple of doses of modified *Chai Hu Gui Zhi Tang* 柴胡桂枝汤 .

The patient's temperature gradually returned to normal on September 1st. However, the patient felt that only the abdominal pain was alleviated, while other symptoms still remained. The patient presented with drowsiness, chest distress, poor appetite and dizziness. On September 3rd, the temperature rose again, with symptoms of aversion to cold, fever and aching pain of the entire body. The patient did not respond to any of the antibiotics, and her temperature rose continuously, day by day. On September 7th, it reached 39.7℃ . After consultation, the doctors concluded that the postnatal infection had not yet been controlled. According to examination, the inflammation was not confined to the endometrium, but had already spread to the muscular layer and the connective tissue. The placenta still remained in the uterus. Doctors proposed surgical removal of the uterus, but the patient and her family members did not give consent.

On September 8th, they requested a consultation with Dr. Pu. Temperature: 39.7℃ . The patient reported that she experienced alternating fever and aversion to cold for several days. When she was chilled she had cold limbs, and when she was feverish she had sweating that was not thorough. She also had chest distress, slight abdominal fullness, pain of the lesser abdomen upon palpation, headache without dizziness, aching pain of the entire body, poor appetite, dryness and bitter taste in the mouth with no desire to drink, one bout of nausea and vomiting, difficult defecation of dry stools followed by loose stools, yellow urine, a small quantity of pus-like lochia, a vague pulse which was forceless when pressed lightly and heavily, dark red tongue with thick, foul, yellow and white coating, and a clear voice. Her mental state and the pain upon palpation both indicate an excess pattern, while the pulse reveals a deficiency pattern. Therefore, the diagnosis should be determined according to the symptoms rather than the pulse manifestation.

The deficiency of right qi as a result of the miscarriage, combined with latent damp-heat, caused recurrent fever that resembles the *Chai Hu* syndrome, but without wiry pulse and rib-side fullness. Although Zhang Zhongjing declared that "diagnosis can be decided according to only one symptom of *Xiao Chai Hu Tang* pattern" , the chief symptoms do not belong to foot lesser yang channel pattern, but is more like the hand lesser channel yang pattern, presenting with the manifestations of binding constraint of san jiao qi.

【Pattern Differentiation】 Binding constraint of san jiao qi due to damp-heat

【Treatment Principle】 Regulate san jiao qi and resolve damp-heat.

【Prescription】

茯苓皮	fú líng pí	9g	Cortex Poriae
杏仁	xìng rén	6g	Semen Armeniacae Amarum
薏苡仁	yì yǐ rén	12g	Semen Coicis
白豆蔻	bái dòu kòu	3g	Amomum Cardamomum
茵陈蒿	yīn chén hāo	9g	Herba Artemisiae Scopariae
猪苓	zhū líng	6g	Polyporus
法半夏	fǎ bàn xià	6g	Rhizoma Pinelliae Praeparatum

滑石块	huá shí kuài	12g	Talcum
黄芩	huáng qín	3g	Radix Scutellariae
蚕沙	cán shā	12g	Faeces Bombycis
白通草	bái tōng cǎo	4.5g	Medulla Tetrapanacis
淡竹叶	dàn zhú yè	6g	Herba Lophatheri

2 bags of this formula were given. Each bag was decocted twice, yielding a total of 300 ml of liquid, and divided into four portions.

【Second Visit on September 10ʰ 】 After taking the decoction, the patient's sweating was more thorough. Gradually, the patient felt relieved. Cold and fever was alleviated and temperature decreased. On the morning of September 9th, her temperature reached 35.8 ℃ , and in the evening it reached 36℃ . The patient defecated six times. The stools were loose, of curd-like color with bloody pus, which contained the following – Gram positive bacilli; Erythrocyte: 30-50/HP; and Leukocyte: 15-20/HP. Today, her body temperature is 36.6℃ . The patient defecated only once, and still felt the need to defecate again. Abdominal distention was alleviated, however, slight pain with discomfort remained. There was continuous slight sweating of the entire body. The patient felt well enough to eat a bowl of thin porridge. She still felt nauseous and was unable to taste her food. Dryness and bitter taste in the mouth was alleviated. The pulse was deep, wiry and slow. The tongue coating has decreased in thickness. The patient's condition has improved since the last visit. This second phase of treatment involved regulating san jiao qi and clearing damp-heat. *Huáng qín* (Radix Scutellariae), *cán shā* (Faeces Bombycis) and *dàn zhú yè* (Herba Lophatheri) were removed from the first formula. *Hòu pò* (Cortex Magnoliae Officinalis) 3g, the stem of *huò xiāng* (Herba Pogostemonis) 3g and *shén qū* (Massa Medicata Fermentata) 6g were added. *Fú líng pí* (Poria) was replaced by *fú líng* (Poria) with exodermis (*lían pí fú líng*). 2 doses of this formula were given internally, following the same instructions as before.

【Third Visit on September 12 th】 After taking the decoction, the patient's temperature was stabilized. Headache and body aches were alleviated. There was slightly dryness and bitter taste in the mouth. The patient has recovered some of her ability to taste food. The patient's mental state seems more vibrant. The patient defecated 4 times the day before yesterday, and 3 times yesterday. The stools were thin and contained mucosal fluid. The pulse is now deep, slow and forceful. The tongue showed further decrease in foul, greasy coating. The disease condition has improved dramatically, but the remaining evil has not been fully expelled. The next treatment step is to regulate and harmonize the functions of the spleen, stomach and san jiao in order to eliminate the lingering pathogen.

【Prescription】

连皮茯苓	fú líng	9g	Poria
扁豆衣	biǎn dòu yī	9g	Pericarpium Lablab Album
苡仁	yǐ rén	12g	Semen Coicis
白豆蔻	bái dòu kòu	3g	Fructus Amomi Rotundus
广陈皮	guǎng chén pí	4.5g	Pericarpium Citri Reticulatae Chachiensis
厚朴	hòu pò	4.5g	Cortex Magnoliae Officinalis
藿香梗	huò xiāng gěng	4.5g	Herba Pogostemonis
茵陈蒿	yīn chén hāo	9g	Herba Artemisiae Scopariae
滑石	huá shí	12g	Talcum
生稻芽	shēng dào yá	9g	Fructus Oryzae Germinatus Recens
神曲	shén qū	3g	Massa Medicata Fermentata

A total of 3 bags were given. Each bag was decocted twice, which yielded a total of 200 ml of liquid, and divided into three portions for oral intake.

【Second Visit on September 10 th】 The patient's temperature has returned to normal. She now has one bowel movement a day, is eating more, and can taste her food. Her mental state is improving gradually. She has slight abdominal distention and occasional gas. The pus-like vaginal discharge has stopped. She has a moderate pulse and a red tongue. The tongue coating has returned to normal. The next phase of the treatment process involved stopping Chinese herbal therapy, monitoring the patient's health, and instructing the patient to build up her health with a good diet and rest for approximately 10 days. Soon afterwards, she left the hospital and returned to work.

Comments:

This is a case of secondary infection after surgical removal of the uterine contents. The inflammation was not confined to the endometrium, but involved the connective tissue of the myometrium. There was retention of the placenta. The patient did not respond to the antibiotics. After the consultation, the doctors had recommended a hysterectomy.

The Chinese medical diagnosis was identified according to pattern differentiation of the signs and symptoms. The doctor concluded that it was not the heat entering the blood chamber after abortion, but the latent damp-heat that caused this disease. The patient has had 8 miscarriages. In order to prevent having another miscarriage, the patient slept more and exercised less during this pregnancy. This was during late summer when the weather was often cloudy and rainy. The weather combined with the damp living environment caused damage to right qi and the interior generation of latent damp-heat. Then, the patient suffered an accidental fall, which injured the fetus. Tocolysis and the surgery to clear out the uterine contents caused further damage to right qi. The latent dampness took advantage of the right qi deficiency and attacked the san jiao, causing the binding constraint of qi and the impaired circulation of nutritive and defensive qi. Although the patient presented with a vague pulse that was weak when pressed lightly and heavily, the patient did not exhibit mental lassitude. Therefore, the diagnosis should be determined according to the symptoms rather than the pulse condition.

The patient presented with sweating without alleviation of fever;

feverish sensations without restlessness; drowsiness; aching pain of the entire body; chest oppression; slight fullness of the lesser abdomen; yellow urine; dry stools followed by loose stools during bowel movements; thick foul greasy tongue coating; and thirst without the desire to drink. All the symptoms point to binding constraint of damp-heat. The treatment was designed to regulate and harmonize the function of the san jiao, unblock the exterior and the interior, and expel the evils. Taking 1 dose of the formula unblocked the interior and harmonized the exterior. The external evils lodged in the muscles were released by the tidal sweating. The latent dampness which accumulated in the intestines and stomach was expelled through purging. Consequently, the body temperature returned to normal. From a Chinese medical viewpoint, the binding constraint has been removed; san jiao qi is no longer obstructed, the dampness has been successfully dispersed, and the heat has been cleared. After taking 2 doses of the formula, her body temperature was stabilized. All the symptoms were alleviated, except for nausea, inability to taste food, and slight abdominal pain. Therefore, *huáng qín* (Radix Scutellariae), *cán shā* (Faeces Bombycis) and *dàn zhú yè* (Herba Lophatheri) were removed from the first formula. *Hòu pò* (Cortex Magnoliae Officinalis) 3g, the stem of *huò xiāng* (Herba Pogostemonis) 3g and *shén qū* (Massa Medicata Fermentata) 6g were added to regulate the functions of the spleen and stomach, which is the focus of the next treatment step. After 1 dose of the formula, the patient's appetite and mental state improved. The pulse became deep, slow and forceful. The foul greasy tongue coating has partially receded. Although the damp-heat has decreased in quantity, the lingering pathogen has not been fully cleared.

Xìng rén (Semen Armeniacae Amarum), which is bitter and has the effect of descending, was removed from the formula, as well as *tōng cǎo* (Medulla Tetrapanacis) that is bland and has the effect of leaching out dampness.

He added *chén pí* (Pericarpium Citri Reticulatae) and *dào yá* (Fructus Oryzae Germinatus) to improve the functions of the spleen and stomach. When the spleen and stomach are functioning normally, the san jiao is unobstructed, and the nutritive and defensive qi are in harmony, the pathogenic evil can be eliminated. After taking 3 doses of the formula, the patient's pulse and tongue returned to normal. Her mental state, appetite, urine and stools are also normal. Pu stopped giving the formula to the patient, and continued to monitor her health. He also instructed the patient to adopt a healthy diet in order to nurse herself back to health, to counteract the damage afflicted on the stomach qi as a result of the harsh medicinals. The patient followed the advice, and hence she recovered quickly and was discharged from the hospital.

(Gao Huiyuan: Editor-in-chief. *Pu Fuzhou's Case Studies* 蒲辅周医案 . Beijing: People's Medical Publishing House, 1990.61)

(2) Wang Minghui's Case Studies: Heat Entering The Blood Chamber (Infection During Menstruation)

Xiao, female, 28 years old, worker, married, admitted to hospital on May 4th, 1961. Hospitalization No. 94488

Chief complaint: Fear of cold, fever, and paroxysmal epigastric and abdominal pain for 1 week.

History of Present Illness: 1 week before hospitalization, the patient began experiencing epigastric fullness and distention. The pain has since then migrated to the periumbilical region, and finally spread to the entire abdomen, manifesting as pain that refuses pressure. She has vomited once, and the vomitus did not contain roundworms. In the early stage of her condition, she presented with fear of cold and fever (with fear of cold being more pronounced), absence of sweating, accompanied by slight frontal headache, dizziness, fatigue, constipation (that lasted for 8 days), scanty yellow urine, thirst without the desire to drink, extremely poor appetite and no cough. Before she was hospitalized, she received a consultation at the outpatient department of this hospital, and was given Western pharmaceutical drugs twice (the names of which are unknown), with no improvement . Finally, she was admitted to the Chinese medical department of this hospital.

The patient has a past medical history of similar epigastric and abdominal pain in June, 1960. But she had neither fear of cold nor fever, and the condition was fairly mild.

The patient married in 1950, and had 5 pregnancies, 3 of which were carried to full term. Her husband and her children are all in good health. In recent years, her menstruation has been irregular. She has not had a menstrual period in the past 7 months. She has no leukorrhea.

Physical examination: The patient was conscious and alert. Her body shape appeared normal. Voice and breathing were normal. Development was normal. She was poorly nourished. The patient exhibited a yellowish complexion and slight drowsiness. No jaundice or rash was present. There was slight tenderness of the hypochondria, wiry and slow pulse, red lips and tongue that is dry with white and yellow. Her body temperature was 37℃ , and her pulse was 108 beats per minute.

【Syndrome Characteristics】 Yang brightness channel syndrome (Gastric flu)

【Treatment Principle】 Relieve the exterior with medicinals that are cool and acrid.

【Prescription】 Modified *Bai Hu Tang* 白虎汤

【On May 8 th】 Modified *Bai Hu Tang* was administered, which was used to relieve the exterior, due to the nature of its cool and acrid ingredients. After taking 5 doses, the pain was alleviated and the tongue had more moisture. The patient felt a little better. However, after taking a bath, she was suddenly stricken with chills and strong fever. She had bitter taste in the mouth, mild thirst, dizziness, pain of the entire body, wiry rapid pulse and a pale, moist tongue.

【On May 11ʰ 】 The symptoms still remained after 3 doses of the formula that contained cool acrid medicinals. Therefore, *Ling Qiao Jie Du Wan* 羚翘解毒丸 and *Yu Shu Dan* 玉枢丹 were administered. The patient was suspected to have malaria or an inflammatory condition, so antimalarial medication and antibiotics were also given.

【On May 11ʰ 】 The patient still had a strong fever. The disease was suspected to be triple yang heat syndrome. The medicinals were replaced by *Chai Ge Jie Ji Tang* in an attempt to treat this disease.

【On May 15ᵗʰ 】 After taking 3 doses of *Chai Ge Jie Ji Tang* 柴葛解肌汤 , the patient was still suffering from chills and fever (pronounced chills followed by fever), severe sweating that drenched the sheets, dizziness, poor appetite, dry mouth, bitter taste in the mouth, a red tongue with yellow coating in the center, and a wiry, thready, rapid and forceless pulse. She had intermittent fever. The chills and fever alternated daily, with the fever sometimes reaching 41 ℃ . Sweating would bring down the fever to 36℃ . Since malaria could not be ruled out, *Xiao Chai Hu Tang* 小柴胡汤 combined with *cǎo guǒ* (Fructus Tsaoko) and *cháng shān* (Radix Dichroae) was the administered formula.

【On May 22ᵗʰ 】 After 7 doses, the formula proved to be ineffective. In addition, the Western pharmaceuticals she had been taking since May 11ᵗʰ to control the chills and fever (quinine, mepacrine, sintomycin, penicillin, streptomycin, e.g.) produced side effects such as tinnitus and partial deafness. The patient stopped the medication after 2 taking them twice. Chest fluoroscopy, liver function, widal reaction and blood culture were all negative, except for the white blood cell count, which was slightly high. ESR rate was high. Blood films were also negative for plasmodium. Physical examination revealed that five sensory organs, heart, lung, liver and spleen were all normal. Since May 8ᵗʰ, the patient's condition did not improve after treatment using integrative medicine. Instead, the patient got thinner and weaker day by day and the diagnosis had not yet been identified. Wang carefully investigated the case and discovered that the patient had her menstrual period the day after she was admitted to the hospital (after having amenorrhea for 7 months). On May 8th, after taking a bath, she experienced chills and fever, and the menstrual bleeding stopped. She had lesser abdominal distention and pain and restlessness. After detailed pattern differentiation, Wang concluded that it was deficiency accompanied by heat entering the blood chamber. He told her to stop taking the western pharmaceuticals, and gave her modified *Xiao Chai Hu Tang* 小柴胡汤 and *Qing Gu San* 清骨散 instead.

【Prescription】

柴胡	chái hú	9g	Radix Bupleuri
黄芩	huáng qín	6g	Radix Scutellariae
党参	dǎng shēn	9g	Radix Codonopsis
秦艽	qín jiāo	9g	Radix Gentianae Macrophyllae
鳖甲	biē jiǎ	9g	Carapax Trionycis
知母	zhī mǔ	9g	Rhizoma Anemarrhenae
青蒿	qīng hāo	9g	Herba Artemisiae Annuae
玉竹	yù zhú	12g	Rhizoma Polygonati Odorati
地骨皮	dì gǔ pí	6g	Cortex Lycii
甘草	gān cǎo	3g	Radix et Rhizoma Glycyrrhizae

Take 1 dose (divided into 2 portions) every day.

【On May 25 th】 After taking 3 doses of the formula mentioned above, the fever was reduced to below 38℃ . The patient no longer experienced subjective chills or fever, and her appetite was greatly improved. Urination and bowel movement were smooth. She had a wiry slow pulse and a red tongue with white moist coating.

【On May 29 th】 After taking 4 doses of the previously prescribed formula, the chills and fever vanished. The patient felt that her health has been restored. Only dizziness and weakness remained. She was instructed to continue taking the formula.

【On June 3 】 A total of 10 doses of the previous formula proved to have a good curative effect and resulted in no relapse of the illness. However, the long-term disease weakened the patient, giving rise to diarrhea before dawn. For this, modified *Si Shen Wan* 四神丸 and *Tong Xie Yao Fang* 痛泻要方 was administered.

【On July 7ᵈ 】 After 1 month of rehabilitation, the patient gradually recovered and was discharged from the hospital on this day. Various examinations revealed that everything was normal except for discoloration of the skin caused by the mepacrine.

Comments:

According to the pulse and the symptoms, at the time the patient was first admitted to the hospital, the diagnosis was yang brightness channel syndrome. Cool acrid medicinals for releasing the exterior were given. Due to the sudden onset of the disease, the patient's condition escaped careful analysis and observation, which lead to an incomplete diagnosis and delay of proper treatment. It was not until half a month later that the disease was finally diagnosed as heat entering the blood chamber, and the formula for removing stagnation and clearing blood heat was given. The last 4 doses were especially effective in resolving the problem. We can learn from this case that pattern differentiation is indeed an important but yet difficult process.

Diagnosis was made as yang brightness channel pattern when the patient was just admitted to hospital. It was mentioned in *Treatise on Febrile Diseases <Shāng Hán Lùn>* 伤寒论 that "Yang brightness disease should lead to great sweating, but there is no sweating. … It is long-term deficiency that causes this." From this, we know that great sweating is due to the excessive dryness-heat of the Yang brightness syndrome. In certain cases there is absence of sweating accompanied by itchiness, which is caused by the deficiency of fluid, and therefore an insufficiency of the source of sweat. The patient contracted cold-induced disease that lasted several days. She presented with pronounced fever, mild chills, thirst, anihydrosis, dark-colored urine, constipation, a red tongue with yellow coating, and a rapid pulse. The disease was the Yang brightness channel dryness-heat syndrome, for which cool acrid medicinals to clear heat were prescribed. The appropriateness of the formula resulted in a quick resolution of the patient's symptoms.

During the hospital stay, the patient was afflicted by external pathogenic evil during menstruation when the yang brightness syndrome was just cured, which caused heat entering the blood chamber. *Treatise on Febrile Diseases* <*Shang Han Lun*> 伤寒论 said, "A woman was afflicted by wind cold. She suffered from fever and aversion to cold at the onset of menstruation. After 7 or 8 days, the external pathogenic heat was eliminated and she presented with a slow pulse and cool skin, fullness below the chest and hypochondria (as if there is retention of evils in the thorax), and delirium. This is heat entering the blood chamber caused by the external pathogenic heat invading the blood chamber at the beginning of menstruation."

By comparison, the symptoms of the two cases are very similar, except for the delirium which is not a symptom of heat entering the blood chamber. It is also mentioned in *Treatise on Febrile Diseases* <*Shang Han Lun*> 伤寒论 that "A woman was afflicted by wind cold. After 7 or 8 days, she suffered from intermittent chills and fever. At that point, her menstrual bleeding stopped. This is heat entering the blood chamber. The heat combined with the blood, and the binding constraint of blood heat caused alternating chills and fever, which is similar to malaria." With reference to this quote, the patient in this case had cold-induced menstrual block for 7 months. Later, the binding constraint of blood heat caused menstrual bleeding, which lasted only 1 day. The patient suffered from the malaria-like symptom of alternating chills and fever, which caused the doctor to suspect that the disease was indeed malaria.

Heat entering the blood chamber is caused by external pathogenic evils which often invades the body during the arrival and departure of menstruation. The heat evil combines with blood, causing the struggle between right qi and evil qi, giving rise to symptoms of alternating chills and fever, similar to that of malaria. Since the liver stores blood and the static blood causes binding constraint of the qi of the reverting yin channel, there may be fullness and oppression or pain in the chest and hypochondria. Since blood combines with evils in the uterus, there may be epigastric and abdominal pain, scanty menses or interrupted menstruation. Since the heart stores the spirit, the blood heat will upwards to disturb the mind, and may cause impaired consciousness that is mild during day and severe at night. Some cases may not involve binding constraint of blood, but excessive ying-level heat instead. Symptoms of this may include scorching hot sensation of the entire body, restlessness, insomnia and a red crimson tongue. If heat enters the blood level, there may be coma and delirium. If the heat evil forces the blood to move recklessly, there may be profuse menses, spitting of blood, bloody stools, and a dark crimson tongue. This case has all the symptoms except heat disturbing the spirit and the blood level.

After being admitted to the hospital, the biomedical diagnosis was suspected to be malaria, ileotyphus, pulmonary tuberculosis or hepatitis. However, there was insufficient evidence to confirm any of these possible diagnoses. Considering the fact that the patient suffered from repeated fever with high white cell and neutrophil count; elevated ESR; and the relation between the symptoms mentioned above and the ebb and flow of menstruation, there is enough evidence to suggest the diagnosis of infection during menstruation.

From the ingredients of the chief formula used to treat heat entering the blood chamber, we can see that the application of *Xiao Chai Hu Tang* 小

柴胡汤 combined with *Qing Gu San* 清骨散 actually followed the treatment principle, but did not utilize all of the medicinals. As we know, *Xiao Chai Hu Tang* 小柴胡汤 is the empirical formula for the treatment of the lesser yang syndrome and *Qing Gu San* 清骨散 is commonly used to treat consumptive disease. Since the patient suffered from alternating chills and fever due to heat entering the blood chamber, *Xiao Chai Hu Tan* 小柴胡汤 was selected to combat this malaria-like symptom. Since the patient was deficient in original qi and fluid as a result of the prolonged disease, *Qing Gu San* 清骨散 was selected to treat tidal fever caused by yin deficiency, which included medicinals for treating type kind of disease -- such as *zhī mǔ* (Rhizoma Anemarrhenae), *dì gǔ pí* (Cortex Lycii), *qīng hāo* (Herba Artemisiae Annuae) and *yù zhú* (Rhizoma Polygonati Odorati). From this case study, we can see the importance of "Learning from the experience of the ancients but not adhering rigidly to them." This quote refers to the significance of clinical guidance.

This disease occurs most frequently among young and middle-aged women. In the modern day, it is commonly seen in the Chinese medical department and gynecological department, but is easily ignored by the doctors. The case mentioned above, where the patient was misdiagnosed for half a month, is a good example. Therefore, it is imperative to pay attention to the theory and application of heat entering the blood chamber.

Sui Dianjun. *Handpicked Medical Records and Notes of Famous Contemporary Chinese Doctors* (中国当代名医医案医话选). Changchun: Jilin Science and Technology Publishing House, 1995.76-80

(3) Li Hengzhi's Case Studies: Pelvic Inflammatory Mass

Case 1: Jian, female, 27 years old.

【Initial Visit】June 18th, 1966.

【Chief Symptoms】Infertility for 5 years after marriage. In the past 6 months, she experienced lower back pain, distention and pain in the right lesser abdomen, and heaviness and distention in the anus. Menstruation was normal.

【Physical Examination】 The uterus was retroverted, small in size, and had limitation of motion. At the right rear of the uterus, a cystic mass was palpated, as big as a male fist, with obscure boundaries. The left adnexa was normal. The uterine cervix was smooth. She had a deep pulse and a thin white tongue coating.

【Pattern Differentiation】 Long-term binding constraint of damp-heat in the lower jiao causing qi stagnation and blood stasis, and resulting in lower abdominal masses.

【Treatment Principle】 Regulate qi and invigorate blood; remove stasis and soften hard masses.

【Prescription】 *Ju He Kun Zao Tang* 橘核昆藻汤 (a self-composed formula)

橘核	jú hé	12g	Semen Citri Reticulatae
昆布	kūn bù	10g	Thallus Laminariae; Thallus Eckloniae
海藻	hǎi zǎo	10g	Sargassum
鳖甲	biē jiǎ	12g	Carapax Trionycis
夏枯草	xià kū cǎo	10g	Spica Prunellae
当归	dāng guī	10g	Radix Angelicae Sinensis
赤芍	chì sháo	10g	Radix Paeoniae Rubra
川楝子	chuān liàn zǐ	10g	Fructus Toosendan
延胡索	yán hú suǒ	10g	Rhizoma Corydalis
香附	xiāng fù	6g	Rhizoma Cyperi
茯苓	fú líng	10g	Poria
海蛤粉	hǎi gé fěn	12g	Concha Meretricis seu Cyclinae

During the course of treatment, *guī bǎn* (Carapax et Plastrum Testudinis), *mǔ lì* (Concha Ostreae), *yì mǔ cǎo* (Herba Leonuri), *baí shí yīng* (Quartz Album) and *é zhú* (Rhizoma Curcumae) were added during modification of the formula. In addition, vine medicinals were used in the external application. After the patient was treated on and off for over

3 months, the symptoms disappeared. The patient was on a business trip in Shanghai, and received a follow-up examination in Guangci Hospital, where the pelvic inflammatory mass was found to have completely disappeared. After 10 years, the patient visited the outpatient department of our hospital for profuse menstruation. She reported no relapse of the pelvic inflammation. Gynecological examination revealed no palpable masses.

Case 2: Ren, female, 25 years old.

【Initial Visit】June 20th, 1978.

【Chief Symptoms】Infertility for more than 3 years after marriage. She has frequent lower abdominal pain. Menstruation was normal.

【Physical Examination】The uterus was retroverted, normal-sized, of medium texture and with no limitation of motion. The left adnexauteri was thickened and there was a cystic mass, which was bigger than a goose egg. It was slightly mobile and adhered to the uterus. The right adnexauteri was thickened and there was a cystic mass, which was bigger than a pigeon egg. The cystic mass was mobile. The cervix was smooth. The pulse was thready and wiry. The tongue was slightly dusky with thin white coating.

【Pattern Differentiation】Qi stagnation and blood stasis which caused abdominal masses

【Treatment Principle】Regulate qi and invigorate blood. Transform blood stasis and soften hard mass.

【Prescription】The patient was taking *Ju He Kun Zao Tang* 橘核昆藻汤. *Chē qián zǐ* (Semen Plantaginis), *guā zǐ jīn* (Herba Polygalae Japonicae) and *bai shí yīng* (Quartz Album) were added to the formula. She took 45 doses of this formula, and received 50 injections of biostimulin and 50 injections of *yú xīng cǎo* (Herba Houttuyniae). After the treatment, the symptoms disappeared. Gynecological examination revealed that the uterus was prostrated. The uterine volume was slightly small. No mass was palpated in both sides of the adnexauteri. The right adnexauteri was slightly thickened. The cervix was smooth.

Comments:

Chronic pelvic inflammatory mass is a common gynecological disease, which belongs to the category of lower abdominal masses in Chinese medicine. It features a long course of disease, a low cure rate and a high recurrence rate. The symptoms that frequently occur are lower abdominal pain, low back pain and profuse leukorrhea. Severe cases may include infertility. Gynecological signs always include thickening of the peritoneum or thickening of the mass, which are found in the adnexa, the tissues near the uterus, the posterior fornix, or pelvic cavity; and accompanied by tenderness.

In Chinese medicine, PID can be categorized to be three patterns:

(1) Damp-heat: It is most frequently seen in acute PID or subacute PID. It is proper to clear heat and drain dampness in the treatment. It is appropriate to use *baí shí yīng* (Quartz Album) and *zǐ huā dì dīng* (Herba Violae) in addition to *Long Dan Xie Gan Tang* 龙胆泻肝汤 or *Dan Zhi Xiao Yao San* 丹栀逍遥散 as treatment.

(2) Qi Constraint: Most commonly seen in chronic PID. Thickening of the adnexa or pelvic cavity is the chief symptom. It is appropriate to course the liver and regulate qi. Use *jú hé* (Semen Citri Reticulatae), *chuān liàn zǐ* (Fructus Toosendan), *yán hú suǒ* (Rhizoma Corydalis) and *xiāng fù* (Rhizoma Cyperi) in addition to *Xiao Yao San* 逍遥散 in the treatment.

(3) Stagnation and Stasis: Most frequently seen in pelvic inflammatory masses and hydrosalpinges. It is proper to regulate qi, invigorate blood, remove blood stasis and soften hard masses. For pelvic inflammatory masses, modified *Ju He Kun Zao Tang* 橘核昆藻汤 is usually prescribed. For hydrosalpinges, modified *Gui Zhi Fu Ling Wan* 桂枝茯苓丸 is usually prescribed. Both diseases can be treated with external application using vine medicinals.

Both Case 1 and Case 2 belong to the stasis and stagnation pattern of pelvic inflammatory masses. The masses were caused by qi stagnation and blood stasis due to long-term binding constraint of damp-heat in the lower jiao. The patient was prescribed *Ju He Kun Zao Tang*. The formula consisted of *jú hé* (Semen Citri Reticulatae), *hǎi zǎo* (Sargassumas Monarch) and *kūn bù* (Thallus Laminariae; Thallus Eckloniae) as the chief medicinals since *jú hé* (Semen Citri Reticulatae) is warm in nature and can transform and dissipate nodules; and *hǎi zǎo* (Sargassumas monarch) and *kūn bù* (Thallus Laminariae; Thallus Eckloniae) that are salty and cold, and can soften hard masses, promote water flow and disperse swelling. The assistant medicinals used were *dāng guī* (Radix Angelicae Sinensis) and *chì sháo* (Radix Paeoniae Rubra) to invigorate blood and transform blood stasis; *biē jiǎ* (Carapax Trionycis), *hǎi gé fěn* (Concha Meretricis seu Cyclinae) and *xià kū cǎo* (Spica Prunellae) to soften hard masses and dissipate nodules, *chuān liàn zǐ* (Fructus Toosendan); *yán hú suǒ* (Rhizoma Corydalis) and *xiāng fù* (Rhizoma Cyperi) to move qi and alleviate pain; and *fú líng* (Poria) to strengthen the spleen and drain dampness.

(Dong Jianhua: Editor-in-chief. *The Essence of the Case Studies of Famous Contemporary Chinese Doctors* 中国现代名中医医案精华 . Beijing: Beijing Publishing House, 1990.515-516)

(4) Yu Yingtao's Case Studies: Postpartum Fever

Wang, female, 24 years old, married, worker.

5 days after labor, the patient had a fever. Axilla temperature: 40℃ . She suffered from delirium and alternating chills and fever. Then, she was treated at an unnamed hospital for 7 days and left the hospital after the fever was abated. Later, the initial problem returned with a high fever of 41℃ - 42℃ . She visited the hospital again, and was treated with all kinds of antibiotics, to no avail. The patient's condition worsened, and she developed delirium and convulsion.

She came in for treatment on August 19th, 1974. She had a pale complexion and flushed cheeks, a crimson tongue with dark yellow coating, restlessness, convulsions, shortness of breath, frequent sighing, speech difficulties, retention of lochia, thirst, no appetite, preference for cool drinks, constipation, yellow urine, difficult urination, and a surging rapid pulse. Axilla temperature: 40℃ .

【Pattern Differentiation】 Heat entering the blood chamber and lochiostasis affecting the heart.

【Treatment Principle】 Harmonize the lesser yang and relieve convulsions.

【Prescription】

党参	dǎng shēn	15g	Radix Codonopsis
柴胡	chái hú	15g	Radix Bupleuri
半夏	bàn xià	15g	Rhizoma Pinelliae
黄芩	huáng qín	15g	Radix Scutellariae
甘草	gān cǎo	15g	Radix et Rhizoma Glycyrrhizae
当归	dāng guī	25g	Radix Angelicae Sinensis
白芍	bái sháo	15g	Radix Paeoniae Alba
木瓜	mù guā	15g	Fructus Chaenomelis
桂枝	guì zhī	15g	Ramulus Cinnamomi
钩藤	gōu téng	15g	Ramulus Uncariae Cum Uncis
川芎	chuān xiōng	15g	Rhizoma Chuanxiong
生地黄	shēng dì huáng	15g	Radix Rehmanniae Recens
没药	mò yào	15g	Myrrha
金银花	jīn yín huā	25g	Flos Lonicerae Japonicae
桑叶	sāng yè	15g	Folium Mori
琥珀面	hǔ pò miàn	2.5g	Succinum
朱砂	zhū shā	2.5g	Cinnabaris

Internal Use: The patient was instructed to take 1 dose, after decocting the medicinals in water. *Hǔ pò miàn* (Succinum) and *zhū shā* (Cinnabaris) were taken separately with water.

【Second Visit on August 20th】 Temperature: 38 ℃ . She was conscious but still had restlessness, convulsions and delirium, flushed complexion, a crimson tongue with moist yellow coating, and a surging large pulse. This is postpartum blazing heat. Therefore, drying medicinals were replaced by ones that promote the production of fluid and moisten dryness.

【Prescription】

柴胡	chái hú	15g	Radix Bupleuri
党参	dǎng shēn	15g	Radix Codonopsis
黄芩	huáng qín	15g	Radix Scutellariae
半夏	bàn xià	10g	Rhizoma Pinelliae
当归	dāng guī	25g	Radix Angelicae Sinensis
白芍	bái sháo	15g	Radix Paeoniae Alba
木瓜	mù guā	15g	Fructus Chaenomelis
桂枝	guì zhī	15g	Ramulus Cinnamomi
钩藤	gōu téng	15g	Ramulus Uncariae Cum Uncis
川芎	chuān xiōng	10g	Rhizoma Chuanxiong
生地黄	shēng dì huáng	25g	Radix Rehmanniae Recens
没药	mò yào	15g	Myrrha
金银花	jīn yín huā	25g	Flos Lonicerae Japonicae
桑叶	sāng yè	15g	Folium Mori
石斛	shí hú	15g	Caulis Dendrobii
甘草	gān cǎo	7.5g	Radix et Rhizoma Glycyrrhizae

Internal Use: The patient was instructed to take 1 dose after decocting the medicinals in water.

【Second Visit on August 22 nd】 After taking the prescribed formula, the patient began to have bowel movements. She had difficult urination, and her urine was yellow. Temperature: 38℃ . She had occasional restlessness, dance-like movement of the limbs, deafness, insomnia, preference for cool drinks, flushed complexion, red tongue tip with dry peeled coating in the center, and yellow and white coating on the tongue margins. This is a pattern of heart yin deficiency and the spirit having no residence. The treatment involves clearing heart fire and resolving heat, expelling blood stasis and invigorating blood.

【Prescription】

柴胡	chái hú	15g	Radix Bupleuri
党参	dǎng shēn	15g	Radix Codonopsis
黄芩	huáng qín	15g	Radix Scutellariae
生地黄	shēng dì huáng	15g	Radix Rehmanniae Recens
法半夏	fǎ bàn xià	15g	Rhizoma Pinelliae Praeparatum
金银花	jīn yín huā	50g	Flos Lonicerae Japonicae
当归	dāng guī	20g	Radix Angelicae Sinensis
牡丹皮	mǔ dān pí	15g	Cortex Moutan
麦冬	mài dōng	15g	Radix Ophiopogonis
桑叶	sāng yè	25g	Folium Mori
没药	mò yào	15g	Myrrha
延胡索	yán hú suǒ	15g	Rhizoma Corydalis
刘寄奴	liú jì nú	15g	Herba Artemisiae Anomalae
蒲黄	pú huáng	15g	Pollen Typhae
川芎	chuān xiōng	15g	Rhizoma Chuanxiong
枳壳	zhǐ qiào	15g	Fructus Aurantii
甘草	gān cǎo	7.5g	Radix et Rhizoma Glycyrrhizae
琥珀末	hǔ pò mò	2.5g	Succinum
朱砂末	zhū shā mò	2.5g	Cinnabaris

Internal Use: The patient was advised to take 1 dose. The medicinals were decocted with water. *Hǔ pò mò* (Succinum) and *zhū shā mò* (Cinnabaris) were taken separately with water.

The patient was examined 14 times during the 40-day course of treatment. The chief formula was *Xiao Chai Hu Tang* 小柴胡汤 and *Xiao Tiao Jing Tang* 小调经汤 with heat-clearing and anticonvulsive medicinals. The chief formula was modified in accordance with the variation of the symptoms. After taking a total of 32 doses, the patient's condition was stabilized. The subsequent treatment centered on clearing liver heat, nourishing yin, and tonifying qi and blood, which resulted in alleviation of the condition.

Comments:

This is a case of postpartum fever that had been treated with many kinds of antibiotics which were unsuccessful. According to the identification of etiologic factors based on differentiation, the disease was diagnosed as heat entering the blood chamber and treated accordingly. *Xiao Chai Hu Tang* 小柴胡汤 and *Xiao Tiao Jing Tang* 小调经汤 combined with the medicinals such as *shēng dì huáng* (Radix Rehmanniae Recens), *jīn yín huā* (Flos Lonicerae Japonicae), *mǔ dān pí* (Cortex Moutan) and *lián qiào* (Fructus Forsythiae) were prescribed to clear heat and resolve toxins. In the intermediate stage of the disease, the lingering heat consumed the yin. Medicinals such as *shí hú* (Caulis Dendrobii), *mài dōng* (Radix Ophiopogonis), *biē jiǎ* (Carapax Trionycis) and *pí pá yè* (Folium Eriobotryae) were added to the formula to nourish yin fluid. *Golden Mirror of Medicine <Yī Zhōng Jīn Jiàn>* 医宗金鉴 states, "The external pathogenic heat which invades the blood chamber at the onset of menstruation causes consciousness during the day and delirium at night. The disease should be treated with caution in order to avoid harming the stomach qi, the upper jiao and the middle jiao. When the heat goes away with the bleeding, the disease will be resolved automatically. " Therefore, on the fourth visit, *yì mǔ cǎo* (Herba Leonuri), *liú jì nú* (Herba Artemisiae Anomalae), *yán hú suǒ* (Rhizoma Corydalis) and *mò yào* (Myrrha) were added to the formula to invigorate blood and transform stasis. After taking the formula, the patient passed a small quantity of blood in the stools, and the other symptoms improved significantly. The last symptoms to manifest were pain of the entire body, pain in the eyes and difficulty in walking. The patient did not contract an exterior invasion after childbirth, so from this we know that it is the qi and blood deficiency combined with the insufficiency of the channels and collaterals that caused these symptoms. Therefore, the subsequent treatment focused on clearing liver heat, nourishing yin, and tonifying qi and blood, which brought complete resolution to the complicated condition. 1 year later, a follow-up consultation revealed that the patient had fully recovered and returned to work.

(Ke Liming: Editor-in-chief. The Anthology of Medical Records of Senior Doctors of Chinese Medicine 老中医医案选 . Harbin: Heilongjiang Science and Technology Publishing House, 1981.303-305)

(5) Ma Longbo's Case Studies in Chronic PID

Liu, female, 38 years old, married.

Initial Visit: January 3rd, 1960.

Chief symptoms: The patient suffered from acute PID in the Spring of 1956. She gave birth to a boy in January, 1959. She had another attack of acute PID 8 months after labor. Since then, she has had continuous mild lower abdominal pain; fullness and distention in the epigastrium and hypochondria; poor appetite, aversion to greasy food, and preference for a liquid diet (e.g., porridge); frequent constipation that can only be alleviated by taking purgatives; scanty yellow urine; difficult and occasionally painful urination with a burning sensation; continuous dull pain in the lesser abdomen; and a cool sensation in the chest, hypochondria and upper back when angry. Menstruation was fairly normal, except for scanty, dark-colored menses, and prolonged menstrual periods (which would last approximately 10 days). The abdominal pain is worse during menstruation. The tongue was pale red. The pulse was wiry and almost rapid. Only the cun positions of the pulse in both wrists were faint.

Gynecological examination: Vulva: multiparous type; vagina: unobstructed; the cervix was smooth; the uterus was anteverted, normal-sized, of medium texture and with limitation of motion. Both sides of adnexa were thickened.

【Pattern Differentiation】 Heat from liver constraint; dual deficiency of qi and blood.

【Treatment Principle】 Regulate liver qi and clear heat; tonify qi and blood.

【Prescription】

制黄精	zhì huáng jīng	18g	Rhizoma Polygonati Praeparata
当归	dāng guī	12g	Radix Angelicae Sinensis
茯苓皮	fú líng pí	15g	Cortex Sclerotii Poriae
木通	mù tōng	6g	Caulis Akebiae
车前子	chē qián zǐ	9g	Semen Plantaginis
滑石块	huá shí kuài	12g	Talcum
淡竹叶	dàn zhú yè	12g	Herba Lophatheri
炒栀子	chǎo zhī zǐ	6g	Fructus Gardeniae Praeparata
淡肉苁蓉	dàn ròu cōng róng	12g	Herba Cistanches Recens
甘草梢	gān cǎo shāo	9g	Cacumen Radix Glycyrrhizae
生橘核	shēng jú hé	9g	Semen Citri Reticulatae Recens
枯黄芩	huáng qín	9g	Radix Scutellariae
灯芯	dēng xīn	1g	Medulla Junci Praeparata

Internal Use: The patient was told to take 2 doses in succession. *Chē qián zǐ* (Semen Plantaginis) was separated in a gauze bag from the other medicinals before decocting.

【Second Visit on January 6 th】 After taking the medicinals mentioned above, the patient felt movement of qi in the abdomen, and the fullness and distention were slightly alleviated. The abdominal pain and constipation was the same as before. There was difficult urination with scanty yellow urine. The pulse was the same. The formula was slightly modified based on the previous formula.

【Prescription】

制黄精	zhì huáng jīng	18g	Rhizoma Polygonati Praeparata
茯苓皮	fú líng pí	15g	Cortex Sclerotii Poriae
生橘核	shēng jú hé	12g	Semen Citri Reticulatae Recens
木通	mù tōng	6g	Caulis Akebiae
滑石块	huá shí kuài	12g	Talcum
秦当归	qín dāng guī	12g	Radix Angelicae Sinensis
淡肉苁蓉	dàn ròu cōng róng	15g	Herba Cistanches Recens
车前子	chē qián zǐ	9g	Semen Plantaginis

炒栀子	chǎo zhī zǐ	9g	Fructus Gardeniae Praeparata
枯黄芩	kū huáng qín	9g	Radix Scutellariae
淡竹叶	dàn zhú yè	9g	Herba Lophatheri
嫩石苇	nèn shí wěi	9g	Folium Pyrrosiae
甘草梢	gān cǎo shāo	9g	Cacumen Radix Glycyrrhizae
灯芯	dēng xīn	1g	Medulla Junci Praeparata

Internal Use: The patient was instructed to take 3 doses in succession. *Chē qián zǐ* (Semen Plantaginis) was separated with a gauze bag from the other medicinals before decocting.

【**Third Visit on January 11ᵗʰ** 】 After taking 1 dose of the previous formula, all of the symptoms were alleviated. On January 8ᵗʰ, the patient's menstruation arrived. This time, the symptoms including abdominal pain, restlessness and frequent, painful, burning urination were less severe. The color of the menses was not as dark as before. Although the abdominal pain of unfixed location and intervals still remained, the patient felt qi movement in the abdomen. The fullness and distention seemed to be lessened. Constipation and frequent, difficult, painful, scanty urination had also improved. The cool sensation in the chest, hypochondria, and upper back still occurred during fits of rage. This cool sensation is considered to be related to the patient's psychological activity, because it is worse when the patient paid more attention to it. The patient had poor appetite, sighing, aversion to greasy food, preference for a liquid diet, a feeling of comfort after drinking beverages, a slightly yellow tongue coating, and a wiry and almost rapid pulse.

【**Prescription**】

制黄精	zhì huáng jīng	18g	Rhizoma Polygonati Praeparata
玉竹	yú zhú	18g	Rhizoma Polygonati Odorati
茯苓皮	fú líng pí	15g	Cortex Sclerotii Poriae
生橘核	shēng jú hé	12g	Semen Citri Reticulatae Recens
滑石块	huá shí kuài	12g	Talcum
甘草梢	gān cǎo shāo	9g	Cacumen Radix Glycyrrhizae

炒栀子	chǎo zhī zǐ	9g	Fructus Gardeniae Praeparata
黄芩	huáng qín	9g	Radix Scutellariae
竹叶	zhú yè	12g	Folium Phyllostachydis Henonis
秦当归	qín dang guī	9g	Radix Angelicae Sinensis
柴胡	chái hú	3g	Radix Bupleuri
焦白术	jiāo bái zhú	3g	Rhizoma Atractylodis Macrocephalae Praeparata
砂仁壳	shā rén qiào	3g	Fructus Amomi
灯芯	dēng xīn	1.5g	Medulla Junci Praeparata

Internal Use: The patient was instructed to take 3 to 6 doses.

【**Fourth Visit on February 9** ᵗʰ】 After taking the formula, the previous menstruation lasted 6 days and the abdominal pain had disappeared for the most part. Bowel movement and urination were almost normal. On February 5th, her menstruation came 3 days early. Before and during menstruation, the patient had no symptoms. The menses color was normal, and the bleeding stopped after 5 days, as opposed to the prolonged bleeding that occurred before. The patient no longer felt cool sensations in the chest, hypochondria, and upper back when during fits of anger. Since the patient needed to travel to Shenyang for a job, she asked for a follow-up formula that can be taken during the week to consolidate the curative effect.

【**Prescription**】

制黄精	zhì huáng jīng	30g	Rhizoma Polygonati Praeparata
玉竹	yú zhú	18g	Rhizoma Polygonati Odorati
茯苓	fú líng	12g	Poria
生橘核	shēng jú hé	12g	Semen Citri Reticulatae Recens
冬瓜子	dōng guā zǐ	15g	Semen Benincasae
滑石块	huá shí kuài	12g	Talcum
龙胆草	lóng dǎn cǎo	4.5g	Radix Gentianae
秦当归	qín dāng guī	12g	Radix Angelicae Sinensis
焦白术	jiāo bái zhú	9g	Rhizoma Atractylodis Macro-cephalae Praeparata

丝瓜络	sī guā luò	9g	Retinervus Luffae Fructus
淡肉苁蓉	dàn ròu cōng róng	12g	Herba Cistanches Recens
砂蔻衣	shā kòu yī	9g	Amomum Cardamomum L.
柴胡	chái hú	3g	Radix Bupleuri
竹叶	zhú yè	9g	Folium Phyllostachydis Henonis
川楝子	chuān liàn zǐ	9g	Fructus Toosendan

Internal Use: The patient was advised to take the decoction regularly if it is effective. *Chǎo zhī zǐ* (Fructus Gardeniae Praeparata) 9g is made into honey pills. Take 9 grams of the honey pills in addition to the above formula.

Gynecological examination: Vulvae: normal. Vagina: normal. The uterus was slightly anteverted, normal in size, medium in texture and with limitation of motion. The left adnexa was normal. The right adnexa was slightly thickened with mild tenderness.

The patient suffered from acute PID three years ago which was not completely cured. Labor induced the relapse of the acute PID, and it gradually developed into chronic PID with symptoms of unremitting dull pain in the lesser abdomen, fullness and distention in the epigastrium, poor appetite, irregularities of the urine and stools, and menstrual disorders. After taking five doses, all of these symptoms declined. After 3 visits, the patient was considered cured and all the symptoms disappeared.

Comments:

Chronic PID always results from untreated or incomplete treatment of acute PID, or untreated inflammation which is inconspicuous in the acute stage and later develops into chronic inflammation. The course of disease varies from several months to several years, and may be more than 10 years. Chronic PID has a very damaging effect on women's health and reproduction, which causes long-term suffering.

Cases of subacute PID are occasionally encountered in the clinic.

Chinese medicine divides PID into five patterns based on the current symptoms. They are qi deficiency, heat from constraint, cold-damp, blood stasis, and kidney deficiency. Each pattern is more or less accompanied by qi stagnation from liver constraint. In addition, there is a simple pattern of qi stagnation from liver constraint, which accounts for a fairly large proportion of patterns. Based on personal experience, patients of chronic PID diagnosed by gynecological examination in biomedicine have some symptoms in common, such as: (1) leukorrhea, (2) pain in the lower abdomen, and (3) menstrual disorders. Each symptom varies in a certain patterns. For example:

1) Leukorrhea

Although each pattern presents with leukorrhea (known as *dai sheng* 带盛 in Chinese medicine), the leukorrhea varies in quantity, quality, color and odor.

2) Pain in the lesser abdomen

The pain varies case by case. Sometimes it may radiate from the sacral vertebrae. Some are located in the lesser abdomen, and are accompanied by distention and aching pain in the lumbosacral area. Some are spontaneous pain located in the bilateral aspects of the lower abdomen. Some are unremitting and dull. Some are only tenderness, and aggravated by taking a long walk or walking in a fast pace. Some are transitory pain that occur every once in a while. Some are more severe in one side than the other. Some manifest as unbearable pain during sexual intercourse.

3) Menstrual disorders

All of the chronic PID patients suffer from painful menstruation to different degrees, which can occur before or after menstruation. Some suffer from early menstruation (caused by qi deficiency, or heat from constraint). Some suffer from delayed menstruation (caused by cold-damp). Some suffer from menstruation at irregular intervals (caused by blood stasis). Some suffer from profuse, pale-colored menstrual flow (caused by qi deficiency). Some suffer from profuse, purple-red menses (caused by heat from constraint). Some menses is dark-colored, normal in quantity and accompanied with purple clots (caused by cold-dampness). Some patients will have menses of abnormal quantity that is accompanied by fairly big clots (caused by blood stasis). However, most PID patients' menstrual volume is decreased, and there is always discomfort during menstrual flow. Throughout the course of the disease, most patients are unable to conceive.

4) Pulse

Nearly all patients with chronic PID have a wiry pulse, which may also be slippery, thready, rapid, slow, or weak.

In treatment, we should not only pay attention to the common variables, but also to the variability during the progression of the disease, in order to resolve presenting issues. According to the principle of seeking common ground while accepting the existing differences, I conclude the experience of treating chronic PID as follows: chronic PID includes two main clinical manifestations -- lesser abdominal pain and wiry pulse. Based on the theory that pathological changes of a channel will manifest as disease on that channel's pathway, the lesser abdominal pain is considered to be caused by the pathological changes of the penetrating and conception vessels. Obstruction always leads to pain, and there are several factors that can cause obstruction. Those factors include deficiency, excess, cold, heat, blood stasis due to the impaired qi flow, congealed blood and qi stagnation. The etiological factor should be identified according to the accompanying symptoms, signs and pulse. Furthermore, the foot reverting yin liver channel passes through the lower abdominal region. Thus, this disease is also related to the liver channel. The wiry pulse indicates liver dysfunction or pain. It is regarded as a sign of the binding constraint of liver qi, which results in pain. According to the two chief clinical manifestations mentioned above, chronic PID is generally caused by the irregularities of the penetrating and conception vessels, and qi stagnation from liver constraint. In addition, leukorrhea is associated with spleen and kidney deficiency. The slippery and irregular pulse is connected to the stagnation of qi and blood, or to congealing phlegm; the thready and irregular pulse is related to qi and blood deficiency; the rapid and irregular pulse should be related to heat caused by the binding constraint of qi; the moderate and irregular pulse is a sign of cold-damp; and the weak and irregular pulse is related to the long-term deficiency of original qi.

(*Compilation of the Experience of Famous Senior Chinese Medical Doctors*. 老中医经验汇编 . Beijing: People's Medical Publishing House. 1977.174-176)

(6) Li Liyun's Case Studies: Acute PID

Liang, female, 39 years old, worker, 1 pregnancy and 1 childbirth, initial visit on July 26th, 1992.

History of Present Illness: The patient suffered from lower abdominal pain and distention for more than 2 months, and has not yet been checked up nor treated, due to her busy work schedule. Her last menstrual period was on June 10th. The quantity of menses was normal. In the past 5 days, the lower abdominal pain worsened, with profuse, yellow, foul-smelling leukorrhea. The pain was accompanied by fear of cold and fever for 5 days, constipation for 3 days, dryness and bitter taste in the mouth, restlessness, poor appetite, red tongue with yellow greasy coating, and slippery rapid pulse.

Physical examination: Temperature: 39℃ .Pulse rate: 94 beats per minute. Blood pressure: 110/50 mm Hg. There was muscular tension in the lower abdomen, with tenderness (+ +), and rebound tenderness (+).

Gynecological examination: Vulvae: normal. Vagina: unobstructed. The cervix was smooth. There was thick yellow pus-like, foul-smelling discharge. The uterus was retroverted and was the size of a gravid uterus in the 6th month of pregnancy. The uterus was fairly immovable, with cervical tenderness. There were palpable masses in both sides of the adnexa, with obscure boundary and tenderness (+ +).

Ultrasound revealed an enlarged uterus. Mixed adnexal masses: right mass was 4.5 cm×4 cm×4cm in size, and the left mass was 3.5 cm×3 cm× 2.7cm in size, and considered to be adnexal inflammation with masses

Laboratory examination: Blood routine examination: WBC 16.0×109/L, N% 85%, ESR 90mm/h.

【Pattern Differentiation】 Binding constraint of damp-heat toxins; obstruction of bowel qi.

【Treatment Principle】 Clear heat and resolve toxins; drain dampness and unblock the bowels.

【Prescription】 Modified combination of *Wu Wei Xiao Du Yin* 五味消毒饮 and *Da Cheng Qi Tang* 大承气汤

蒲公英	pú gōng yīng	20g	Herba Taraxaci
金银花	jīn yín huā	20g	Flos Lonicerae Japonicae
野菊花	yě jú huā	15g	Flos Chrysanthemi Indici
穿心莲	chuān xīn lián	15g	Herba Andrographis
鱼腥草	yú xīng cǎo	20g	Herba Houttuyniae
牡丹皮	mǔ dān pí	15g	Cortex Moutan
冬瓜仁	dōng guā rén	30g	Semen Benincasae
大黄	dà huáng	12g	Radix et Rhizoma Rhei
枳实	zhǐ shí	15g	Fructus Aurantii Immaturus
芒硝	máng xiāo	9g	Natrii Sulfas
厚朴	hòu pò	15g	Cortex Magnoliae Officinalis
败酱草	bài jiàng cǎo	30g	Herba Patriniae

Internal Use: The patient was instructed to take 1 bag a day. The following instructions were given: Cook the medicinals in water, and strain the decoction. The same medicinals are then cooked a second time. Add *dà huáng* (Radix et Rhizoma Rhei) in the last 5 to 10 minutes of cooking. Take *máng xiāo* (Natrii Sulfas) with water.

At the same time, venous transfusion was administered once a day, which contained 5% glucose with *Shuang Huang Lian Zhu She Ji* 双黄连泘射剂 and 5% glucose saline with *Chuang Hu Ning* 穿琥宁 20ml. *Fu Fang Mao Dong Qing Guan Chang Ye* 复方换懈青灌肠液 was given as retention enema twice a day. *Si Huang Shui Mi* 四黄水蜜 (Four Yellow Liquid Honey) was applied externally on the lower abdomen twice a day. After 3 days of treatment, the patient began having bowel movements. The stool was rotten and foul-smelling. Temperature dropped to normal. She had profuse menstrual bleeding. *Máng xiāo* (Natrii Sulfas) and *dà huáng* (Radix et Rhizoma Rhei) were removed from the formula; and *yì mǔ cǎo* (Herba Leonuri) 30g and *dì yú* (Radix Sanguisorbae) 15g were added. The menstruation lasted 5 days and all the symptoms were alleviated. The treatment was continued for another 12 days, after which the general symptoms disappeared. Gynecological examination: Vulva: normal. Vagina: normal. Cervix: smooth. The uterus was of normal size, without tenderness and limitation of motion. Both sides of adnexa were normal. Ultrasound: The uterus was normal in size and shape. No masses were found. Blood routine: ESR was normal. The patient was considered cured and was discharged from the hospital.

Comments:

Acute pelvic peritonitis induced by acute PID is a severe gynecological disease. Several steps in the treatment process should be noted. They are:

1) Control the infection as soon as possible

Preventing septicemia and infectious shock is one of the main steps. Damp-heat toxins are the chief etiological factor that causes acute pelvic peritonitis. In the early stage of the disease, using large doses of medicinals that clear heat, resolve toxins and drain dampness can quickly control the infection and prevent further disease progression.

The formula includes *jīn yín huā* (Flos Lonicerae Japonicae), *pú gōng yīng* (Herba Taraxaci), *yě jú huā* (Flos Chrysanthemi Indici), *chuān xīn lián* (Herba Andrographis), *huáng bǎi* (Cortex Phellodendri Chinensis), *zhī zǐ* (Fructus Gardeniae), *bài jiàng cǎo* (Herba Patriniae), *mián yīn chén* (Herba Artemisiae Scopariae) and *mǔ dān pí* (Cortex Moutan). These medicinals that clear heat, resolve toxins, drain dampness and cool blood have a fairly strong inhibitory effect on many types of pathogenic bacteria. In addition, *chuān xīn lián* (Herba Andrographis) can increase phagocytosis of the bacteria by leukocytes, which is effective in eliminating inflammation and bacterial growth.

2) Purge the bowels to clear heat

The method of purging the bowels to clear heat provides the evils with an exit out of the body, which is the second step of the treatment. In the clinic, we find that many patients of acute PID have the accompanying symptoms of bowel qi obstruction, such as abdominal distention and constipation. The medicinals for purging the bowels to clear heat, such as *dà huáng* (Radix et Rhizoma Rhei), *máng xiāo* (Natrii Sulfas) and *zhǐ shí* (Fructus Aurantii Immaturus), can promote gastrointestinal peristalsis and increase gastrointestinal volume for purging, which will clear the obstruction, loosen the constraint, provide an exit route for the evils, and decrease bacterial growth. Furthermore, the medicinals can also improve microcirculation and decrease capillary permeability. Thus, they have the ability to invigorate blood, transform blood stasis and alleviate pain.

3) Multiple-route medication.

Multiple-route medication is an indispensable step in the treatment of acute PID.

a. There needs to be an adequate concentration of medication in the blood for the internal medication to be effective. Therefore, patients of acute PID require larger formulas and heavier doses, which will facilitate the elimination of the evils and increase the curative effect. They should take 2 to 3 doses, at least once during the day and once at night.

b. *Qing Kai Ling Zhu She Ji* 清 开 灵 注 射 剂 and *Shuang Huang Lian Zhu She Ji* 双 黄 连 注 射 剂 have the functions of clearing heat, resolving toxins and purging pathogenic fire. They are in the list of mandatory Chinese patent medicines used in emergencies by all medical hospitals throughout China. Venous transfusion allows the medicine to act directly on the infected area, which can increase the effective concentration of antibiotic medicine, and control the disease quickly and effectively.

c. The medicinal *máo dōng qīng* (Radix Ilecis Pubescens) can invigorate blood, transform stasis, clear heat and resolve toxins. Using the decoction of *máo dōng qīng* (Radix Ilicis Pubescentis) for retention enema (which can be directly assimilated by the mucous membrane of the rectum and has a distinct curative effect) can control the infected lesion, alleviate pain, increase the blood flow in the infected lesion, improve blood circulation, increase the absorption and transformation of the inflamed hyperplastic tissue. On the whole, combining different Chinese medical treatment modalities can greatly enhance the curative effect.

(Li Liyun, Wang Xiaoyun. *Pattern Differentiation and Treatment of Chinese Medical Gynecology <Zhong Yi Fu Ke Lin Zheng Zheng Zhi>* 中 医 妇 科 临 证 证 治 . Guangzhou: People's Publishing House of Guangdong. 1999: 209-210, 216-217)

(7) Ban Xiuwen's Case Studies: Salpingemphraxis

Wei, 28 years old, female, administrator, initial visit on October 10th, 1990.

【Chief Symptoms】 The patient got married in 1986. The couple has been living together ever since, and has been having normal sexual intercourse without the use of contraception. So far, the patient has not been able to get pregnant. Her menstruation was fairly normal, with menses of normal color, quantity and quality. However, before menstruation, the patient would experience pain and distention in the lesser and lower abdomen. She reported no other daily discomforts.

【Physical Examination】 Gynecological examination revealed mild inflammation in both fallopian tubes. On October 8th, 1990, the patient received hydrotubation in the municipal hospital, which revealed salpingitides (inflammation in both fallopian tubes). She had a pale red tongue with thin white coating, and a deep thready pulse.

【Pattern Differentiation】 Qi stagnation and blood stasis; obstruction in the uterine vessels.

【Treatment Principle】 Nourish and invigorate blood; transform stasis and unblock the vessels.

【Prescription】

鸡血藤	jī xuè téng	20g	Caulis Spatholobi
丹参	dān shēn	15g	Radix et Rhizoma Salviae Miltiorrhizae
当归	dāng guī	10g	Radix Angelicae Sinensis
赤芍	chì sháo	10g	Radix Paeoniae Rubra
路路通	lù lù tōng	10g	Fructus Liquidambaris
桃仁	táo rén	6g	Semen Persicae
皂角刺	zào jiǎo cì	10g	Spina Gleditsiae
穿破石	chuān pò shí	10g	Radix Cudraniae
川红花	chuān hóng huā	6g	Flos Carthami
香附	xiāng fù	6g	Rhizoma Cyperi
炒山甲	chǎo shān jiǎ	10g	Squama Manis Praeparata

Internal Use: The patient was instructed to decoct the medicinals in water. 7 bags were prescribed weekly.

【Second Visit on January 29th】 The patient took 1 bag of the previous formula every day for more than 2 months. The pain and distention in the lesser and lower abdomen were alleviated. The patient currently experiences fullness and distention in the right hypochondria. There was also occasional dull pain in the lesser and lower abdomen. The patient had a pale red tongue with thin white coating and a thready pulse. For chronic disease always leads to binding constraint, the next treatment step is to course the liver, regulate qi and unblock collaterals.

【Prescription】

柴胡	chái hú	6g	Radix Bupleuri
当归	dāng guī	10g	Radix Angelicae Sinensis
赤芍	chì sháo	10g	Radix Paeoniae Rubra
茯苓	fú líng	10g	Poria
白术	bái zhú	10g	Rhizoma Atractylodis Macrocephalae
丹参	dān shēn	15g	Radix et Rhizoma Salviae Miltiorrhizae
路路通	lù lù tōng	10g	Fructus Liquidambaris
皂角刺	zào jiǎo cì	10g	Spina Gleditsiae
郁金	yù jīn	10g	Radix Curcumae
炙甘草	zhì gān cǎo	6g	Radix et Rhizoma Glycyrrhizae Praeparata cum Melle

Internal Use: The patient was told to decoct the medicinals in water. 7 bags were prescribed weekly.

【Third Visit on March 19 ᵗʰ】 The patient took a total of 30 bags. All of the symptoms disappeared. The patient received hydrotubation in the municipal hospital yesterday, which revealed that both fallopian tubes were unobstructed. After the operation, the patient had slight lumbago, loose stools, a pale red tongue with thin white coating, and a thready pulse. The treatment principle for this session was to nourish original qi with warm medicinals.

【Prescription】

当归	dāng guī	10g	Radix Angelicae Sinensis
熟地黄	shú dì huáng	15g	Radix Rehmanniae Praeparata
赤芍	chì sháo	10g	Radix Paeoniae Rubra
党参	dǎng shēn	15g	Radix Codonopsis
白术	bái zhú	10g	Rhizoma Atractylodis Macrocephalae
覆盆子	fù pén zǐ	10g	Fructus Rubi
菟丝子	tù sī zǐ	20g	Semen Cuscutae
枸杞子	gǒu qǐ zǐ	10g	Fructus Lycii

路路通	lù lù tōng	6g	Fructus Liquidambaris
仙茅	xiān máo	6g	Rhizoma Curculiginis
红花	hóng huā	10g	Flos Carthami
素馨花	sù xīn huā	10g	Flos Jasmini

Internal Use: The patient was instructed to take 7 doses, after decocting the medicinals in water.

Comments:

Although there is no equivalent disease name in Chinese medicine for salpingitides (inflammation of the fallopian tubes), it is still considered the main pathogenic factor of infertility according to the pulse manifestation and pattern differentiation of qi stagnation and blood stasis with obstruction in the uterine vessels. The treatment should be centered on regulating qi, nourishing blood, removing blood stasis, softening hard masses and unblocking the uterine collaterals.

The first formula was a modification of *Tao Hong Si Wu Tang* 桃红四物汤 . It consisted of medicinals that can remove blood stasis without harming right qi, such as *jī xuè téng* (Caulis Spatholobi), *dān shēn* (Radix et Rhizoma Salviae Miltiorrhizae) and *dāng guī* (Radix Angelicae Sinensis). These herbs function to nourish blood, invigorate blood and unblock the uterine collaterals. *Xiāng fù* (Rhizoma Cyperi) moves the qi of the blood and invigorates qi dynamic to promote blood circulation. *Lù lù tōng* (Fructus Liquidambaris) is acrid and bitter in flavor, neutral and non-toxic in property, and has the ability to unblock the twelve channels and collaterals. *Chuān pò shí* (Radix Cudraniae) is slightly bitter and sweet in flavor, has neutral and non-toxic properties, and can invigorate blood and unblock the channels. *Chuān pò shí* (Radix Cudraniae), which is slightly bitter, slightly sweet and non-toxic, and invigorates blood and unblocks the channels, is used together with *zào jiǎo cì* (Spina Gleditsiae), which is warm and acrid, to powerfully enhance the effects of opening the orifices and expelling phlegm and stasis. *Chuān shān jiǎ* (Squama

Manis Praeparata) is salty in flavor and slightly cold in property, and is used to soften hardness and dissipate nodules. It is also used as an envoy to guide the effects of other medicinals to the disease location, because of its moving nature.

This formula primarily uses the acrid medicinals for dispersing and the bitter medicinals for downbearing, thereby relieving the stagnation and promoting the circulation of qi and blood. To treat fullness and distention in the right hypochondria caused by liver constraint, *Xiao Yao San* 逍遥散 is prescribed as main formula, modified by the addition of medicinals that can unblock the channels and promote the circulation of qi and blood.

The patient was cured after continuously taking several dozens of doses of this formula. The medicinals were successful in targeting the location of the disease, regulating qi and blood, and dredging the uterine collaterals.

(Sui Dianjun. *Handpicked Medical Records and Notes of Famous Contemporary Chinese Doctors <Zhong Guo Dang Dai Ming Yi Yi An Yi Hua Xuan>* 中国当代名医医案医话选 . 长春 . Changchun: Jilin Science and Technology Publishing House, 1995.470-471)

3. Discussions

(1) Ha Litian treated PID by resolving toxins, eliminating dampness, regulating qi and removing blood stasis.

The chief clinical manifestations of acute PID include fever; abdominal pain that refuses pressure or a sensation of heaviness in the abdomen; profuse thick, yellow, pus-like leukorrhea that is occasionally mixed with blood; or turbid foul-smelling leukorrhea which resembles water after rinsing rice; a red tongue with yellow or greasy coating, and a surging slippery rapid or wiry rapid pulse. This is a result of the interior invasion of damp toxins that obstruct the channels and blood vessels, causing excessive heat and rotten flesh. Therefore, the treatment involves clearing heat, resolving toxins, regulating qi and harmonizing blood.

Ha Litian often uses *jīn yín huā* (Flos Lonicerae Japonicae), *pú gōng yīng* (Herba Taraxaci), *bài jiàng cǎo* (Herba Patriniae), *qīng dài* (Indigo Naturalis), *hǔ zhàng* (Rhizoma et Radix Polygoni Cuspidati), *hóng téng* (Caulis Sargentodoxae), *chuān liàn zǐ* (Fructus Toosendan), *yán hú suǒ* (Rhizoma Corydalis), *tǔ fú líng* (Rhizoma Smilacis Glabrae), *qú mài* (Herba Dianthi), *cāng zhú* (Rhizoma Atractylodis), *huáng bǎi* (Cortex Phellodendri Chinensis) and *gān cǎo* (Radix et Rhizoma Glycyrrhizae) to modify the formula according to the symptoms.

For fever, reddish complexion and constipation, consider adding *huáng lián* (Rhizoma Coptidis), *huáng qín* (Radix Scutellariae) and *dà huáng* (Radix et Rhizoma Rhei) to purge the bowels and clear heat.

For painful abdominal masses, nausea and vomiting, consider adding *xiāng yuán* (Fructus Citri), *zhú rú* (Caulis Bambusae in Taenia) and *jiāng bàn xià* (Rhizome Pinelliae Praeparata) to regulate stomach qi.

This formula includes *qīng dài* (Indigo Naturalis), which is not usually used to treat gynecological inflammation, but is used here because according to personal experience, *qīng dài* (Indigo Naturalis) can not only effectively treat the heat toxins in the upper jiao but also acute PID, for it has the functions of cooling blood and resolving toxins.

Hǔ zhàng (Rhizoma et Radix Polygoni Cuspidati), which clears heat, drains dampness, invigorates blood and resolves toxins, as well as *hóng téng* (Caulis Sargentodoxae), which clears heat, resolves toxins, expels wind and invigorates blood, are both clinically proven to be good choices for treating the binding constraint of turbid dampness, heat toxins, and the stagnation of qi and blood.

If there is formation of abscesses (which are caused by the binding constraint of damp-heat and belongs to "*Nei Yong* 内 痈 " in Chinese medicine), accompanied by high body temperature in the early stage, the treatment should focus on clearing heat, resolving toxins and expelling dampness. We can add *dāng shēn* (Radix et Rhizoma Salviae Miltiorrhizae) and *chì sháo* (Radix Paeoniae Rubra) to invigorate blood and transform stasis. However, in cases of high body temperature, one should not suddenly use mass-breaking medicinals such as *sān léng* (Rhizoma Sparganii), *é zhú* (Rhizoma Curcumae), *shān jiǎ* (Squama Manis), and *zào cì* (Spina Gleditsiae), for they can cause the proliferation of heat toxins and endanger the patient's health. The expelling method should be administered only after the body temperature has returned to normal.

The chief clinical manifestations of chronic PID include lower abdominal pain and heaviness; masses accompanied by sharp pain or continuous dull pain; aching pain in the lumbosacral area; profuse white or yellow and white leukorrhea; blue dusky tongue or a tongue with stasis maculae; moist white coating, greasy coating, or yellow coating in the tongue root; a wiry-thready, thready-rough, or deep-thready pulse. The disease is caused by lingering pathogenic evils, deficiency of right qi, and blood stasis accumulating in the uterus. Therefore, the treatment should focus on regulating qi, transforming blood stasis and dissipating nodules. Moreover, the treatment should include strengthening right qi and expelling evil qi. Ha Litian often uses *xiāng fù* (Rhizoma Cyperi), *wū yào* (Radix Linderae), *zhì mò yào* (Myrrha Praeparata), *cù biē jiǎ* (Carapax Trionycis Praeparata), *shēng mǔ lì* (Concha Ostreae Recens), *dǎng shēn* (Radix Codonopsis), *dāng guī* (Radix Angelicae Sinensis), *chǎo bái zhú* (Rhizoma Atractylodis Macrocephalae Praeparata), *chē qián zǐ* (Semen Plantaginis), *hǔ zhàng* (Rhizoma et Radix Polygoni Cuspidati), *hóng téng* (Caulis Sargentodoxae) and *gān cǎo* (Radix et Rhizoma Glycyrrhizae) to modify the formula according to the symptoms.

Due to the long course of disease, chronic PID will usually manifest as a combined pattern of excess and deficiency in the clinic. Therefore, we should not use acrid and dry medicinals for expelling evils to treat qi and blood stagnation, because they will further consume qi and blood and harm the spleen and stomach. Instead, we should take all factors into consideration when designing a treatment plan.

For cases accompanied by feverish palms and soles, flushed cheeks and night sweats, consider adding *shēng dì huáng* (Radix Rehmanniae Recens), *dì gǔ pí* (Cortex Lycii) and *qīng hāo* (Herba Artemisiae Annuae) to nourish yin and clear heat. For cases accompanied by soreness and weakness of the low back and knees, mental fatigue and physical lassitude, consider adding *gǒu jǐ* (Rhizoma Cibotii), *dù zhòng* (Cortex Eucommiae) and *chuān xù duàn* (Radix Dipsaci) to strengthen the waist and tonify the kidney. For cases accompanied by lesser abdominal pain with cold sensation, preference for warmth, fear of cold and lack of warmth in the limbs, consider replacing *hóng téng* (Caulis Sargentodoxae) and *hǔ zhàng* (Rhizoma et Radix Polygoni Cuspidati) with *bā jǐ tiān* (Radix Morindae Officinalis), *xiǎo huí xiāng* (Fructus Foeniculi) and *ròu guì* (Cortex Cinnamomi) to warm yang and disperse cold. For cases accompanied by dizziness, restlessness, breast distention, and discomfort in the chest and hypochondria, consider adding *chái hú* (Radix Bupleuri) and *qīng pí* (Pericarpium Citri Reticulatae Viride) to course the liver and regulate qi. For cases accompanied by epigastric fullness, nausea and vomiting, consider adding *jiāng bàn xià* (Rhizome Pinelliae Praeparata) and *chén pí* (Pericarpium Citri Reticulatae) to regulate stomach qi. For poor appetite and loose stools, consider replacing *hóng téng* (Caulis Sargentodoxae) and *hǔ zhàng* (Rhizoma et Radix Polygoni Cuspidati) with *shā rén* (Fructus Amomi) and *bái biǎn dòu* (Semen Lablab Album) to strengthen the spleen and treat diarrhea.

Fumigation is often administered as an auxiliary treatment for acute and chronic PID with profuse leukorrhea, and is clinically proven to have great results. The formula contains:

蛇床子	shé chuáng zǐ	9g	Fructus Cnidii
黄柏	huáng bǎi	6g	Cortex Phellodendri Chinensis
淡吴茱萸	dàn wú zhū yú	3g	Fructus Evodiae

For foul-smelling yellow leukorrhea, add *pú gōng yīng* (Herba Taraxaci) 12g. For thin white leukorrhea, add *xiǎo huí xiāng* (Fructus Foeniculi) 6g. For severe pruritis, add *dì fū zǐ* (Fructus Kochiae) 9g. First, wrap the medicinals mentioned above with a cloth and soak them in warm water for 15 minutes. Next, bring to a boil, then pour the warm decoction into a bathtub for a medicated hip bath. The medicinals can be used again several times by re-boiling. This treatment is carried out once during the day and once at night. Each bath should last from 5 to 10 minutes. After bathing, dry the vulva with a towel. The treatment should be suspended during menstruation.

(Song Zujing. *Compilation of Pattern and Treatment in Contemporary Chinese Medicine <Dang Dai Zhong Yi Zheng Zhi Hui Cui>* 当代中医证治汇粹 . Shijiazhuang: Hebei Science & Technology Publishing House. 1990. 631-632)

(2) Luo Yuan Kai's experience in treating PID

Pelvic inflammatory disease (PID) is a common gynecological disease. It refers to the inflammation of the female internal genital organs (including the uterus, the fallopian tube and the ovaries), the surrounding connective tissue and pelvic peritoneum, which is caused by the infection of pathogenic bacteria or virus. If the inflammation is confined to the fallopian tube and the ovaries, it is usually called "adnexitis". In the clinic, PID may be divided into three stages -- acute, subacute, and chronic. The chief symptom of PID is lower abdominal pain, which is always accompanied by profuse leukorrhea. Patients of acute or subacute PID may also experience aversion to cold, fever, and severe abdominal pain. Patients of chronic PID often suffer from dull lower abdominal pain and lumbago, often accompanied by menstrual irregularities, infertility, and lower abdominal masses.

There is no equivalent term for PID in Chinese medicine. According to the syndrome manifestations, PID can be categorized as leukorrhea, painful menstruation or abdominal masses. In *Detailed Outline for Women · Regulation of the Menses <Ji Yin Gang Mu·Tiao Jing Men>* 济阴纲目·调经门, there is a disease called "*Jin Bing Teng Tong* 经病疼痛", which translates as "pain of menstrual diseases" and resembles PID. A passage from Dai's speech states "All abdominal pain that occurs during menstruation is caused by irregularities of the blood." Therefore, in order to regulate blood, we should first regulate qi." Zhu Danxi writes: "Abdominal pain occurring during the onset of menstruation is caused by excessive blood or the stagnation of blood or qi. Use *Si Wu Tang* 四物汤, which is modified by adding *táo rén* (Semen Persicae), *xiāng fù* (Rhizoma Cyperi) and *huáng lián* (Rhizoma Coptidis) to treat this." The abdominal pain of PID is not associated with the menstrual cycle at all, as opposed to the pain of painful menstruation which can occur before, during, or after menstruation. In terms of pathogenesis, both of the two diseases have the manifestation of qi stagnation and blood stasis. Inflammation is defined in biomedicine as redness, swelling, heat sensation, pain and loss of function. However, according to Chinese medical pattern differentiation, the inflammation can not only be attributed to heat but also to cold, dampness, or blood stasis. In addition, there is also excess and deficiency.

This disease is often induced by two factors. One of these factors is the deficiency of right qi. For instance, the blood chamber is open during menstruation -- this is a regular, normal phenomenon known as the period of deficiency within the month. This is also seen after induced abortion, miscarriage or normal delivery, when the qi and blood have been consumed, and the cervical os has not yet closed. The other factor is the invasion of the external pathogenic evils which accumulate in the uterus, the uterine channels, and the uterine collaterals. This may occur due to unhealthy practices during menstruation or after childbirth (when there is still lochia), such as sexual intercourse, or taking a tub bath, swimming or wading. The external invasion may also occur as a result of improper sterilization during induced abortion or delivery, which result in the infection of evil toxins.

Evil toxins accumulate in the lower jiao and obstruct the qi dynamic, causing qi stagnation and blood stasis, which blocks the uterine channels and collaterals. The stagnation results in pain, hence patients with this disease will often present abdominal pain. The invasion of external dampness and the generation of internal damp turbidity due to cold evil congealing and stagnating in the channels may result in the downward flow of watery dampness into the yin orifices, causing leukorrhea. Moreover, excessive heat toxins obstructing the uterine collaterals may produce carbuncles and abscesses, causing bowel excess syndrome, which is characterized by high fever, abdominal fullness and constipation. If acute PID is treated incompletely, the disease will develop into chronic PID. However, some cases have no apparent symptoms at the acute stage of PID before the patient is admitted to the hospital. Therefore, they are diagnosed as chronic PID from the very beginning. In addition, long-term accumulation of evil qi and blood stasis may cause the binding constraint of evil and blood stasis, resulting in the formation of masses. The stagnation of evil and blood stasis obstructing the uterine channels and collaterals may lead to menstrual irregularities and infertility.

PID is often encountered in the clinic as a chronic recurrent disease with a prolonged course. The primary treatment for PID should focus on invigorating blood, removing blood stasis and moving qi in accordance with pattern differentiation. For acute or subacute PID, the treatment should involve first clearing heat, resolving toxins and expelling evils. For chronic PID, the treatment should revolve around promoting the circulation of qi and blood, or warming and unblocking the channels and collaterals.

Acute PID often presents as the pattern of heat toxins in the lower abdomen, which is characterized by strong fever; aversion to cold; headache; dryness and bitter taste in the mouth; irritability and thirst; intense lower abdominal pain that refuses pressure or awareness of a scorching sensation in the lower abdomen; heaviness, distention and discomfort in the anus; yellowish or reddish urine; frequent painful urination; constipation; profuse, yellow, thick, foul-smelling leukorrhea; a red tongue with yellow thick greasy coating, and a wiry rapid or slippery rapid pulse.

The treatment principle should focus on clearing heat and resolving toxins, as well as regulating qi and transforming stasis. Use *Hao Pu Jie Du Tang* 蒿蒲解毒汤 (a self-composed formula).

青蒿	qīng hāo (add towards the end)	12g	Herba Artemisiae Annuae
蒲公英	pú gōng yīng	30g	Herba Taraxaci
白薇	bái wēi	20g	Radix et Rhizoma Cynanchi Atrati
丹参	dān shēn	20g	Radix et Rhizoma Salviae Miltiorrhizae
牡丹皮	mǔ dān pí	12g	Cortex Moutan
赤芍	chì sháo	15g	Radix Paeoniae Rubra
黄柏	huáng bǎi	12g	Cortex Phellodendri Chinensis
桃仁	táo rén	15g	Semen Persicae
连翘	lián qiào	20g	Fructus Forsythiae
青皮	qīng pí	10g	Pericarpium Citri Reticulatae Viride
川楝子	chuān liàn zǐ	10g	Fructus Toosendan

Internal Use: Add *qīng hāo* (Herba Artemisiae Annuae) in the last 5 to 10 minutes of cooking. Take 1 or 2 bags a day. Repeatedly decoct each bag of medicinals. Take in intervals, several times a day.

For constipation, add *dà huáng* (Radix et Rhizoma Rhei) 12g. Add *dà huáng* (Radix et Rhizoma Rhei) to the decoction in the last 5 to 10 minutes of cooking.

For nausea, vomiting and poor appetite, add *xiān zhú rú* (Caulis Bambusae in Taenia Recens) 15g and *huò xiāng* (Herba Pogostemonis) 10g.

For urination with sharp pain, add *Liu Yi San* 六一散 20g.

For masses in the lesser abdomen, add *bài jiàng cǎo* (Herba Patriniae) 30g and *zǐ huā dì dīng* (Herba Violae) 15g.

For impaired consciousness, delirious speech, and cold limbs, immediately administer *Zi Xue Dan* 紫雪丹 or *An Gong Niu Huang Wan* 安宫牛黄丸 .

Patients with subacute PID always have a history of chronic PID and symptoms which are like those of acute PID (but milder than acute PID). They often present with binding constraint of damp-heat, with symptoms such as moderate fever that is difficult to rid of, chest fullness, nausea, and ungratifying defecation. One could also add medicinals that powerfully remove dampness based on the previous formula, such as *dōng guā rén* (Semen Benincasae) 30g, *shēng yì yǐ rén* (Semen Coicis Recens) and *chē qián zǐ* (Semen Plantaginis). When pathogenic heat is cleared away, treat the disease as you would chronic PID, in order to strengthen the curative effect.

Chronic PID commonly occurs in the form of qi stagnation and blood stasis, which manifests as lower abdominal pain and distention with heaviness; or pain radiating to the lumbosacral area that worsens before and after menstruation, or after exertion. It is often accompanied by profuse leukorrhea, menstrual irregularities, painful menstruation, and infertility. Gynecological examination reveals lesser abdominal masses or thickening of tissues with tenderness; salpingemphraxis (obstruction of the fallopian tube) or sactosalpinx (fluid in the fallopian tube) in some cases; a dark red tongue, and a wiry pulse.

The treatment principle should focus on invigorating blood and transforming stasis, while moving qi and alleviating pain. Use *Dan Shen Huo Xue Xing Qi Tang* 丹芍活血行气汤 (a self-composed formula)

丹参	dān shēn	20g	Radix et Rhizoma Salviae Miltiorrhizae
赤芍	chì sháo	15g	Radix Paeoniae Rubra
牡丹皮	mǔ dān pí	10g	Cortex Moutan
乌药	wū yào	15g	Radix Linderae
川楝子	chuān liàn zǐ	10g	Fructus Toosendan
延胡索	yán hú suǒ	12g	Rhizoma Corydalis
香附	xiāng fù	9g	Rhizoma Cyperi
桃仁	táo rén	15g	Semen Persicae
败酱草	bài jiàng cǎo	30g	Herba Patriniae
当归	dāng guī	9g	Radix Angelicae Sinensis

Internal Use: Decoct each package of medicinals twice. Take 1 package of medicinals a day, in 2 intervals throughout the day.

For pronounced stagnation of blood stasis resulting in severe lower abdominal pain, add *wǔ líng zhī* (Faeces Togopteri) 12g.

For cold signs and symptoms, add *xiǎo huí xiāng* (Fructus Foeniculi) 10g and *guì zhī* (Ramulus Cinnamomi) 12g.

For kidney deficiency, replace *táo rén* (Semen Persicae) with *hé shǒu wū* (Radix Polygoni Multiflori) 15g and *jī xuè téng* (Caulis Spatholobi) 20g.

For constipation, add *shēng dì huáng* (Radix Rehmanniae Recens) 25g.

For scanty painful urination, add *chē qián cǎo* (Herba Plantaginis) 30g and *shēng yì yǐ rén* (Semen Coicis Recens) 30g

For salpingemphraxis (obstruction of the fallopian tubes), add *qīng pí* (Pericarpium Citri Reticulatae Viride) 10g, *lù lù tōng* (Fructus Liquidambaris) 15g, *chuān pò shí* (Radix Cudraniae) 15g and *wáng bù liú xíng* (Semen Vaccariae) 15g.

For pronounced abdominal masses, add *é zhú* (Rhizoma Curcumae)

10g and *sān léng* (Rhizoma Sparganii) 10g.

Patients at the chronic stage of PID may receive a combination of external application and internal medication to increase the curative effect. There are two methods of external application. One is to apply external application on the lower abdomen using approximately 60g of 双柏散 *Shuang Bai San*, which includes equal quantities of *dà huáng* (Radix et Rhizoma Rhei), *huáng bǎi* (Cortex Phellodendri Chinensis), *cè bǎi yè* (Cacumen Platycladi) and *zé lán* (Herba Lycopi). Grind the medicinals into powder, and add boiled water and honey to make a paste. Mix thoroughly, heat the mixture, and then apply externally on the lower abdomen or lesser abdomen. Change dressings once a day. Ten sessions constitutes a treatment course. The other method is to retention enema, using:

大黄	dà huáng	30g	Radix et Rhizoma Rhei
虎杖	hŭ zhàng	30g	Rhizoma et Radix Polygoni Cuspidati
丹参	dān shēn	20g	Radix et Rhizoma Salviae Miltiorrhizae
蒲公英	pú gōng yīng	30g	Herba Taraxaci
枳壳	zhǐ qiào	12g	Fructus Aurantii

External Use: Decoct the medicinals with 600 ml of water until 200 ml of liquid remains. When the temperature of the water cools down to around normal body temperature, it is ready to use. Administer as retention enema once a day. 10 sessions constitute a treatment course. One can opt to use a decoction of *máo dōng qīng* (Radix Ilicis Pubescentis) [as a single dry medicinal, 60g for one session] for retention enema instead.

The treatment of chronic PID also applies to diseases with the biomedical diagnoses of pelvic venous congestion and pelvic endometriosis.

The primary treatment principle of PID is to move qi, invigorate blood and transform blood stasis. The selection of the medicinals varies by patterns and individual cases. Generally speaking, clearing heat and resolving toxins is stressed to treat excessive heat toxins, and the medicinals include *qīng hāo* (Herba Artemisiae Annuae), *lián qiào* (Fructus Forsythiae) and *huáng bǎi* (Cortex Phellodendri Chinensis). In addition, one may select other medicinals that can not only resolve toxins, but also disperse carbuncles and swellings, cool blood and transform blood stasis, such as *pú gōng yīng* (Herba Taraxaci) and *bài jiàng cǎo* (Herba Patriniae). *Compendium of Materia Medica <Ben Cao Gang Mu>* 本草纲目 elucidates, "The medicinal *bài jiàng cǎo* (Herba Patriniae) specializes in expelling pus and removing blood stasis, which is always used in the treatment of gynecological diseases in ancient times. But it is not used by people of later generations, for they do not know of its effect." For the case accompanied by the symptoms of bowel excess, add *dà huáng* (Radix et Rhizoma Rhei), which can not only purge the stools to disperse the binding constraint of heat, but also invigorates blood and transforms blood stasis. The medicinals like *dān shēn* (Radix et Rhizoma Salviae Miltiorrhizae) and *chì sháo* (Radix Paeoniae Rubra) can be used in different stages, for they are neutral in nature.

Lower abdominal pain is the chief symptom of PID, so the prescribed formula should include medicinals that move qi and alleviate pain. The selection of pain-relieving medicinals varies by pattern. For heat patterns, add cool medicinals such as *yù jīn* (Radix Curcumae) and *chuān liàn zǐ* (Fructus Toosendan). For cold patterns, add warm medicinals such as *xiǎo huí xiāng* (Fructus Foeniculi) and *wū yào* (Radix Linderae). Since medicinals that move qi and alleviate pain are usually warm in nature, they should not be used excessively. One should not select too many of those medicinals at one time. Generally, one or two medicinals are enough. Also, the dosage of these medicinals should not be too high lest they strengthen heat due to their acrid and warm nature. In addition, there are some medicinals that move qi, alleviate pain and invigorate blood, such as *yù jīn* (Radix Curcumae) and *yán hú suǒ* (Rhizoma Corydalis); and some medicinals for transforming blood stasis and alleviating pain, such as *tiān qī* (Radix et Rhizoma Notoginseng), *wǔ líng zhī* (Faeces Togopteri) and *pú huáng* (Pollen Typhae). These medicinals can treat the causes as well as the symptoms of this disease.

Chronic PID patients who have been treated for the condition tend to experience relapses when fatigued or weak. Since the expulsion of evils damage right qi, we should pay attention to strengthening right qi during the treatment. In addition, we should encourage patients to exercise, or practice *qi gong* 气功 or *dao yin* 导引 to strengthen the constitution and prevent the recurrence of disease.

After treatment, some patients will no longer exhibit positive signs during gynecological examinations, and thus they can return to work and daily life. However, they will occasionally experience dull pain in the lower abdomen that disappears during exercise and movement. This symptom is caused by liver qi constraint and the disruption of the qi dynamic, and occurs frequently in some introverted and anxious women. *Xiao Yao San* 逍遥散 is prescribed, with the addition of other medicinals such as *mǔ dān pí* (Cortex Moutan) and *zhī zǐ* (Fructus Gardeniae) to resolve constraint. In addition, the patient should be given psychological counseling or suggestive therapy, which can lead to an automatic resolution of the symptom.

In short, Chinese medical treatment of PID should not follow the conventional biomedical mode of thinking and its fixed medical prescriptions; but rather, we should alter the treatment approach in accordance with specific situations. And when the treatment takes effect, we should consolidate the curative effect to prevent recurrence.

(Luo Yuankai. *Luo Yuankai's Treatise on Chinese Medical Treatment <Luo Yuan Kai Lun Yi Ji>* 罗元恺论医集 . Beijing: People's Medical Publishing House, 1987.60-61)

(3) Wang Ziyu treats acute and chronic PID based on the identification of primary and secondary patterns:

PID is a common and frequently-occurring disease. It can be separated into two types – acute and chronic PID. Based on Chinese medical etiology and pathomechanism, both of these conditions involve blood stasis in varying degrees. Acute PID presents as exuberant heat toxins or the stagnation of blood heat. Chronic PID occurs mostly as qi stagnation and blood stasis or congealing cold-damp. Therefore, in treatment we should identify the primary and secondary patterns.

For acute PID, I use clearing heat and resolving toxins as the main treatment principle, and activating blood and transforming stasis as the assisting treatment principle.

Commonly used medicinals:

连翘	lián qiào	15g	Fructus Forsythiae
金银花	jīn yín huā	15g	Flos Lonicerae Japonicae
红藤	hóng téng	15g	Caulis Sargentodoxae
败酱草	bài jiàng cǎo	15g	Herba Patriniae
红药子	hóng yào zǐ	10g	Radix Pteroxygoni Giraldii
丹皮	dān pí	10g	Cortex Moutan
柴胡	chái hú	10g	Radix Bupleuri
赤芍	chì sháo	10g	Radix Paeoniae Rubra
桃仁	táo rén	10g	Semen Persicae
枳实	zhǐ shí	12g	Fructus Aurantii Immaturus
野菊花	yě jú huā	12g	Flos Chrysanthemi Indici
川军	chuāng jūn	6g	Radix et Rhizoma Rhei
生甘草	shēng gān cǎo	6g	Radix et Rhizoma Glycyrrhizae Recens

Internal Use: Add *chuāng jūn* (Radix et Rhizoma Rhei) in the last 5 to 10 minutes of decocting.

For abdominal distention, add *chuān liàn zǐ* (Fructus Toosendan) 10g and *mù xiāng* (Radix Aucklandiae) 6g.

For severe pain, add *zhì rǔ xiāng* (Olibanum Praeparata) 10g and *zhì mò yào* (Myrrha Praeparata) 10g.

For profuse, foul-smelling leukorrhea, add *tǔ fú líng* (Rhizoma Smilacis Glabrae) 15g.

Decoct the medicinals with water for internal use. Take 2 packages a day. Take 1 package a day when symptoms are alleviated. 7 to 10 sessions constitute one treatment course. The treatment should be continuously carried out for 3 treatment courses but suspended during menstruation.

For chronic PID, one should primarily apply the methods of activating blood and removing blood stasis. Clearing heat and resolving toxins are secondary. For qi stagnation and blood stasis, one should move qi and invigorate blood.

Commonly Used Medicinals:

柴胡	chái hú	10g	Radix Bupleuri
枳实	zhǐ shí	10g	Fructus Aurantii Immaturus
赤芍	chì sháo	10g	Radix Paeoniae Rubra
当归	dāng guī	10g	Radix Angelicae Sinensis
桃仁	táo rén	10g	Semen Persicae
延胡索	yán hú suǒ	10g	Rhizoma Corydalis
川楝子	chuān liàn zǐ	10g	Fructus Toosendan
没药	mò yào	10g	Myrrha
丹参	dān shēn	15g	Radix et Rhizoma Salviae Miltiorrhizae
败酱草	bài jiàng cǎo	15g	Herba Patriniae
木香	mù xiāng	6g	Radix Aucklandiae
生甘草	shēng gān cǎo	6g	Radix et Rhizoma Glycyrrhizae Recens

Internal Use: Take 1 bag a day. The treatment may be continuously carried out for 6 treatment courses but suspended during menstruation.

For the stagnation of cold-damp and the congealing constraint of blood stasis, which are always accompanied by masses, apply the methods of warming channels, dispersing cold, drying dampness, transforming blood stasis and dispersing masses.

Commonly Used Medicinals:

桂枝	guì zhī	10g	Ramulus Cinnamomi
炒小茴香	chǎo xiǎo huí xiāng	10g	Fructus Foeniculi Praeparata
乌药	wū yào	10g	Radix Linderae
桃仁	táo rén	10g	Semen Persicae
牡丹皮	mǔ dān pí	10g	Cortex Moutan
赤芍	chì sháo	10g	Radix Paeoniae Rubra
五灵脂	wǔ líng zhī	10g	Faeces Togopteri
当归	dāng guī	10g	Radix Angelicae Sinensis
延胡索	yán hú suǒ	10g	Rhizoma Corydalis
葫芦巴	hú lú bā	15g	Semen Trigonellae
苍术	cāng zhú	15g	Rhizoma Atractylodis
茯苓	fú líng	15g	Poria
广木香	guǎng mù xiāng	6g	Radix Aristolochiae

For severe abdominal pain with cold, replace *guì zhī* (Ramulus Cinnamomi) with *ròu guì* (Cortex Cinnamomi) 6g. For severe distention, add *lì zhī hé* (Semen Litchi) 12g.

For abdominal masses, add *sān léng* (Rhizoma Sparganii) 10g, *é zhú* (Rhizoma Curcumae) 10g and *hái zǎo* (Sargassum) 15g.

For chronic PID accompanied by qi deficiency or no improvement after long-term treatment, add shēng huáng qí (Radix Astragali Recens) 30g to replenish right qi.

The treatment may be continuously carried out for 9 treatment courses but suspended during menstruation.

For qi stagnation and blood stasis in acute and chronic PID, Wang prescribes modified *Si Ni San* 四逆散 because both conditions include lower abdominal pain as the main symptom. Since the liver channel passes through the lower abdomen, lower abdominal pain is caused by the binding constraint of liver qi resulting in the stagnation of channel. Therefore, *Si Ni San* 四逆散 is used to course the liver, resolve constraint, move qi and invigorate blood. Furthermore, the combination of *bái sháo*

(Radix Paeoniae Alba) and *gān cǎo* (Radix et Rhizoma Glycyrrhizae) is very effective in relieving spasm and alleviating pain.

(Song Zujing. *Compilation of Patterns and Treatment in Contemporary Chinese Medicine <Dang Dai Zhong Yi Zheng Zhi Hui Cui>* 当代中医证治汇粹. Shijiazhuang: Heibei Science & Technology Press. 1990.637-638)

(4) Meng Yumei emphasizes congenital and acquired factors in the treatment of chronic PID:

In Chinese medical classics, there is no corresponding term for PID. The descriptions of the chief manifestations of PID were mentioned randomly in the chapters of abdominal pain, heat entering the blood chamber, and leukorrhea. *Treatise on the Causes and Symptoms of All Diseases · The Symptoms of Eight Kind of Masses <Zhu Bin Yuan Hou Lun>* 诸病源候论 · 八瘕候 explains, "Sexual intercourse during menstruation will lead to the spasm of channels and blood vessels, lower abdominal pain with heaviness and fullness, …The binding constraint of static blood and menstrual irregularities cause masses." *Detailed Analysis of Warm Febrile Diseases <Wen Bin Tiao Bian>* 温病条辨 records, "Heat entering the blood chamber … is caused by the interior invasion of heat evil. The evil combined with blood stasis causes stagnation and pain (which refuses pressure) in the chest, abdomen and lower abdomen. "

Meng Yumei understands this perspective in accordance with the symptoms (which include lower abdominal pain as the requisite symptom, prolonged disease course, and difficult recovery) and the Chinese medical theories of "pain is caused by obstruction" and "long-term disease enters the collaterals." She considers the location of this disease to be in the lower abdomen, the uterus, and the penetrating and conception vessels. It is often caused by blood stasis and qi stagnation. Dampness evil invades the body when right qi is deficient, which is often caused by unhealthy habits. The evil accumulating in the penetrating and conception vessels and the uterus leads to the struggle between evil qi and right qi and the binding constraint of blood stasis. Thus, blood stasis and qi stagnation is the key pathomechanism of PID. The progression of this disease varies according to the congenital constitution of the patient, the damage caused by long-term medication, and the changes in pathomechanism. The condition may be complicated by the following: congealed cold; binding constraint of damp-heat; damage to both the spleen and the kidney; or the formation of masses due to chronic disease. However blood stasis and qi stagnation is undoubtedly the core of the pathomechanism. Even during acute episodes of chronic PID when there is blazing of heat toxins , the stagnation of qi and blood caused by the accumulation of evil toxins still exists as part of the pathophysiology. Therefore, Meng views the method of invigorating blood, regulating qi and alleviating pain as the primary principle in the treatment of PID.

The spleen and stomach are the root of acquired foundation and the source of qi and blood generation. The five solid yin organs, the six hollow yang bowels, the four limbs and bones of the body all depend on the nourishment of the essence of water and grain. Moreover, the transportation of medicinals also depends on the spleen and stomach for them to take effect. Patients of chronic PID often suffer from worry and mental burden because of the recurrent disease. It is known in Chinese medicine that "worry and excessive contemplation damages the spleen." In addition, prolonged disease and the binding constraint of evils will further consume right qi. Therefore, approximately one third of all patients present with symptoms of spleen and stomach deficiency and insufficiency of right qi, such as fatigue and decreased appetite. Most patients tend to relapse when tired and overworked, which is considered a characteristic of chronic PID.

In *Treatise on the Spleen and Stomach·Fluctuation of Spleen and Stomach <Pi Wei Lun·Pi Wei Sheng Shuang Lun>* 脾胃论·脾胃胜衰论, Li Dongyuan raised, "Most diseases are caused by the deficiency of the spleen and stomach." If the spleen and stomach are heavily damaged from harsh medicinals, the qi and blood will lack a production source and the deficiency of right qi will be unable to conquer the pathogen, resulting in the refusal of medicinals (pain and discomfort in the stomach duct, nausea and vomiting). Therefore, Meng constantly warns us that stomach qi should be protected during the course of treatment and we should not abuse the usage of bitter and cold medicinals (to expel evils whenever we see inflammation), which she regards as the behavior of an amateur doctor. The treatment varies by pattern and individual case. Some patients need medicinals that warm channels and transform blood stasis. Some need herbs that replenish right qi and expel blood stasis. Some need purgatives preceding tonification. Those who need medicinals for clearing heat and resolving toxins such as *huáng qín* (Radix Scutellariae), *huáng lián* (Rhizoma Coptidis), *huáng băi* (Cortex Phellodendri Chinensis), *pú gōng yīng* (Herba Taraxaci) and *bài jiàng căo* (Herba Patriniae) are less than one tenth of all cases. These medicinals are used only to treat exuberant heat toxins with symptoms of fever, aversion to cold, foul-smelling leukorrhea, dry mouth, reddish urine, yellow coating and constipation.

Meng will often add qi-moving medicinals to the basic formula for treating chronic PID to strengthen stomach qi and improve appetite, such as *shā rén* (Fructus Amomi), *mù xiāng* (Radix Aucklandiae) and *chén pí* (Pericarpium Citri Reticulatae). For deficiency of spleen and stomach qi with fatigue and poor appetite, combine *yún fú líng* (Poria), *jiāo bái zhú* (Rhizoma Atractylodis Macrocephalae Praeparata), *huáng qí* (Radix Astragali) and *dăng shēn* (Radix Codonopsis) with medicinals that regulate qi and invigorate blood, in order to tonify right qi and strengthen the patient's resistance to disease. This can effectively improve the general symptoms.

Pelvic inflammatory masses are caused by the accumulation of stagnant qi and the retention of static blood in the penetrating and conception vessels and the uterus due to long-term illness. Meng Yumei uses *rǔ xiāng* (Olibanum), *mò yào* (Myrrha), *sān léng* (Rhizoma Sparganii) and *é zhú* (Rhizoma Curcumae) to move qi, alleviate pain, expel blood stasis and disperse accumulations. These bitter medicinals can cause diarrhea because of their strong qi-moving and evil-expelling effects. Therefore, she will often add *shān yào* (Rhizoma Dioscoreae Praeparata) 30g to tonify spleen qi, replenish stomach yin, transform dampness and arrest diarrhea, which enhances the therapeutic effect.

In treatment, Meng Yumei does not only emphasize the protection of acquired constitution (spleen and stomach qi), but also the tonification of congenital constitution (kidney qi). She is of the opinion that the methods of tonifying the kidney, invigorating blood, regulating qi and alleviating pain, can significantly shorten the treatment course and increase curative effect, which amounts to half the work with double the results.

The kidney resides in the lower jiao. It is "the root of original qi and the residence of water and fire", the foundation of life, and the root of the penetrating and conception vessels and the uterus. Kidney deficiency may result in damage to the penetrating and conception vessels in women, causing problems with menstruation, leukorrhea, the fetus and childbirth. Conversely, long-term static blood and stagnant qi accumulating in the lower jiao may influence the diffusion of kidney yin and the warming function of kidney yang, causing damage to the kidney. This is why most chronic PID patients present with symptoms of kidney deficiency, such as soreness and discomfort of the lumbus and back, dizziness, and tinnitus. Furthermore, the longer the course of disease, the more severe the symptoms of kidney deficiency will be. After evaluation of the symptoms, Meng selectively adds *gǒu jǐ* (Rhizoma Cibotii), *bā jǐ tiān* (Radix Morindae Officinalis), *sāng jì shēng* (Herba Taxilli), *chuān xù duàn* (Radix Dipsaci), *nǚ zhēn zǐ* (Fructus Ligustri Lucidi) and *hàn lián cǎo* (Herba Ecliptae) to warm yang, replenish kidney essence, strengthen lumbus and bones, strongly reinforce original qi, assist right qi and expel evils. This will not only alleviate the symptoms such as discomfort of the lumbus and back, but also speed up the dissipation of inflammation and shorten the medication time.

(Bi Huanying, Jin Lin. *Journal of Beijing University of Traditional Chinese Medicine* 北京中医药大学学报 . 2000. 23(3):48-49)

PERSPECTIVES OF INTEGRATIVE MEDICINE

1. Challenges and Solutions

Pelvic inflammatory disease is a common gynecological disease. Acute pelvic inflammatory disease is quite serious, and if not controlled in time, it can quickly lead to septicemia, pyemia, septic shock, and can even be life-threatening. Chronic PID often has a long course of disease, and recurrent attacks tend to occur. Treatment becomes relatively difficult in both acute pelvic inflammatory disease and chronic pelvic inflammatory disease if there are masses. The frequently encountered challenges are: how to quickly control acute pelvic inflammation, how to prevent and treat chronic pelvic inflammatory disease, and how to treat pelvic inflammatory masses.

Challenge #1: How to quickly control acute PID

Since acute PID is a severe condition that attacks suddenly and develops quickly, integrative medicine is the best treatment approach.

1) Treatment with Chinese medicinals

Chinese medicine considers damp-heat toxins to be the main cause of acute PID, and the encumbrance of heat toxins to be the main pattern of acute PID. Therefore, the treatment should concentrate on clearing heat, resolving toxins and draining dampness. The usual selection of medicinals include *bài jiàng cǎo* (Herba Patriniae), *rěn dōng téng* (Caulis Lonicerae Japonicae), *bái huā shé shé cǎo* (Herba Hedyotis), *hŭ zhàng* (Rhizoma et Radix Polygoni Cuspidati) and *huáng băi* (Cortex Phellodendri Chinensis). *Bài jiàng căo* (Herba Patriniae) is acrid, bitter and slightly cold. It can clear heat, resolve toxins, expel pus, disperse carbuncles, invigorate blood, transform blood stasis and alleviate pain. *Rěn dōng téng* (Caulis Lonicerae Japonicae) is sweet, bitter and cold. It can clear heat, resolve toxins, unblock the channels and collaterals, and is especially effective in clearing damp-heat in the collaterals. *Bái huā shé shé căo* (Herba Hedyotis) is sweet, bland and slightly cold. It can clear heat, resolve toxins and drain damp-heat. *Hŭ zhàng* (Rhizoma et Radix Polygoni Cuspidati) is bitter and cold. It can clear heat, resolve toxins and expel pathogenic heat to unblock the stools. *Huáng băi* (Cortex Phellodendri Chinensis) is bitter and cold. It can clear heat and drain dampness, and powerfully clears damp-heat in the lower jiao. All of these medicinals are clinically proven to be effective in treating acute PID.

Purging the bowels to clear heat, which provides an exit route for the pathogens, is another key to treating PID. In the clinic, we may find that acute PID patients often suffer from distention, constipation, or diarrhea with discomfort, which are symptoms of bowel qi obstruction. Therefore, we use *dà huáng* (Radix et Rhizoma Rhei) to purge the bowels, clear heat, invigorate blood and transform blood stasis, accompanied by *hòu pò* (Cortex Magnoliae Officinalis) and *zhǐ shí* (Fructus Aurantii Immaturus) to purge the bowels, move qi and disperse stagnation. This treatment can unblock the bowels, clear heat, and alleviate all symptoms.

The method and the route of medication are other problems in the treatment of acute PID that should not be ignored. The main active ingredients of *Qing Kai Ling Zhu She Ji* 清开灵注射剂 (medicinal injection) are *niú huáng* (Calculus Bovis), *shuǐ niú jiǎo* (Cornu Bubali), *huáng qín* (Radix Scutellariae), *jīn yín huā* (Flos Lonicerae Japonicae) and *zhī zǐ* (Fructus Gardeniae). The main active ingredients of *Shuang Huang Lian Zhu She Ji* 双黄连注射剂 are *jīn yín huā* (Flos Lonicerae Japonicae), *lián qiào* (Fructus

Forsythiae) and *huáng qín* (Radix Scutellariae). Both of these formulas can clear heat, resolve toxins and purge fire, which make up the first batch of medicinals listed in the mandatory Chinese patent medicines used in emergency cases in hospitals throughout China. Venous transfusion is used to treat acute PID, which proves to be fairly effective. Venous transfusion can help the medicine target the lesions directly and quickly control the disease. At the same time, we should prescribe adequate dosages of internal medicinals. We advise that patients should take a least 2 doses a day, which are divided into three to four portions, for maximum efficacy. In addition, medicinals that clear heat, resolve toxins, invigorate blood and transform blood stasis are prescribed for retention enema and external application on the lower abdomen. The combination of internal and external use of medicinals in addition to multiple–route medication can increase the clinical curative effect and quickly control pelvic inflammation.

2) Using Antibiotics

For general toxic symptoms of acute PID, patients should be prescribed the maximum dosage of broad-spectrum antibiotics immediately. Generally, we prescribe a combination of bigeminy or trigeminy medication, which are effective in treating gram-positive bacteria, gram-negative bacteria, aerobic bacteria and anaerobic bacteria. The combination should be compatible, and venous transfusion is the main route of administration. The antibiotics should be continued until 2 weeks after the cessation of symptoms.

3) Application of adrenocorticoids

For severe infection and high fever that does not go down, one can combine broad-spectrum antibiotics with adrenocorticoids. Generally, we administer 5 to 10 mg of dexamethasone mixed with 500 ml of 5% or 10% Glucose for venous transfusion. After 3 to 5 days, the symptoms will be alleviated, at which time we can prescribe oral prednisone (decrease dosage gradually).

Challenge #2: How to prevent and treat chronic PID

Chronic PID has a prolonged course with recurrent attacks, which can adversely affect patient health. How to prevent and cure chronic PID is another challenge in the treatment of PID.

For chronic PID, biomedical treatment usually produces mild effects, while Chinese medical treatment has distinct advantages. In recent years, many effective formulas and methods of treating chronic PID have been reported. Regarding medicinals for internal use, some people use formulas and medicinals according to pattern differentiation; some make patents for specific patterns, such as powders (infusions), pills, tablets and liquid formulas for long-term use. Besides, the route of medication should be diverse, such as venous transfusion with Chinese medicinal injection, intramuscular injection, Chinese medicinal retention enema, Chinese medicinal external application, and Chinese medicinal ion therapy. Overall, the combination of Chinese medical treatment modalities has advantages in efficacy over the usage of a single treatment modality. We have prescribed *Pen Yan Fang* 盆炎方 (a self-composed formula) for internal use, combined with *Fu Fang Mao Dong Qing Guan Chang Ye* 复方毛冬青灌肠液 for retention enema and *Si Huang Shui Mi* 四黄水蜜 for external application on the lower abdomen to treat 148 cases of chronic PID, with an effectiveness rate of 99.3%.

Since "prolonged disease often leads to blood stasis", patients of chronic PID will frequently present with symptoms of stasis and stagnation regardless of what the pattern is. Therefore, in treatment, we always select medicinals for invigorating blood and transforming stasis, such as *chì sháo* (Radix Paeoniae Rubra), *dān pí* (Cortex Moutan) and *dāng guī* (Radix Angelicae Sinensis). Since "prolonged disease often leads to deficiency", patients with chronic PID will also present with symptoms of deficiency. Therefore, in the clinic, we always select medicinals for strengthening the spleen and tonifying the kidney to strengthen the constitution, such as *fú líng* (Poria), *bái zhú* (Rhizoma Atractylodis Macrocephalae), *huái shān yào* (Rhizoma Dioscoreae), *zhì gān cǎo* (Radix et Rhizoma Glycyrrhizae Praeparata cum Melle) and *sāng jì shēng* (Herba Taxilli).

Preventing the recurrence of chronic PID is also a key to treating this disease. First, the treatment of acute PID should be quick and thorough. Second, patients of chronic PID should pay attention to lifestyle modification and personal hygiene, especially during menstruation, pregnancy and after childbirth. Keep personal sanitary supplies clean and avoid the use of contaminated substitutions. Avoid excessive or unclean intercourse. Third, pay attention to receiving adequate nutrition in the diet. Avoid the intake of fatty, sweet, acrid or spicy foods such as shrimp and crab. Fourth, patients should pay attention to emotional regulation. Avoid excessive worry and anger and keep a positive outlook on life. Last but not least, participate in physical exercise. "Right qi protects the body" so that "evil qi cannot do harm."

Challenge #3: How to treat PID masses

If there is formation of inflammatory masses, the treatment of acute and chronic PID becomes fairly difficult.

In acute PID with masses, if there are clear and evident general symptoms of toxicity and unremitting high fever, one should consider that there may be formation of pelvic abscesses. The treatment may follow the integrative medical treatment introduced in the discussion of challenge # 1. After the inflammation is controlled for 2 to 3 weeks and the masses have been confined, surgical excision and drainage of the nidus can be performed.

Chronic PID accompanied by masses may be caused by incomplete treatment of abscesses in the fallopian tube and the ovaries, which can lead to the formation of pus. In addition, salpingo-oophoritis adheres to the surrounding pelvic peritoneum and can form inflammatory masses. In Chinese medicine, the mass formation belongs to the category of lower abdominal masses. The etiology and pathomechanism is within the scope of qi stagnation, blood stasis and phlegm dampness. As Zhu Danxi said, "Masses are substances with physical form, which are produced by phlegm, food retention and static blood." Based on this concept, the treatment should involve invigorating blood, breaking stasis and dispersing masses, using medicinals such as *sān léng* (Rhizoma Sparganii), *é zhú* (Rhizoma Curcumae), *chì sháo* (Radix Paeoniae Rubra), *dān shēn* (Radix et Rhizoma Salviae Miltiorrhizae), *dà huáng* (Radix et Rhizoma Rhei) and *biē jiǎ* (Carapax Trionycis).

Sān léng (Rhizoma Sparganii) is bitter and neutral, while *é zhú* (Rhizoma Curcumae) is bitter, acrid and warm. Both of them can break blood stasis, regulate qi, alleviate pain, disperse masses and dissipate nodules. In the clinic, they are used in combination to enhance the curative effect. *Chì sháo* (Radix Paeoniae Rubra) is bitter and slightly cold, and can clear heat, cool blood, invigorate blood and transform blood stasis. *Dān shēn* (Radix et Rhizoma Salviae Miltiorrhizae) is bitter and slightly cold, and its function is to invigorate blood, transform blood stasis, clear heat and relieve restlessness. *Dà huáng* (Radix et Rhizoma Rhei) is bitter and cold, and it can invigorate blood, transform blood stasis and purge the bowels to expel heat. *Biē jiǎ* (Carapax Trionycis), which is salty and slightly cold, can nourish yin to suppress yang, dissipate nodules and disperse masses. These medicinals are quite effective in treating pelvic inflammatory masses.

In addition to medicinals for internal use, we should also administer venous transfusion of Chinese medicinals, Chinese medicinal retention enema, external application on the lower abdomen, and physical therapy.

If the masses do not diminish from the treatments mentioned above, one could consider laparoscopic surgery or laparotomy.

2. Insight From Empirical Wisdom

(1) The Chinese medical treatment of acute PID should be carried out in stages:

During the early stage of acute PID, patients often exhibit symptoms of excessive heat toxins such as aversion to cold, fever, shivering and high fever (if severe), lower abdominal pain that refuses pressure, dryness and bitter taste in the mouth, constipation, scanty yellow urine, a red tongue with yellow coating and a rapid pulse. At this stage of the Chinese medical treatment, it is best to clear heat and resolve toxins using *huáng bǎi* (Cortex Phellodendri Chinensis), *huáng qín* (Radix Scutellariae), *jīn yín huā* (Flos Lonicerae Japonicae), *lián qiào* (Fructus Forsythiae), *bài jiàng cǎo* (Herba Patriniae), *pú gōng yīng* (Herba Taraxaci), *bái huā shé shé cǎo* (Herba Hedyotis) and *hǔ zhàng* (Rhizoma et Radix Polygoni Cuspidati), in conjunction with *dà huáng* (Radix et Rhizoma Rhei), *hòu pò* (Cortex Magnoliae Officinalis) and *zhǐ shí* (Fructus Aurantii Immaturus) to unblock the bowels and drain heat.

In the middle stage, patients often have symptoms of binding constraint of damp-heat and blood stasis, such as fever dissipation, fluctuation of low-grade fever, distending pain of the lower abdomen, dry mouth, chest oppression, greasy taste in the mouth, extremely poor appetite, rotten stools, a dusky red tongue with yellow greasy coating, and a soggy rapid pulse. Treatment should be focused on clearing heat and draining dampness, using *bài jiàng cǎo* (Herba Patriniae), *máo dōng qīng* (Radix Ilicis Pubescentis), *yú xīng cǎo* (Herba Houttuyniae) and *huáng bǎi* (Cortex Phellodendri Chinensis). In addition, select *chì sháo* (Radix Paeoniae Rubra), *dān pí* (Cortex Moutan) and *dān shēn* (Radix et Rhizoma Salviae Miltiorrhizae) to assist the processes of invigorating blood and transforming stasis. By this phase, patients have used antibiotics (especially metronidazole) for a period of time, and therefore will present with symptoms caused by damp turbidity, such as yellow thick greasy tongue coating. One may select *pèi lán* (Herba Eupatorii), *yīn chén* (Herba Artemisiae Scopariae), *chē qián zǐ* (Semen Plantaginis) and *bì xiè* (Rhizoma Dioscoreae Septemlobae) to transform damp turbidity.

In the late stage of the disease, patients present with complete dissipation of fever, dull pain in the lower abdomen or no pain, often accompanied by symptoms of qi deficiency and yin deficiency such as poor appetite, lassitude, fatigue, dry mouth, greasy taste in the mouth, and a thready, wiry pulse. Gynecological examination or ultrasound may still reveal pelvic masses. It is best to invigorate blood, transform blood stasis, tonify qi and nourish yin, using *chì sháo* (Radix Paeoniae Rubra), *mǔ dān pí* (Cortex Moutan), *dān shēn* (Radix et Rhizoma Salviae Miltiorrhizae), *sān léng* (Rhizoma Sparganii), *é zhú* (Rhizoma Curcumae), *tài zǐ shēn* (Radix Pseudostellariae), *bái zhú* (Rhizoma Atractylodis Macrocephalae) and *fú líng* (Poria), combined with one or two medicinals that clear heat and drain dampness, such as *bài jiàng cǎo* (Herba Patriniae), *máo dōng qīng* (Radix Ilicis Pubescentis), *rěn dōng téng* (Caulis Lonicerae Japonicae) and *yú xīng cǎo* (Herba Houttuyniae), in order to support right qi and expel evils. This method protects the body without harming right qi.

(2) Complexity of the patterns of chronic PID:

Chronic PID features a prolonged course, an obstinate condition, and frequently-occurring complex mutable patterns that are always combined patterns of cold and heat, or of excess and deficiency. Therefore, we should pay attention to pattern differentiation in the clinic.

For binding constraint of damp-heat and blood stasis, taking the medicinals for a certain amount of time may cause symptoms of spleen deficiency, such as bland taste in the mouth, poor appetite, lassitude and fatigue. We should discontinue the usage of excessively cold and cool medicinals such *huáng bǎi* (Cortex Phellodendri Chinensis), *zhī zǐ* (Fructus Gardeniae) and *yīn chén* (Herba Artemisiae Scopariae) and add spleen-invigorating, qi-replenishing and blood-nourishing medicinals such as *fú líng* (Poria), *dāng guī* (Radix Angelicae Sinensis) and *bái zhú* (Rhizoma Atractylodis Macrocephalae) instead. If there is spleen and kidney deficiency with the symptoms of severe lower abdominal pain and profuse yellow leukorrhea caused by damp-heat (which can be caused by eating too much shrimp or crab), we should remove warm and dry medicinals such as *dǎng shēn* (Radix Codonopsis) and *dāng guī* (Radix Angelicae Sinensis), and add *bài jiàng cǎo* (Herba Patriniae), *máo dōng qīng* (Radix Ilicis Pubescentis) and *rěn dōng téng* (Caulis Lonicerae Japonicae) to clear heat, relieve toxins and drain dampness. The treatment should be adjusted according to the specific situation.

The ancients observed that the vital activities of women are dominated by blood. Since blood belongs to yin, it is important to protect yin fluid when prescribing medicinals for gynecological disorders. In order to avoid the consumption of yin, doctors should not use too many bitter and cold medicinals. Long-term intake of medicinals that clear heat, resolve toxins, invigorate blood and remove blood stasis will harm the spleen. Especially for those who have congenital deficiency of the spleen or a history of stomach disease, we should stop using these medicinals when the disease is cured. In addition, we add medicinals like *fú líng* (Poria), *bái zhú* (Rhizoma Atractylodis Macrocephalae) and *shā rén* (Fructus Amomi) to strengthen the spleen and regulate stomach qi.

(3) Clinical experience in the use of medicinals for arresting leukorrhea:

Both acute and chronic PID present with profuse leukorrhea. How to treat the leukorrhea? First, we should differentiate cold from heat, and deficiency from excess. Dark-colored (yellow, red, green), thick, foul-smelling leukorrhea is usually attributed to excess and heat. Pale-colored (light white, light yellow, colorless), thin, odorless leukorrhea is usually attributed to deficiency and cold. For excess type leukorrhea, we should clear heat and drain damp with *huáng bǎi* (Cortex Phellodendri Chinensis), *bài jiàng cǎo* (Herba Patriniae), *yú xīng cǎo* (Herba Houttuyniae), *chē qián zǐ* (Semen Plantaginis), *bì xiè* (Rhizoma Dioscoreae Septemlobae), *tǔ fú líng* (Rhizoma Smilacis Glabrae), *yì yǐ rén* (Semen Coicis) and *zé xiè* (Rhizoma Alismatis). For deficiency type leukorrhea, we should differentiate between spleen and kidney deficiency. For spleen deficiency, select *cāng zhú* (Rhizoma Atractylodis), *bái zhú* (Rhizoma Atractylodis Macrocephalae), *huái shān yào* (Rhizoma Dioscoreae) and *qiàn shí* (Semen Euryales). For kidney deficiency, select *jīn yīng zǐ* (Fructus Rosae Laevigatae), *sāng piāo xiāo* (Oötheca Mantidis), *wū zéi gǔ* (Endoconcha Sepiae) and *fù pén zǐ* (Fructus Rubi).

(4) Understanding the clinical application of hemostatic medicinals:

PID patients, especially those with acute PID, will always present with profuse menstruation, prolonged menstruation, or irregular vaginal bleeding (often occurring after childbirth or miscarriage, with dark-colored, profuse or constantly-dripping lochia). We consider this the internal blockage of blood stasis, or the binding constraint of blood stasis and heat causing the accumulation of static blood and poor distribution of fresh blood, resulting in profuse menstruation, prolonged menstruation, and leukorrhea after childbirth or miscarriage.

For profuse menstruation associated with this disease, we often select *yì mǔ cǎo* (Herba Leonuri), *guàn zhòng tàn* (Rhizoma Dryopteridis Crassirhizomatis Carbonisatum), *sān qī* (Radix et Rhizoma Notoginseng), *dì yú* (Radix Sanguisorbae), *qiàn cǎo gēn* (Radix et Rhizoma Rubiae) and *jīng jiè tàn* (Herba Schizonepetae Carbonisatum). *Yì mǔ cǎo* (Herba Leonuri) invigorates blood, transforms blood stasis and regulates menstruation. Modern pharmacological research reveals that *yì mǔ cǎo* has the effect of contracting the uterus. *Guàn zhòng* (Rhizoma Dryopteridis Crassirhizomatis) is bitter and cold, and it can clear heat, resolve toxins, cool blood and arrest bleeding. It is commonly used to treat profuse uterine bleeding. In its decocted and refined form, it contains active constituents that significantly stimulate the uterus of rabbits and boost tensile force and contraction. *Sān qī* (Radix et Rhizoma Notoginseng), *dì yú* (Radix Sanguisorbae) and *qiàn cǎo gēn* (Radix et Rhizoma Rubiae) all have the functions of expelling blood stasis and arresting bleeding. *Dì yú* (Radix Sanguisorbae) and *qiàn cǎo gēn* (Radix et Rhizoma Rubiae) have the added function of cooling blood. Modern pharmacological research shows that *jīng jiè tàn* (Herba Schizonepetae Carbonisatus) can eliminate inflammation and arrest bleeding. All of the medicinals mentioned above have good effects on the alleviation of profuse and prolonged menstruation caused by endometritis.

For leukorrhea associated with this disease, we often select *yì mǔ cǎo* (Herba Leonuri), *pú huáng* (Pollen Typhae), *táo rén* (Semen Persicae), and *zhǐ qiào* (Fructus Aurantii). According to modern pharmacological research, all of these can contract the uterus. *Yì mǔ cǎo* (Herba Leonuri), *pú huáng* (Pollen Typhae) and *táo rén* (Semen Persicae) are especially effective at invigorating blood and transforming blood stasis. When static blood is eliminated, the leukorrhea will be cured.

In addition, liver and kidney yin deficiency causes internal heat, especially during menstruation. Internal heat forces blood to move recklessly, causing profuse and prolonged menstruation. To treat patients with these symptoms, we often select medicinals for nourishing yin, clearing heat, cooling blood and arresting bleeding, such as *nǚ zhēn zǐ* (Fructus Ligustri Lucidi), *mò hàn lián* (Herba Ecliptae) and *dì yú* (Radix Sanguisorbae). We also use *jīn yīng zǐ* (Fructus Rosae Laevigatae), which can tonify the kidney and stanch bleeding. We should not use medicinals that clear heat, drain dampness, invigorate blood and transform stasis, for they will only exacerbate the weakness.

3. Summary

Pelvic inflammatory disease is a common gynecological disease. Acute pelvic inflammatory disease is quite severe, and if not controlled in time, can quickly lead to septicemia, pyemia, septic shock, and may even be life-threatening. For chronic pelvic inflammatory disease, there is always a prolonged course with recurrent attacks and a difficult cure. It may lead to serious complications such as salpingemphraxis (obstruction of the fallopian tubes), pelvic adhesions and infertility, causing patients a great deal of suffering.

In the treatment of PID, biomedicine stresses disease differentiation, while Chinese medicine emphasizes pattern differentiation. Acute PID is an acute gynecological abdominal disease, which is a severe condition. We should determine the diagnosis using biomedical examinations to rule out other acute abdominal diseases, and administer prompt treatment and medication. Once diagnosed with acute PID, patients should be treated with integrative treatment immediately. Antibiotics of maximum dosage should be administered promptly in order to control the spread of inflammation and prevent further development of disease. Meanwhile, prescribing Chinese medicinals based on pattern differentiation can not only work together with antibiotics to reinforce the anti-inflammatory effect, but can also alleviate the side effects of antibiotics and strengthen the immune system. Integrative treatment has the advantages of producing good curative effect, short course of disease, and rapid rate of recovery.

The pathogens responsible for chronic PID are not easily detected for mild toxicity due to the prolonged course of disease and a weak body constitution. Thus, treatment with antibiotics has more disadvantages than advantages. By comparison, Chinese medical treatment has distinct advantages over antibiotic use because it is a combination of therapies that include medication based on pattern differentiation, Chinese medicinal retention enema, Chinese medicinal external application, acupuncture, moxibustion, and physical therapy. Moreover, it places emphasis on the regulation of the emotions, the diet and lifestyle, in order to improve quality of life and the effectiveness of therapy.

SELECTED QUOTES FROM CLASSICAL TEXTS

Yellow Emperor 's Internal Classic - Basic Questions • Treatise on Bone Interval Chapter 60 <Huang Di Nei Jing Su Wen • Gu Kong Lun Pian Di Liu Shi> 黄帝内经素问 • 骨空论篇第六十 :

"The disorder of the conception vessel causes leukorrhea and abdominal masses in women."

Synopsis of Prescriptions of the Golden Chamber • Volume 2 • Treatment of Miscellaneous Gynecological Diseases Based on Patterns and Pulse - Chapter 22 < Jin Kui Yao Lue Fang Lun • Juan Xia • Fu Ren Za Bing Mai Zheng Bing Zhi Di Er Shi Er > 金匮要略方论 · 卷下 · 妇人杂病脉证并治第二十二 :

"A woman was attacked by wind cold. After 7 or 8 days, she suffered from intermittent chills and fever, at which time her menstruation stopped suddenly. This is heat entering the blood chamber and combining with the blood; the binding constraint of blood heat caused chills and fever similar to that of malaria, which occurred at regular intervals. Use *Xiao Chai Hu Tang* 小柴胡汤 to treat the disease."

Treatise on the Causes and Symptoms of All Diseases • Volume 37 • Symptoms of Miscellaneous Gynecological Diseases 1 (32 Kinds of Symptoms) • Leukorrhea <Zhu Bing Yuan Hou Lun•Juan Zhi San Shi Qi•Fu Ren Za Bing Zhu Hou Yi (Fang San Shi Er Lun)•Dai Xia Hou > 诸病源候论 · 卷之三十七 · 妇人杂病诸候一（凡三十二论）· 带下候 :

"Excessive fatigue and exertion will damage menstrual blood, causing constitutional deficiency and wind cold. Wind cold invades the uterine collaterals and combines with the ill blood, causing leukorrhea. The penetrating and conception vessels are the sea of the channels. Diseases of the conception vessel will lead to leukorrhea. … The combination of foul fluid and blood flows downward, which is white if caused by cold, and red if caused by heat. Therefore, it is called leukorrhea."

Treatise on Three Causes of Diseases with Syndromes and Remedies • Volume 18 • Syndromes and Remedies of All Kinds of Gynecological Diseases <San Yin Ji—Bing Zheng Fang Lun • Juan Zhi Shi Ba • Fu Ren Nv Zi Zhong Bing Lun Zheng Zhi Fa> 三因极一病证方论 · 卷之十八 · 妇人女子众病论证治法 : Masses (concretions and conglomerations)

"…are caused by impaired regulation of the channels, poor healthcare after childbirth, internal damage of the seven emotions, six pathogenic factors of disease, exhaustion from excessive intercourse and a diet of cold and raw foods. All of these can cause failure of the *ying* and *wei* to be transported. The new evils combine with old evils, resulting in rotten turbidity, profuse leukorrhea and congealing stagnation of blood stasis, and causing concretions and conglomerations."

Revisions and Notes of Effective Formulae for Gynecological Diseases • Formulae for Treating Static Blood in the Abdomen of Women - Chapter 10 <Jiao Zhu Fu Ren Liang Fang • Fu Ren Fu Zhong Yu Xue Fang Lun Di Shi> 校注妇人良方 · 妇人腹中瘀血方论第十 :

"Static blood in the female abdomen is caused by the suppression of menses, remnant blood after childbirth or wind cold stagnation. If it is not removed, and remains in the body for a long period of time, it will cause accumulations, gatherings, concretions and conglomerations."

Abstracts on Gynecological Diseases • Volume 1 • Heat Entering the Blood Chamber <Nv Ke Cuo Yao • Juan Shang• Re Ru Xue Shi> 女科撮要 · 卷上 · 热入血室 :

"Women who were subjected to damage by cold, have suffered excessive physical labor, or were angry or had a fever during menstruation, are prone to heat entering the blood chamber. They may also suffer from static blood or incessant bleeding, and present with consciousness during the day and delirious speech at night (as if she had seen a ghost). Use *Xiao Chai Hu Tang* 小柴胡汤 with *shēng dì huáng* (Radix Rehmanniae Recens). For blood deficiency, use 四物汤 plus *shēng dì huáng* (Radix Rehmanniae Recens) and *chái hú* (Radix Bupleuri). Do not harm the stomach qi. If the disease is cured but the bleeding has not stopped, or the fever has not gone down, and there is deficiency of original qi, use *Bu Zhong Yi Qi Tang* 补中益气汤. For qi and blood deficiency, use *Shi Quan Da Bu Tang*."

Abstracts on Gynecological Diseases • Volume 1 • Leukorrhea <Nv Ke Cuo Yao • Juan Shang • Dai Xia> 女科撮要·卷上·带下：

"...caused by the six pathogenic factors, the seven emotions, excessive consumption of alcohol, overeating, a rich and fatty diet, exhaustion from excessive intercourse, or the intake of drying medicinals. The deficiency of the spleen and stomach causes the sinking of yang qi. The downward flow of dampness and phlegm accumulates in the lower jiao. Both of these conditions can lead to leukorrhea."

The Complete Works of Jingyue • The Regulation of Women's Health • Turbid Leukorrhea, Profuse Leukorrhea • Leukorrhea <Jing Yue Quan Shu • Fu Ren Gui • Dai Zhuo Yi Lin Lei • Dai Xia> 景岳全书·妇人规·带浊遗淋类·带下：

"The downward flow of damp-heat causes turbid leukorrhea with slippery and rapid pulse. For patients that present with red leukorrhea, restlessness, thirst and other heat symptoms, use *Bao Yin Jian* 保阴煎, *Jia Wei Xiao Yao San* 加味逍遥散 or *Jing Yan Zhu Du Wan* 经验猪肚丸; all of these are effective. For excessive heat with profuse red leukorrhea, use *Long Dan Xie Gan Tang* 龙胆泻肝汤."

The Complete Works of Jingyue • The Regulation of Women's Health • Lower Abdominal Masses (Concretions and Conglomerations) • Blood Masses <Jing Yue Quan Shu • Fu Ren Gui • Zheng Jia Lei • Xue Jia> 景岳全书·妇

人规 · 癥瘕类 · 血瘕：

"The retention of static blood causes masses, which are seen only in women; this condition arises during menstruation or after childbirth. The static blood can be caused by internal damage from cold and raw foods, the external contraction of wind cold, the stagnation of liver qi due to anger and grudges, constant overwork, long-standing weakness, or the aggravation of qi deficiency. The static blood will combine with internally accumulated evils and eventually form masses."

The Complete Works of Jingyue • Miscellaneous Diseases • Abdominal Masses (Accumulations and Gatherings) • Pattern Differentiation <Jing Yue Quan Shu • Za Zheng Mo • Ji Ju • Lun Zheng> 景岳全书 · 杂证谟 · 积聚 · 论证：

"Masses…should be carefully identified….Those which have physical form, the retention of purulent blood, or the congealed gathering of fluid that form lumps, all belong to accumulations. This disorder is in the blood level. "

Variorum of Yellow Emperor 's Spiritual Pivot • Volume 9 • Carbuncle and Abscess, Chapter 81 < Huang Di Nei Jing Ling Shu Ji Zhu • Juan Jiu • Yong Ju Di Ba Shi Yi> 黄帝内经灵枢集注 · 卷九 · 痈疽第八十一：

"Nutritive qi and protective qi continuously remain in the meridians, causing the stagnation of blood. The stagnation of blood causes the blockage of protective qi, giving rise to strong heat. The long-lasting heat rots the flesh, leading to the formation of pus."

Golden Mirror of Medicine • The Essence of Gynecological Diseases • Leukorrhea <Yi Zong Jin Jian • Fu Ke Xin Fa Yao Jue • Dai Xia Men> 医宗金鉴 · 妇科心法要诀 · 带下门：

"All types of leukorrhea are caused by dampness. For lesser abdominal pain with profuse foul leukorrhea due to damp-heat, use *Dao Shui Wan* 导水丸 , which contains *qiān niú zǐ* (Semen Pharbitidis), *huá shí* (Talcum), *huáng qín* (Radix Scutellariae) and *dà huáng* (Radix et Rhizoma

Rhei); this formula is used to treat excessive heat. For damp-cold, use *Wan An Wan* 万安丸 , which contains *qiān niú zǐ* (Semen Pharbitidis), *hú jiāo* (Fructus Piperis), *xiǎo huí xiāng* (Fructus Foeniculi) and *mù xiāng* (Radix Aucklandiae) to treat excessive cold."

Secret Transmissions of Gynecology in the Inner Mansion • Volume 2 • Red Leukorrhea <Nei Fu Mi Zhuan Jing Yan Nv Ke • Juan Er • Chi Bai Dai> 内府 秘传经验女科 · 卷二 · 赤白带 :

"Red belongs to blood, and white belongs to qi. Uterine bleeding and leukorrhea are all caused by damp-heat. The accumulation of phlegm in the stomach flows downward and seeps into the bladder, forming a thick and sticky substance. Some of it is like white soup, and is called white turbidity. The treatment is to dry dampness first, and then lift qi. In severe cases, the treatment is to lift qi and avoid the consumption of greasy and cloying foods and medicinals."

Fu Qingzhu's Gynecology • Gynecological Diseases Volume 1 • Leukorrhea <Fu Qing Zhu Nv Ke • Nv Ke Shang Juan • Dai Xia> 傅青主女科 · 女科上卷 · 带下 :

"All types of leukorrhea belong to dampness pattern. Since this disease arises from failure of the girdling vessel (*dài mài* 带 脉) to bind and hold, we call this disease *dài xià* 带 下 . …In addition, spleen qi deficiency, liver qi constraint, the invasion of dampness, and the force of heat can all cause leukorrhea. White leukorrhea is caused by excessive dampness, decline of original qi, the liver qi constraint, and qi deficiency. Use *Wán Dài Tāng* 完带汤 ."

"Green leukorrhea is caused by damp-heat in the liver channel. Use *Jiā Wèi Xiāo Yáo Sǎn* 加味逍遥散 ."

"Yellow leukorrhea is caused by damp-heat in the conception vessel. Use *Yì Huáng Táng* 易黄汤 ."

"Black leukorrhea is caused by extreme fire and heat. Use *Lì Huǒ Tāng* 利火汤 ."

"Red leukorrhea is caused by fire-heat. Use *Qīng Gān Zhǐ Lín Tāng* 清 肝止淋汤 ."

Compendium of Epidemic Febrile Diseases • Volume 3 • Ye Xiangyan's Experience with Epidemic Febrile Diseases <Wen Re Jing Wei • Juan San • Ye Xiang Yan Wai Gan Wen Re Pian> 温热经纬 · 卷三 · 叶香岩外感温热篇 :

"Xiong's commentary: There are 3 patterns of warm evil entering the blood chamber. For invasion of heat evil causing stagnation at the onset of menstruation, it is appropriate to disperse the binding constraint of blood. For evil attacking the empty and deficient blood chamber when menstruation is over, it is appropriate to nourish nutritive qi to clear heat. For evil heat invading ying (nutritive) phase and forcing blood to move recklessly during mid-cycle, it is appropriate to clear heat and calm ying (nutritive)."

MODERN RESEARCH

1. Clinical Research

(1) Pattern Differentiation and Corresponding Treatment

1) Gao Yuhua conducted a study on the etiology, pathogenesis, and clinical symptoms of pelvic inflammatory disease. He divided the disease into the following four patterns:

A. Exuberant Heat Toxins with Congealed Qi and Blood:

Clinical signs and symptoms include high fever and aversion to cold; abdominal pain that refuses pressure; profuse, yellow, thick, pus-like, foul-smelling leukorrhea; dryness and bitter taste in the mouth; constipation; yellowish or reddish urine; a red tongue with yellow greasy or yellow rough coating; and a slippery rapid pulse. The treatment for this pattern is to clear heat, resolve toxins, regulate qi and transform blood stasis. Modified *Yin Qiao Hong Jiang Tang* 银翘红酱汤 is often selected for this pattern. It consists of *jīn yín huā* (Flos Lonicerae Japonicae), *lián qiào* (Fructus Forsythiae), *pú gōng yīng* (Herba Taraxaci), *bài jiàng cǎo* (Herba Patriniae), *hóng téng* (Caulis Sargentodoxae), *mǔ dān pí* (Cortex Moutan), *chì sháo* (Radix Paeoniae Rubra), *dōng guā rén* (Semen Benincasae), *yán hú suŏ* (Rhizoma Corydalis) and *chuān liàn zĭ* (Fructus Toosendan). This pattern is commonly seen in acute PID or during acute attacks of chronic PID.

B. Damp-heat Pouring Downward combined with Qi Stagnation and Blood Stasis:

Common clinical features include lesser abdominal pain; lumbago; profuse, yellow, sticky leukorrhea; frequent urination; pain in the lower abdomen that worsens during menstruation; profuse menses of red color; a red tongue with yellow coating; and a wiry, rapid pulse. Treatment requires clearing heat, draining dampness, moving qi and invigorating blood. Modified *Qing Re Li Shi Tang* 清热利湿汤 is used for this pattern, which consists of *pú gōng yīng* (Herba Taraxaci), *lián qiào* (Fructus Forsythiae), *qú mài* (Herba Dianthi), *biăn xù* (Herba Polygoni Avicularis), *mù tōng* (Caulis Akebiae), *chē qián zĭ* (Semen Plantaginis), *chái hú* (Radix Bupleuri), *zhì xiāng fù* (Rhizoma Cyperi Praeparata) and *yán hú suŏ* (Rhizoma Corydalis). These signs and symptoms are typical of chronic PID patients with damp-heat pouring downward.

C. Stagnation of Congealing Cold-dampness and Internal Retention of Static Blood:

Clinical manifestations include lesser abdominal pain with cold sensation that is alleviated by warmth, or lesser abdominal pain with heaviness and distention; profuse, white, thin leukorrhea; delayed menstruation; dark-colored menses with blood clots; a dusky tongue with white coating; and a deep slow pulse. The treatment principle involves warming the channels, dispelling cold, invigorating blood and transforming blood stasis. Modified *Shao Fu Zhu Yu Tang* 少腹逐瘀汤 is often used for this pattern. It includes *xiăo huí xiāng* (Fructus Foeniculi), *pào jiāng* (Rhizoma Zingiberis Praeparatum), *guì zhī* (Ramulus Cinnamomi), *dāng guī* (Radix Angelicae Sinensis), *chì sháo* (Radix Paeoniae Rubra), *chuān xiōng* (Rhizoma Chuanxiong), *zhì xiāng fù* (Rhizoma Cyperi Praeparata), *wū yào* (Radix Linderae), *yán hú suǒ* (Rhizoma Corydalis) and *wǔ líng zhī* (Faeces Togopteri). This presentation is usually seen in chronic PID patients with downward flow of cold-damp.

D. Qi Stagnation and Blood Stasis with Obstruction and Stagnation in the Channels:

The clinical signs and symptoms include distending sharp pain in the lesser abdomen that worsens during menstruation; downbearing sensation of the anus; lumbago; profuse white leukorrhea (possibly combined with yellow leukorrhea); pre-menstrual breast distention and pain; depression and moodiness; a dusky tongue with stasis maculae, stasis spots and thin coating; and a wiry, thready pulse or wiry, rough pulse. The treatment is to move qi, invigorate blood, transform blood stasis and unblock the channels. Modified *Ge Xia Zhu Yu Tang* 膈下逐瘀汤 is usually chosen for this particular pattern. It includes *zhì xiāng fù* (Rhizoma Cyperi Praeparata), *wū yào* (Radix Linderae), *yù piàn* (Semen Arecae), *dāng guī* (Radix Angelicae Sinensis), *chuān xiōng* (Rhizoma Chuanxiong), *mò yào* (Myrrha), *hóng huā* (Flos Carthami), *táo rén* (Semen Persicae), *yán hú suǒ* (Rhizoma Corydalis) and *wǔ líng zhī* (Faeces Togopteri). This pattern is commonly seen in patients with pelvic inflammatory disease accompanied by abdominal masses.

The four patterns mentioned above are commonly seen in the clinic. In addition, one may apply treatment based on the chief signs and symptoms. For pronounced abdominal masses, add *sān léng* (Rhizoma Sparganii), *é zhú* (Rhizoma Curcumae), *chuān shān jiǎ* (Squama Manis), *zào jiǎo cì* (Spina Gleditsiae), *hǎi zǎo* (Sargassum) and *kūn bù* (Thallus Laminariae; Thallus Eckloniae) to disperse masses. For severe lumbago, add *xù duàn* (Radix Dipsaci), *tù sī zǐ* (Semen Cuscutae), *sāng jì shēng* (Herba Taxilli), *dù zhòng* (Cortex Eucommiae) and *gǒu jǐ* (Rhizoma Cibotii) to strengthen the lumbus and tonify the kidney. For pronounced yin deficiency, add *shí hú* (Caulis Dendrobii), *Dì gǔ pí* (Cortex Lycii), *qīng hāo* (Herba Artemisiae Annuae), *xuán shēn* (Radix Scrophulariae) and *mài dōng* (Radix Ophiopogonis) to nourish yin and clear heat. [1]

2) Gao Hui treats chronic PID of blood stasis pattern:

A. Qi Stagnation and Blood Stasis

Clinical manifestations include fixed lesser abdominal pain of sharp or dull nature; profuse leukorrhea; irregular menses; painful menstruation; dizziness and fatigue; a dusky red tongue (possibly with stasis maculae on the margins of the tongue) with white coating; and a deep or wiry pulse. The treatment principle is to move qi, invigorate blood and transform blood stasis. This pattern is often treated with *Dan Shao Huo Xue Xing Qi Tang* 丹芍活血行气汤 (a self-composed prescription), which consists of *dān shēn* (Radix et Rhizoma Salviae Miltiorrhizae), *chì sháo* (Radix Paeoniae Rubra), *wū yào* (Radix Linderae), *mǔ dān pí* (Cortex Moutan), *chuān liàn zǐ* (Fructus Toosendan), *yán hú suǒ* (Rhizoma Corydalis), *táo rén* (Semen Persicae), *bài jiàng cǎo* (Herba Patriniae), *dāng guī* (Radix Angelicae Sinensis) and *xiāng fù* (Rhizoma Cyperi).

B. Stagnation of Cold-damp

Clinical features include a long course of disease; fear of cold and cold limbs; distending pain and cold sensation in the lower abdomen; aching pain in the lumbosacral portion that is exacerbated by menstruation and fatigue; delayed menstruation; scanty dark-colored menses; profuse, thin leukorrhea; a pale tongue (possibly with stasis maculae) with white thin coating, and a deep slow pulse. The treatment principle is to warm the channels, disperse cold, transform stasis and remove dampness. Use *dāng guī* (Radix Angelicae Sinensis), *chuān xiōng* (Rhizoma Chuanxiong), *chì sháo* (Radix Paeoniae Rubra), *yán hú suǒ* (Rhizoma Corydalis), *xiāng fù* (Rhizoma Cyperi), *shēng pú huáng* (Pollen Typhae Recens), *xiǎo huí xiāng* (Fructus Foeniculi), *guì xīn* (Cortex Cinnamomi), *fú líng* (Poria) and *cāng zhú* (Rhizoma Atractylodis). For cases accompanied by blood clots, add *sān léng* (Rhizoma Sparganii) and *é zhú* (Rhizoma Curcumae).

C. Stagnation of Damp-heat

Clinical signs and symptoms include soreness of the lower back; lower abdominal pain; profuse yellow thick foul-smelling leukorrhea; menstrual irregularities or early menstruation; yellow urine and dry stools; a red tongue with yellow greasy coating; and a slippery rapid pulse. The treatment principle is to clear heat, drain dampness, invigorate blood and transform stasis. Use *xuán shēn* (Radix Scrophulariae), *zhú yè* (Folium Phyllostachydis Henonis), *biǎn xù* (Herba Polygoni Avicularis), *qú mài* (Herba Dianthi), *yán hú suǒ* (Rhizoma Corydalis), *pú gōng yīng* (Herba Taraxaci), *bài jiàng cǎo* (Herba Patriniae), *dān shēn* (Radix et Rhizoma Salviae Miltiorrhizae), *shēng pú huáng* (Pollen Typhae Recens), *mù xiāng* (Radix Aucklandiae), *zhì rǔ xiāng* (Olibanum Praeparata) and *zhì mò yào* (Myrrha Praeparata). [2]

3) Zhu Aimei believes that the treatment of chronic PID should comply with the main pathomechanism, and should be focused on invigorating blood and transforming stasis. In addition, one should treat the branch (*biao*) and root (*ben*) simultaneously, support the right qi and dispel evils. Since blood stasis is the main pathomechanism, the primary treatment principle is to invigorate blood and transform stasis, assisted by clearing heat, dispersing cold, dispelling dampness, regulating qi and tonifying deficiency. When dispelling evils, it is necessary to support the right qi, strengthen the spleen and stomach, soften the liver, nourish blood, tonify the kidney and strengthen the root (*ben*).

Zhu Aimei divides PID into three patterns:

A. Stagnation of Blood Heat

The clinical features of this pattern are fever and aversion to cold; headache; lower abdominal pain that refuses pressure; rebound tenderness; profuse thick, yellow, pus-like and foul-smelling leukorrhea; excessive thirst; nausea with the desire to vomit; poor appetite; dry or loose stools; frequent urination with reddish urine; a red tongue with yellow greasy coating, and a slippery rapid pulse. The treatment principle is to clear heat, resolve toxins, invigorate blood and transform blood stasis. Use *jīn yín huā* (Flos Lonicerae Japonicae) 15g, *lián qiào* (Fructus Forsythiae) 15g, *hóng téng* (Caulis Sargentodoxae) 15g, *shēng yì yǐ rén* (Semen Coicis Recens) 15g, *mǔ dān pí* (Cortex Moutan) 10g, *shēng gān cǎo* (Radix et Rhizoma Glycyrrhizae) 10g, *chái hú* (Radix Bupleuri) 10g, *zhǐ shí* (Fructus Aurantii Immaturus) 10g, *hóng yào zǐ* (Radix Pteroxygoni Giraldii) 10g, *táo rén* (Semen Persicae) 10g and *dà huáng* (Radix et Rhizoma Rhei) 6g (add in the end). For loose foul-smelling stools, replace *dà huáng* (Radix et Rhizoma Rhei) with *gé gēn* (Radix Puerariae Lobatae) 10g and *huáng lián* (Rhizoma Coptidis) 10g. For abdominal distention and pain, add *chuān liàn zǐ* (Fructus Toosendan) 10g. For severe pain, add *rǔ xiāng* (Olibanum) 10g and *zhì mò yào* (Myrrha Praeparata) 10g. For pelvic abscesses, add *bài jiàng cǎo* (Herba Patriniae) 15g.

B. Qi Stagnation and Blood Stasis

Clinical manifestations include lower abdominal distending pain with heaviness during menstruation; aching pain in the lumbosacral area; profuse, yellow, pus-like, foul-smelling leukorrhea; early menstruation; profuse dark purple menses with blood clots; a red tongue with yellow greasy coating; and a wiry slippery pulse. The treatment principle is to promote qi, invigorate blood and transform blood stasis, assisted by clearing heat and draining dampness. Use *dāng guī* (Radix Angelicae Sinensis) 10g, *chì sháo* (Radix Paeoniae Rubra) 10g, *wū yào* (Radix Linderae) 10g, *lì zhī hé* (Semen Litchi) 10g, *zhì mò yào* (Myrrha Praeparata) 10g, *shēng pú huáng* (Pollen Typhae Recens) 10g (wrap), *guǎng mù xiāng* (Radix Aucklandiae) 6g, *shēng dì huáng* (Radix Rehmanniae Recens) 15g, *bài jiàng cǎo* (Herba Patriniae) 15g, *tǔ fú líng* (Rhizoma Smilacis Glabrae) 15g and *dà fù pí* (Pericarpium Arecae) 15g.

C. Congealing Cold-damp

Clinical signs and symptoms include lower abdominal cold pain and distention during menstruation; delayed menstruation; scanty dark-colored menses with blood clots; lesser abdominal pain with coldness that is alleviated by warmth; profuse, thin, foul-smelling leukorrhea; stasis spots on the tongue with white greasy coating; and a deep slow pulse. The treatment principle is to warm the channels, disperse cold, dry dampness, regulate qi and transform blood stasis. Use *guì zhī* (Ramulus Cinnamomi) 10g, *zhì fù zǐ* (Radix Aconiti Lateralis Praeparata) 10g, *wū yào* (Radix Linderae) 10g, *dāng guī* (Radix Angelicae Sinensis) 10g, *chì sháo* (Radix Paeoniae Rubra) 10g, *cāng zhú* (Rhizoma Atractylodis) 15g, *fú líng* (Poria) 15g, *hú lú bā* (Semen Trigonellae) 15g, *lù jiǎo shuāng* (Cornu Cervi Degelatinatum) 15g and *guǎng mù xiāng* (Radix Aristolochiae) 5g. For severe lower abdominal pain with coldness, replace *guì zhī* (Ramulus Cinnamomi) with *ròu guì* (Cortex Cinnamomi) 10g. For severe distention, add *lì zhī hé* (Semen Litchi) 15g. For qi deficiency, add *huáng qí* (Radix Astragali) 20g. For masses, add *tòu gǔ cǎo* (Caulis Impatientis) 15g and *é zhú* (Rhizoma Curcumae) 10g. [4]

4) Liang Jianping divides PID into four patterns:

A. Stagnation of Blood Heat

Clinical features are fever or aversion to cold; aching pain in the lumbosacral area; intense pain in one or both sides of the lower abdomen that refuses pressure; foul-smelling or sticky yellow leukorrhea; early menstruation; dry mouth without the desire to drink; painful difficult urination; a red tongue with yellow coating, and a slippery rapid pulse. Treatment is to clear heat, cool blood, resolve toxins and disperse stagnation. Use modified *Yin Hong Bai Du Yin*, which consists of *jīn yín huā* (Flos Lonicerae Japonicae) 20g, *hóng téng* (Caulis Sargentodoxae) 30g, *bài jiàng cǎo* (Herba Patriniae) 40g, *chì sháo* (Radix Paeoniae Rubra) 10g, *mǔ dān pí* (Cortex Moutan) 10g, *qīng mù xiāng* (Radix Aristolochiae) 12g, *lián qiào* (Fructus Forsythiae) 15g and *zǐ huā dì dīng* (Herba Violae) 20g. For high fever, add *chái hú* (Radix Bupleuri) 15g and *pú gōng yīng* (Herba Taraxaci) 20g, or *Liu Shen Wan* 六神丸 15 pills. For constipation, add *dà huáng* (Radix et Rhizoma Rhei). For painful urination, add *shēng dì huáng* (Radix Rehmanniae Recens) 15g and *zhú yè* (Folium Phyllostachydis Henonis) 10g. For profuse menses, add *Yun Nan Bai Yao* 云南白药 0.8g, taken with water.

B. Internal Accumulation of Damp Toxins

Clinical manifestations include fever or aversion to wind; distending pain in the lower abdomen; headaches and dizziness; fatigued limbs; soreness and weakness of the lower back and legs; profuse thick yellow leukorrhea or thin watery leukorrhea; vulval pruritis; possible infertility; yellow greasy tongue coating; and a slippery rapid pulse. Treatment is to clear toxins, strengthen the spleen and transform dampness. Use modified *Bi Xie Shen Shi Tang* 萆薢渗湿汤 , which contains *bì xiè* (Rhizoma Dioscoreae) 20g, *chē qián zǐ* (Semen Plantaginis) 15g, *yún líng* (Poria) 15g, *huáng bǎi* (Cortex Phellodendri Chinensis) 10g, *yì yǐ rén* (Semen Coicis) 60g, *tǔ fú líng* (Rhizoma Smilacis Glabrae) 15g, *bài jiàng cǎo* (Herba Patriniae) 30g, *cāng zhú* (Rhizoma Atractylodis) 8g and *bái zhú* (Rhizoma Atractylodis Macrocephalae) 12g. For high fever, add *hóng téng* (Caulis Sargentodoxae) 20g and *zǐ huā dì dīng* (Herba Violae) 20g. For distending pain, add *wū yào* (Radix Linderae) 12g and *yán hú suǒ* (Rhizoma Corydalis) 12g. For profuse foul-smelling leukorrhea, add *lóng dǎn cǎo* (Radix Gentianae) 15g and *ǎi dì chá* (Herba Ardisiae Japonicae) 15g.

C. Qi Stagnation and Blood Stasis

Clinical features include pain in one or both sides of the lower abdomen or lumbosacral area that is worse before and after menstruation; painful menstruation; pre-menstrual breast distention; restlessness; irritability; profuse menses; a dark purple tongue possibly with stasis maculae; a wiry thready pulse; and palpable masses during gynecological examination. The treatment principle is to regulate qi and alleviate pain. Use *dāng guī* (Radix Angelicae Sinensis) 10g, *chuān xiōng* (Rhizoma Chuanxiong) 6g, *yán hú suǒ* (Rhizoma Corydalis) 15g, *wǔ líng zhī* (Faeces Togopteri) 12g, *chuān liàn zǐ* (Fructus Toosendan) 10g, *xiāng fù* (Rhizoma Cyperi) 10g, *liú jì nú* (Artemisiae Anomale) 15g, *shēng pú huáng* (Pollen Typhae Recens) 10g, *hóng téng* (Caulis Sargentodoxae) 30g and *bái zhú* (Rhizoma Atractylodis Macrocephalae) 10g. For severe pain, add *San Qi Fen* 三七粉 (Sanqi Powder) 6g (taken with water), *rǔ xiāng* (Olibanum) 6g and *mò yào* (Myrrha) 6g. For breast distention, add *jú hé* (Semen Citri Reticulatae) 20g and *qīng pí* (Pericarpium Citri Reticulatae Viride) 10g. For masses, add *mǔ lì* (Concha Ostreae) 30g and *chuān shān jiǎ* (Squama Manis) 12g. For hard masses, add *biē jiǎ* (Carapax Trionycis) 15g.

D. Liver and Kidney Deficiency

Clinical manifestations include long-term soreness and heaviness in the lumbosacral area that worsens after movement; dizziness; lassitude; weakness; feverish palms and soles; emaciation; restlessness; insomnia; scorching vulval pain; poor appetite; a pale tongue with thin coating, and a thready rapid pulse. There may be infertility in some cases. Use modified *Zhi Bai Di Huang Tang* 知柏地黄汤 , which consists of *zhī mǔ* (Rhizoma Anemarrhenae) 10g, *huáng bǎi* (Cortex Phellodendri Chinensis) 6g, *shēng dì huáng* (Radix Rehmanniae Recens) 12g, *shú dì huáng* (Radix Rehmanniae Praeparata) 12g, *zǎo pí* (Fructus Corni), *shān yào* (Rhizoma Dioscoreae) 15g, *mǔ dān pí* (Cortex Moutan) 10g, *bài jiàng cǎo* (Herba Patriniae) 30g, *lián qiào* (Fructus Forsythiae) 15g and *shí hú* (Caulis Dendrobii) 10g. For feverish palms and soles, add *guī bǎn* (Carapax et

Plastrum Testudinis) 15g. For low-grade fever, add *bái wéi* (Radix et Rhizoma Cynanchi Atrati) 10g and *dì gǔ pí* (Cortex Lycii) 15g. For qi and blood deficiency, add *huáng jīng* (Rhizoma Polygonati) 15g and *sāng shèn* (Fructus Mori) 15g. For restlessness and insomnia, add *suān zǎo rén* (Semen Ziziphi Spinosae) 15g and *yè jiāo téng* (Caulis Polygoni Multiflori) 15g. [5]

(2) Specific Formulas

a) *Fu You Chong Ji* 妇友冲剂

Contains shēng *huáng qí* (Radix Astragali Recens), *tù sī zǐ* (Semen Cuscutae), *é zhú* (Rhizoma Curcumae), *kūn bù* (Thallus Laminariae; Thallus Eckloniae), *zào jiǎo cì* (Spina Gleditsiae) and *wú zhū yú* (Fructus Evodiae). Results after treating 104 cases of chronic PID: effectiveness rate 83.6%. [6]

b) *Hua Yu Jie Du Tang* 化瘀解毒汤

Contains *chái hú* (Radix Bupleuri) 10g, *cù zhì yán hú suǒ* (Rhizoma Corydalis Praeparata) 20g, *dāng guī* (Radix Angelicae Sinensis) 20g, *chì sháo* (Radix Paeoniae Rubra) 15g, *chuān liàn zǐ* (Fructus Toosendan) 15g, *bài jiàng cǎo* (Herba Patriniae) 30g, *hóng huā* (Flos Carthami) 10g, *fú líng* (Poria) 20g, *pú gōng yīng* (Herba Taraxaci) 30g and *bái huā shé shé cǎo* (Herba Hedyotis) 20g. Results of treating 106 cases of acute and chronic PID: a cure rate of 66.7%, and a total effectiveness rate of 94.5%. [7]

c) *Jia Wei Gui Zhi Fu Ling Tang* 加味桂枝茯苓汤

Contains *guì zhī* (Ramulus Cinnamomi) 20g, *mǔ dān pí* (Cortex Moutan) 20g, *fú líng* (Poria) 30g, *zé xiè* (Rhizoma Alismatis) 30g, *yì mǔ cǎo* (Herba Leonuri) 30g, *chì sháo* (Radix Paeoniae Rubra) 30g, *yì yǐ rén* (Semen Coicis) 30g, *shēng huáng qí* (Radix Astragali Recens) 40g and *táo rén* (Semen Persicae) 10g. Results of treating 36 cases of chronic PID accompanied by pelvic fluid with modified *Jia Wei Gui Zhi Fu Ling Tang*: total effectiveness rate of 97.2%. [8]

d) *Pen Qiang Yan He Ji* 盆腔炎合剂

Contains *chái hú* (Radix Bupleuri), *huáng qín* (Radix Scutellariae), *chì sháo* (Radix Paeoniae Rubra), *yì yǐ rén* (Semen Coicis), *bài jiàng cǎo* (Herba Patriniae), *pú gōng yīng* (Herba Taraxaci), *chén pí* (Pericarpium Citri Reticulatae), *fú líng* (Poria), *lù lù tōng* (Fructus Liquidambaris), *dān shēn* (Radix et Rhizoma Salviae Miltiorrhizae), *chuān liàn zǐ* (Fructus Toosendan), *zé xiè* (Rhizoma Alismatis), *yì mǔ cǎo* (Herba Leonuri), *guā lóu* (Fructus Trichosanthis) and *yù jīn* (Radix Curcumae). Result of treating 200 cases of chronic PID: total effective rate of 100%. [9]

e) *Bai Chun Ke Li* 柏椿颗粒

Contains *huáng bǎi* (Cortex Phellodendri Chinensis), *chūn pí* (Cortex Ailanthi) and *bái tóu wēng* (Radix Pulsatillae). Results of treating 102 cases of damp-heat accumulation type subacute PID: excellent improvement in 72.55% of cases, and a total effectiveness rate of 96.08 %. [10]

f) *Pen Qiang Xiao Yan Jiao Nang* 盆腔消炎胶囊

Contains *jīn yín huā* (Flos Lonicerae Japonicae), *pú gōng yīng* (Herba Taraxaci), *lián qiào* (Fructus Forsythiae), *pú huáng* (Pollen Typhae), *bài jiàng cǎo* (Herba Patriniae), *hóng téng* (Caulis Sargentodoxae), *yīn chén* (Herba Artemisiae Scopariae), *tǔ fú líng* (Rhizoma Smilacis Glabrae), *zǐ huā dì dīng* (Herba Violae), *dà qīng yè* (Folium Isatidis), *biē jiǎ* (Carapax Trionycis) and *yán hú suǒ* (Rhizoma Corydalis). Results of treating 100 cases of damp-heat accumulation type chronic PID: excellent improvement in 87% of cases, and a cure rate of 52%. [11]

g) *Kang Ning Tang* 康宁汤

Contains *zǐ huā dì dīng* (Herba Violae) 50g, *pú gōng yīng* (Herba Taraxaci) 50g, *bài jiàng cǎo* (Herba Patriniae) 30g, *bái huā shé shé cǎo* (Herba Hedyotis) 30g and *kǔ shēn* (Radix Sophorae Flavescentis) 15g. Results of treating 50 cases of chronic PID using *Kang Ning Tang* retention enema: a cure in 38 cases and improvement in 10 cases.

h) *Hong Teng Tang* 红藤汤

Contains *hóng téng* (Caulis Sargentodoxae), *zǐ huā dì dīng* (Herba Violae), *pú gōng yīng* (Herba Taraxaci), *yā zhí cǎo* (Herba Commelinae), *bài jiàng cǎo* (Herba Patriniae), *xiāng fù* (Rhizoma Cyperi) and *táo rén* (Semen Persicae). Results of treating 48 cases of acute PID (combined with western pharmaceuticals): an effectiveness rate of 93.74%. [13]

i) *Dan Shao Huo Xue Xing Qi Tang* 丹芍活血行气汤

Contains *dān shēn* (Radix et Rhizoma Salviae Miltiorrhizae) 20g, *chì sháo* (Radix Paeoniae Rubra) 15g, *wū yào* (Radix Linderae) 15g, *táo rén* (Semen Persicae) 15g, *mǔ dān pí* (Cortex Moutan) 10g, *chuān liàn zǐ* (Fructus Toosendan) 10g, *xiāng fù* (Rhizoma Cyperi) 9g, *dāng guī* (Radix Angelicae Sinensis) 9g, *yán hú suǒ* (Rhizoma Corydalis) 12g and *bài jiàng cǎo* (Herba Patriniae) 30g. Result after treating 50 cases of chronic PID: total effectiveness rate of 88%. [14]

j) *Fu Fang Feng Ling Ke Li* 复方风灵颗粒

Contains *wēi líng xiān* (Radix et Rhizoma Clematidis) 30g, *bái zhǐ* (Radix Angelicae Dahuricae) 10g, *dú huó* (Radix Angelicae Pubescentis) 10g, *hóng téng* (Caulis Sargentodoxae) 15g, *fáng fēng* (Radix Saposhnikoviae) 10g, *niú xī* (Radix Achyranthis Bidentatae) 15g, *shí wéi* (Folium Pyrrosiae) 10g, *gōu téng* (Ramulus Uncariae Cum Uncis) and *bì xiè* (Rhizoma Dioscoreae Septemlobae) 15g. The medicinals mentioned above are in granule form, taken with boiled water. Take 1 dose a day, divided into 2 times, one for morning and the other for evening. Result after treating 65 cases: an effectiveness rate of 85.12%. [15]

(3) Acupuncture and Moxibustion

a) Acupuncture:

Yuan Junyi used acupuncture combined with TDP radiation in the treatment of chronic PID. For spleen and kidney yang deficiency, damp-heat pouring downward, liver and kidney yin deficiency, and dysfunction of the penetrating and conception vessels, RN 3, RN 4, RN 6, SP 6, zǐ gōng, BL 23 and ST 36 were selected. For masses, qi stagnation and blood stasis, RN 3, RN 6, zǐ gōng, BL 23 and SP 10 were selected. 28-gauge filiform needles were used. After the needles were inserted, twirling, rotating, lifting and thrusting were applied moderately and equally. When the needling sensation was obtained, the needles were retained for 30 minutes and then TDP radiation was applied locally for 30 minutes. Results of treating 124 cases: excellent improvement in 62.10% of cases, and an effectiveness rate of 87.9%. [16]

Han Chonghua inserted a 3 cun 28-gauge filiform needle into BL 32 perpendicularly at the depth of 2.5 to 2.8 cun. Then, a 4 cun 28-gauge filiform needle was inserted into BL 54 obliquely, and electric stimulation was applied to BL 32, BL 54 and RN 4. Results of treating 144 cases of chronic PID: excellent improvement in 89 cases (61.81%), improvement in 46 cases (31.94%), and a total effectiveness rate of 99.31%. [17]

Li He used fire needles to treat chronic PID according to pattern differentiation. The treatment group selected RN 3, RN 4, ST 28, SP 6, ST 29, BL 32. For deficiency of kidney and congealing cold, needle BL 23 and apply moxibustion to RN 4. For stagnation of damp-heat, SP 9 and LV 5 were needled. For spleen and stomach deficiency, BL 20 and ST 36 were needled. A medium-gauge needle was selected and burned it until it is glowing white, then quick insertion and removal were performed on the selected points. The needle was not retained. For the points on the abdomen, the needle was inserted to the depth of 3 to 5 cun. For SP 6 and BL 32, the needle was inserted to the depth of 2 to 3 cun. The treatment was carried out every other day, with 7 sessions constituting one treatment course. Each subsequent treatment course was carried out 3 days after the previous one. Treatment was suspended during menstruation. After 3 courses, an assessment of the curative effect was given. Results of treating 90 cases of chronic PID: 70.0% cure rate, 97.8%

effectiveness rate, and 7.9% recurrence rate. [18]

Hong Jianyun needled the abdominal plexus and the sacroiliac plexus to treat chronic PID. The abdominal plexus was located in the following manner: With RN 3 as the midpoint, two points were located -- one on the left of RN 3, the other on the right. The distance from each point to the inside of the anterior superior iliac spine was 2 cun. These two points were connect in a line and the line was equally divided into 8 parts. There were a total of 9 points needled (the two ends of this line plus the meeting points of the 8 parts). The location of the sacroiliac plexus: BL 32 was chosen as two midpoints. Then, the bony suture that is on the superior border of sacrum was linked to the inside of the posterior superior iliac spine. The line was then divided into 4 parts. This revealed a total of 10 points for acupuncture stimulation. Manipulation: The abdominal plexus was needled perpendicularly to the depth of 13 to 25 mm with a 25 to 44mm filiform needle. Care was taken not to penetrate the peritoneum, and lifting and thrusting methods applied only until the needle seemed stuck. Twirling and rotating methods were not used. Needling the sacroiliac plexus required a 40 to 50mm filiform needle. The needle was inserted perpendicularly to the depth of 25 to 40 mm on the superior border of the iliac bone. Lifting and thrusting methods were applied only until there was a needling sensation. Twirling and rotating methods were not used. Result: 75.7% cure rate, 97.1% total effective rate. [19]

Xu Xia used acupuncture on the basis of medication on the Chinese medicinal group. LV 3, SP 6, SP 9 and RN 4 were selected and needled with even method, and the needles were retained for 30 minutes. The treatment was carried out once a day. One menstrual cycle counted as a treatment course. During menstruation, the treatment was suspended. Result: a total effectiveness rate of 97.1%. [20]

b) Moxibustion

Zhao Jianchun applied warming moxibustion to treat 60 cases of chronic PID. RN 4, zǐ gōng (two points) and ST 36 (two points) were selected. A common moxa stick or a medicinal moxa stick was ignite at one end. Moxibustion was applied at the points mentioned above. After 50 days, the results were: a cure in 24 cases, excellent improvement in 26 cases, effective in 8 cases, and ineffective in 2 cases. The therapeutic effect in the trial group is significantly higher than in the control group which used antibiotics. [21]

Du lei used acupuncture to treat 83 cases of chronic PID and evaluated the curative effect. ST 28, SP 6 (two points) and SP 10 (two points) were needled after the points were sterilized. When the needling reaction arrived, even method was applied, and the needle was retained for 30 minutes. The treatment was carried out once a day. Moxibustion was performed at BL 23 and RN 4 with a moxa cone. 3 units of moxa cones were used at each point . The treatment was carried out once a day, with the following result: 88.71 % total effectiveness rate. [22]

(4) Additional Treatment Modalities

a) Herbal Enema:

Wang Zhexiang used *jīn yín huā* (Flos Lonicerae Japonicae) 15g, *lián qiào* (Fructus Forsythiae) 15g, *chì sháo* (Radix Paeoniae Rubra) 15g, *huáng qí* (Radix Astragali) 15g, *sān léng* (Rhizoma Sparganii) 15g, *é zhú* (Rhizoma Curcumae) 15g, *dāng shēn* (Radix et Rhizoma Salviae Miltiorrhizae) 20g, *xià kū cǎo* (Spica Prunellae) 30g and *bài jiàng cǎo* (Herba Patriniae) 30g decocted into 100 ml of thick soup for retention enema on 100 patients. Treatment was administered every night before sleep, once 1 day. The velocity of irrigation was 10 ml/min to 20 ml/min. The longer retention, the better the effect. Results of treating 100 cases of PID after 14 days: a cure in 81 cases, improvement in 16 cases, ineffective in 3 cases. [23]

Wang Yan used anorectal enema to treat 30 cases of PID. For binding constraint of blood stasis and toxins, a mixture of 双黄连粉针 剂 *Shuang Huang Lian Fen Zhen Ji* (Shuanghuanglian Injection) 3.6g and ligustrazine 200 mg, dissolved in 200 ml sodium chloride was used. For qi stagnation and blood stasis, 40 ml of 丹参注射液 *Dan Shen Zhu She Ye* (Danshen Injection) dissolved in 200 ml of sodium chloride and 200 mg of ligustrazine dissolved in 200 ml of sodium chloride were used. For pelvic inflammatory masses, hysteromyoma and endometriosis, *chì sháo* (Radix Paeoniae Rubra), *dāng shēn* (Radix et Rhizoma Salviae Miltiorrhizae), *xià kū cǎo* (Spica Prunellae), *sān léng* (Rhizoma Sparganii), *é zhú* (Rhizoma Curcumae) and *zào jiǎo cì* (Spina Gleditsiae) were decocted into a thick soup. Results: a cure in 15 cases, excellent improvement in 8 cases, effectiveness in 6 cases, ineffective in 1 case. [24]

Wang Kecan prescribed *dāng guī* (Radix Angelicae Sinensis) 15g, *hóng téng* (Caulis Sargentodoxae) 15g, *chì sháo* (Radix Paeoniae Rubra) 15g, *pú gōng yīng* (Herba Taraxaci) 15g, *dān shēn* (Radix et Rhizoma Salviae Miltiorrhizae) 15g, *bài jiàng cǎo* (Herba Patriniae) 30g, *hóng huā* (Flos Carthami) 10g, *xiāng fù* (Rhizoma Cyperi) 10g, *chuān liàn zǐ* (Fructus Toosendan) 10g and *yán hú suǒ* (Rhizoma Corydalis) 10g to treat 47 cases of PID. For masses, *sān léng* (Rhizoma Sparganii) 10g and *é zhú* (Rhizoma Curcumae) 10g were added. For fluid in the pouch of Douglas, *yì yǐ rén* (Semen Coicis) 15g and *zé xiè* (Rhizoma Alismatis) 15g were decocted for retention enema, and *zhì rǔ xiāng* (Olibanum Praeparata) 15g, *zhì mò yào* (Myrrha Praeparata) 15g, *ròu guì* (Cortex Cinnamomi) 15g, *chǎo xiǎo huí xiāng* (Fructus Foeniculi Praeparata) 30g, *gān jiāng* (Rhizoma Zingiberis) 10g and *hú jiāo* (Fructus Piperis) 3g were prescribed for external application. Results of treating 47 cases of PID: a cure in 9 cases, excellent improvement in 18 cases, and improvement in 20 cases. [25]

Wan Jin prescribed *Hong Teng Tang* 红藤汤 for retention enema, which includes *bài jiàng cǎo* (Herba Patriniae) 50g, *zǐ huā dì dīng* (Herba Violae) 50g, *dān shēn* (Radix et Rhizoma Salviae Miltiorrhizae) 30g, *hóng téng* (Caulis Sargentodoxae) 50g and *bái huā shé shé cǎo* (Herba Hedyotis) 50g. Each bottle contained 200 ml. The decoction was warmed to 37 - 39°C and given as retention enema at night before bedtime. 10 sessions constituted one treatment course. Intermission between two treatment courses was 2 days. The treatment was suspended during menstruation. After 2 courses, the results were: a cure in 162 cases, effective in 34 cases, ineffective in 4 cases, and a total effectiveness rate of 98%. [26]

b) External Application of Chinese Medicinals:

Zhu Zhaolian prescribed the following medicinals for external application: *dà huáng* (Radix et Rhizoma Rhei) 6g, *cāng zhú* (Rhizoma Atractylodis) 6g, *xiāng fù* (Rhizoma Cyperi) 6g, *huáng bǎi* (Cortex Phellodendri Chinensis) 10g, *jiāng huáng* (Rhizoma Curcumae Longae) 8g, *hóng huā* (Flos Carthami) 8g, *bái zhǐ* (Radix Angelicae Dahuricae) 8g, *chén pí* (Pericarpium Citri Reticulatae) 8g, *fáng fēng* (Radix Saposhnikoviae) 8g, *hòu pò* (Cortex Magnoliae Officinalis) 8g, *tòu gú cǎo* (Caulis Impatientis) 15g, *cǎo wū* (Radix Aconiti Kusnezoffii) 15g, *tiān huā fěn* (Radix Trichosanthis) 15g, *ài yè* (Folium Artemisiae Argyi) 12g, *zé lán* (Herba Lycopi) 12g, *dān shēn* (Radix et Rhizoma Salviae Miltiorrhizae) 9g, *rǔ xiāng* (Olibanum) 5g and *mò yào* (Myrrha) 5g. Add warm water and a desired quantity of white spirit or liquor. Blend them into a paste for local application. Results of treating more than 300 cases of chronic PID were: 96.7% total effective rate. [27]

Zhang Wen used external application to treat 100 cases of chronic PID by prescribing *xiǎo huí xiāng* (Fructus Foeniculi), *mò yào* (Myrrha), *hóng huā* (Flos Carthami), *dāng guī* (Radix Angelicae Sinensis), *qiān nián jiàn* (Rhizoma Homalomenae), *tòu gú cǎo* (Caulis Impatientis), *chì sháo* (Radix Paeoniae Rubra), *ài yè* (Folium Artemisiae Argyi), *yán hú suǒ* (Rhizoma Corydalis), *máng xiāo* (Natrii Sulfas) and *huáng lián* (Rhizoma Coptidis). In addition, TDP radiation was used. Result: 91% total effective rate. [28]

c) Physical Therapy:

Zheng Hongjun treated 48 cases of chronic PID using *zǐ huā dì dīng* (Herba Violae) 30g, *yě jú huā* (Flos Chrysanthemi Indici) 30g, *sān léng*

(Rhizoma Sparganii) 30g, *é zhú* (Rhizoma Curcumae) 30g, *bài jiàng cǎo* (Herba Patriniae) 24g, *yán hú suǒ* (Rhizoma Corydalis) 24g, *lián qiào* (Fructus Forsythiae) 24g, *xiǎo huí xiāng* (Fructus Foeniculi) 20g, *huó xuě lián* (Aconitum Cavaleriei Var. Vaginatum) 40g and *jīn yín huā* (Flos Lonicerae Japonicae) 40g. Apply ion therapy. After 24 days of treatment, the results were: a cure in 31 cases, excellent improvement in 17cases, which equals a total effectiveness rate of 100%. [29]

Meng Wen treated 82 cases of chronic PID by first applying a sonicator (for 5 minutes, 2 times a day) and then applying iontophoresis for 30 minutes with an audio frequency therapy apparatus, using *tòu gú cǎo* (Caulis Impatientis) 20g, *yì yǐ rén* (Semen Coicis) 20g, *mǔ dān pí* (Cortex Moutan) 20g, *hóng téng* (Caulis Sargentodoxae) 15g, *táo rén* (Semen Persicae) 15g, *hóng huā* (Flos Carthami) 15g, *huáng lián* (Rhizoma Coptidis) 15g, *yán hú suǒ* (Rhizoma Corydalis) 15g and *bài jiàng cǎo* (Herba Patriniae) 20g. After 30 days of treatment, the results were: a cure in 62 cases, excellent improvement in 10 cases and moderate improvement in 10 cases. [30]

Huang Yanzhen applied iontophoresis with audio frequency therapy apparatus, using *dān shēn* (Radix et Rhizoma Salviae Miltiorrhizae), *bái huā shé shé cǎo* (Herba Hedyotis), *mò yào* (Myrrha), *rǔ xiāng* (Olibanum), *xuè jié* (Sanguis Draconis), *hóng huā* (Flos Carthami), *guì zhī* (Ramulus Cinnamomi), *xiāng cǎo* (Herba), *dāng guī* (Radix Angelicae Sinensis), *chì sháo* (Radix Paeoniae Rubra) and *hú jiāo* (Fructus Piperis). The results of the treatment were satisfactory. [31]

Zheng Mingying utilized helium-neon laser therapy on CV 4, ST 29, CV 3, CV 2, ST 28 and zǐ gōng, with an effectiveness rate of 100%. [32]

d) Massage Therapy:
Wang Yanjun selected RN 4, ST 29, RN 3, BL 23, BL 31, BL 32, BL 33, BL 34, SP 6 and SP 9 and applied the following techniques: one-finger method, kneading, pushing, point-pressing and scrubbing. Results: a

cure in 12 cases, improvement in 16 cases and no effect in 2 cases. [33]

e) Lateral Vaginal Fornix Injection Therapy:

Dong Shihua injected 复方败酱注射液 *Fu Fang Bai Jiang Zhu She Ye* (Complex Prescription Baijiang Injection) through the lateral vaginal fornix. The ingredients of the formula included *bài jiàng cǎo* (Herba Patriniae), *dān shēn* (Radix et Rhizoma Salviae Miltiorrhizae), *jīn yín huā* (Flos Lonicerae Japonicae), *chì sháo* (Radix Paeoniae Rubra), *yì yǐ rén* (Semen Coicis), *mù xiāng* (Radix Aucklandiae) and *xià kū cǎo* (Spica Prunellae). An volume of 10 ml was injected once a day. 14 sessions constituted one treatment course. Pharmacological tests proved this medicine can alleviate pain and eliminate inflammation. Injection though the lateral vaginal fornix allows the medicine to directly target the connective tissue of the pelvic cavity, which enhances its pharmacodynamic action. Thus, this method can effectively clear heat, drain dampness, resolve toxins, move qi, invigorate blood and transform blood stasis. [34]

f) Point-blocking Therapy:

Jiang Junwei employed point-blocking therapy to treat 78 cases of chronic PID. The clinical total effectiveness rate reached 98.72%. Zǐ gōng, RN 3, BL 32 and ST 36 selected, and BL 23 was added to the protocol if there was lumbago. A mixture consisting of 6 ml of *Dan Shen Zhu She Ye* 丹参注射液 (Dan Shen Injection) and 6 ml of sodium chloride was injected into zǐ gōng, RN 3 and BL 32. 100mg of vitamin B1, 200ug of VB$_{12}$ and 6 ml of sodium chloride was injected into ST 36. For severe inflammation, replace *Dan Shen Zhu She Ye* 丹参注射液 (Dan Shen Injection) with 4 ml of *Fu Fang Chuan Xin Lian Ye* 复方穿心莲液 (Complex Prescription of Chuan Xin Lian Injection). For lumbago, inject BL 23 (two points) with 4 ml of biostimulin and 6 ml of sodium chloride. Point-blocking therapy combines the advantages of the medicine with the advantages of acupuncture, which can tonify qi and blood, move qi, invigorate blood, transform blood stasis and alleviate pain. [35]

g) Blood-letting Combined with Cupping:

Zhang Yuxin divided chronic PID into two patterns—qi stagnation and blood stasis, and stagnation of congealed cold and dampness. SP 6, BL 23, RN 4 and yāo yǎn were selected. For qi stagnation and blood stasis, blood-letting was performed first, followed by cupping. For stagnation of congealed cold and dampness, cupping was performed first, followed by blood-letting. Results of treating 100 cases of chronic PID: a total effectiveness rate of 95%. This treatment method is based on the principle of channel theory, which is the selection of points along the channel to treat the interior via the exterior. The combination of blood-letting and cupping therapies can improve microcirculation and hemorheological changes, improve metabolism of local tissues, promote the dissipation of inflammation and accelerate the reparation and regeneration of damaged tissues. [36]

h) Point Application:

Qiao Yin administered point application with *Hua Yu Gao* 化瘀膏 to treat 184 cases of chronic PID. Results: total effectiveness rate of 94.02%. Due to long-term exudation and hyperplasia caused by chronic PID, the organs adhere to the surrounding tissues. The adhesion hinders the absorption of medicine, which prolongs the course of disease and results in a difficult recovery. Point application with *Hua Yu Gao* 化瘀膏 can facilitate the absorption of the medicine by the skin. This treatment modality is easy to use, and patients can apply the paste by themselves. [37]

i) Injection of Medical Solution into the Uterine Cavity:

Zhang Xiaoli used the combination of 160,000 units of gentamicin, metronidazole and dexamethasone, and injected the solution using a double-duct tube with the assistance of hysterography to treat 182 cases of chronic PID. Results: a cure in 151 cases, (82.96%), and a total effectiveness rate of 97.8%. Injection of the solution can directly increase the density of the medicine in the local tissues and reinforce the effect of eliminating bacteria due to the synergistic action of medicine. [38]

j) Pelvic Detained Intubation and Instillation:

Yang Huaguang applied pelvic detained intubation and instillation to treat chronic PID. The Chinese medicinal group was given 200 ml of *Pen Qiang Yan Zhu She Ye* 盆腔炎注射液 (Injection for Pelvic Inflammatory Disease), which included *pú gōng yīng* (Herba Taraxaci), *dāng guī* (Radix Angelicae Sinensis), *zǐ huā dì dīng* (Herba Violae), *bài jiàng cǎo* (Herba Patriniae), *hóng téng* (Caulis Sargentodoxae), *chì sháo* (Radix Paeoniae Rubra), *sān léng* (Rhizoma Sparganii), *yán hú suǒ* (Rhizoma Corydalis) and *ròu guì* (Cortex Cinnamomi). Before the drip, add 15 ml of 5% sodium bicarbonate. The Western medicine group was given mixed liquor including 180 ml of sodium chloride, 320,000 units of gentamicin, 50 mg of prednisolone, 20 ml of 1% procaine, and 15 ml of 5% sodium bicarbonate. The liquor was dripped slowly through the tube for the treatment. Results: the Chinese medicinal group (including 36 cases): a cure in 32 cases; improvement in 4 cases. The western medicine group (including 33 cases): a cure in 28 cases; improvement in 4 cases; ineffective in 1 case. Pelvic detained intubation and instillation offers an alternate route of medication, and can directly soak the pelvic inflammatory tissues in liquor, thereby increasing the local density of medicine and enhancing the curative effect. [39]

k) Medicated Pads:

Zhu Jiangai used medicated pats made from medicinals that clear heat, resolve toxins, regulate qi, activate blood stasis, dispel blood stasis and alleviate pain, such as *jīn yín huā* (Flos Lonicerae Japonicae) and *zǐ huā dì dīng* (Herba Violae). The pads are placed on the lower abdomen, so when patients put on their clothes, the pads will press tightly on the skin, around the area of RN 4. Combined with massage, this method can treat the interior via the exterior. The medicinals absorbed by skin can aid right qi, strengthen the root (*ben*), regulate the immune system, promote pelvic blood circulation, increase blood flow, promote cytothesis (cell repair), clear heat, resolve toxins, regulate qi, invigorate blood, dispel blood stasis, alleviate pain, eliminate a broad-spectrum of bacteria, and eliminate viruses. The application of medicated pads on points with massage can accelerate the softening and absorption of inflamed nodules and the breaking apart of adhesions. [40]

l) Suppository:

Li Cuiping gives patients 盆炎栓 *Pen Yan Shuan* (Pelvic Inflammation Suppository):

The patent contains *huáng bǎi* (Cortex Phellodendri Chinensis), *mǎ chǐ xiàn* (Herba Portulacae), *táo rén* (Semen Persicae), *chì sháo* (Radix Paeoniae Rubra), *xià kū cǎo* (Spica Prunellae), *shān cí gū* (Pseudobulbus Cremastrae seu Pleiones) and *ròu guì* (Cortex Cinnamomi). Its functions include eliminating inflammation, alleviating pain, inhibiting bacteria, improving pelvic blood circulation, promoting the absorption of inflammation, and resolving adhesions. Its effect is local and direct, because of its administration route as a suppository, and thus has quick therapeutic effects. In addition, it has a long-standing excellent curative effect, produces no toxic or side effects, and is easy to use. [41]

m) Point Injection Therapy:

Guo Guotian performed point injection therapy to treat chronic PID. Select RN 3 and SP 6 as the main points, SP 8 and BL 32 as the auxiliary points (alternately used). Alternately use *Dang Gui Zhu She Ji* 当归注射液 (Dang Gui Injection) and *Yu Xing CaoZhu She Ji* 鱼腥草注射液 (Yu Xing Cao Injection). Method: Draw 6 ml of *Dang Gui Zhu She Ji* 当归注射液 (Dang Gui Injection) or *Yu Xing Cao Zhu She Ji* 鱼腥草注射液 (Yu

Xing Cao Injection) with a 10 ml syringe. Ask the patient lie down in the prone position. Insert needle into the points perpendicularly at a depth of 1 to 1.5 cun. The patient may experience soreness, numbness, distention or pain. Before injection, make sure there is no bleeding when drawing the syringe back. Slowly inject the medicine into the points (2 ml in each point). After the treatment, have the patient rest for 30 minutes. This treatment is carried out once a day. 7 sessions constitute one treatment course. A total of 2 courses were administered. Results of 56 cases were: a cure in 48 cases (85.7%); excellent improvement in 4 cases (7.2%); moderate effectiveness in 3 cases (5.4%); and no effect in 1 case (1.8%). The total effective rate is 98.21%. [42]

2. Experimental Studies

(1) Research on the Efficacy of Individual Chinese Medicinals

a) Studies on the treatment of salpingemphraxis with ilexonin A

Liu Xiaoyu used ilexonin A, the extract of *máo dōng qīng* (Radix Ilicis Pubescentis), to treat salpingemphraxis in rats. Results revealed: Ilexonin A can inhibit the desmoplasia caused by salpingitis, antagonize the apomorphosis and necrosis of epithelium mucosae, and inhibit inflammatory infiltration. Furthermore, after medication there was significant improvement in blood specific viscosity, erythrocyte electrophoresis rate, and erythrocyte aggregation index. The research demonstrated that ilexonin A may have the ability to improve blood circulation and microcirculation of local lesions, improve the hypoxemic state of its tissues, promote the absorption of inflammation and prevent salpingemphraxis. [43]

b) Research on the treatment of acute and chronic PID with *dān shēn* liquid

Cheng Jing conducted a pharmacological experiment that showed *dān shēn* liquid can inhibit aeruginosus bacillus, and is especially effective in antagonizing staphylococcus aureus. Applying it to the affected area can improve local microcirculation, increase metabolic rate of tissues, reduce exudation, promote the absorption of inflammation, and break up adhesions. [44]

c) *Hong Teng Shui Rong Ye* 红藤水溶液

The extract of 红藤水溶液 *Hong Teng Shui Rong Ye* given to patients via in vivo and ex vivo medication may inhibit platelet aggregation, promote platelet disaggregation and increase coronary artery blood flow in guinea pigs without influencing the heart. It may inhibit thrombogenesis in rats, increase blood plasma cAMP levels (without influencing platelet cAMP levels) in rabbits. In addition, *hóng téng* (Caulis Sargentodoxa) has been shown to have anti-inflammatory and antiviral properties. [45]

(2) Research on the Efficacy of Herbal Prescriptions

a) *Pen Yan Qing Jiao Nang* 盆炎清胶囊

Contains *dān shēn* (Radix et Rhizoma Salviae Miltiorrhizae), *chì sháo* (Radix Paeoniae Rubra), *zhǐ shí* (Fructus Aurantii Immaturus), *máo dōng qīng* (Radix Ilicis Pubescentis) and *yán hú suǒ* (Rhizoma Corydalis). Experiments on animals revealed it can increase pain threshold in mice, inhibit swelling in the auricles of mice, improve microcirculation disturbance of mesenterium caused by norepinephrine, and increase phagocytosis. Experiments also show that this capsule has strong anti-inflammatory and analgesic properties. It can alleviate the symptoms caused by inflammation, such as redness, swelling, heat and pain. In addition, it can improve microcirculation, promote the absorption of inflammation and increase immunity. [46]

b) *Fu You Chong Ji* 妇友冲剂

This formula invented by Yao Yuchen includes *shēng huáng qí* (Radix Astragali Recens), *sān léng* (Rhizoma Sparganii), *hóng huā* (Flos

Carthami), *tù sī zǐ* (Semen Cuscutae), *yì yǐ rén* (Semen Coicis), *wú zhū yú* (Fructus Evodiae) and *kūn bù* (Thallus Laminariae; Thallus Eckloniae). Animal experiments revealed that the medicinal granules can antagonize effusion and proliferating inflammation, reinforce the phagocytosis of monocytes and macrophages. The formula can also antagonize exudative inflammation, relieve pelvic hemostasis, promote the mollification and absorption of proliferative lesions, antagonize proliferating inflammation, increase immune function and achieve the curative effect. [47]

c) *Pen Qiang Yan Pian* 盆腔炎片

This patent contains more than 10 Chinese medicinals, including *yì mǔ cǎo* (Herba Leonuri), *hóng huā* (Flos Carthami), *bái zhú* (Rhizoma Atractylodis Macrocephalae), *dāng guī* (Radix Angelicae Sinensis), *xiāng fù* (Rhizoma Cyperi) and *chuān xiōng* (Rhizoma Chuanxiong). Experiments revealed that it can significantly increase the phagocytosis of peritoneal macrophages in mice, promote the proliferation of the thymus and spleen, strengthen immunity, significantly inhibit metritis in mice, and significantly improve the blood rheological index in rats. This formula can increase immunity, significantly inhibit desmoplasia and the infiltration of inflammatory cells, transform the thick, sticky and aggregated blood state caused by inflammation, and attain the curative effect. [48]

d) *Qi Jie Ke Li* 芪竭颗粒

This formula contains *huáng qí* (Radix Astragali), *xuè jié* (Sanguis Draconis), *zhì jū* (Radix et Rhizoma Rhei), *guì zhī* (Ramulus Cinnamomi), *fú líng* (Poria) and *hóng téng* (Caulis Sargentodoxae). Results of an experiment on mice revealed an abnormal increase in CD_4 and a significant decrease in CD_8. *Qi Jie Ke Li* 芪竭颗粒 can significantly increase CD_8 level, and make the CD_4/CD_8 ratio close to normal. Compared with the control group, there was a significant difference. In addition, it can increase the weight of mice. Studies performed on model rats with metritis (caused by benzene paste) showed that this formula can relieve the inflammatory reaction of the uterus and strongly inhibit swelling of the auricles caused by xylene. However, compared with the control group, there was no significant difference. The toxicity test revealed that the mice had no evident toxic and side effects. Overall results indicated that *Qi Jie Ke Li* 芪竭颗粒 can eliminate inflammation and regulate the immune function in mice with chronic PID. [49]

e) *Fu Yan Kang Tai Chong Ji* 妇炎康泰冲剂

Chief ingredients are *xiāng fù* (Rhizoma Cyperi), *sān léng* (Rhizoma Sparganii), *táo rén* (Semen Persicae), *yán hú suǒ* (Rhizoma Corydalis), *pú gōng yīng* (Herba Taraxaci) and *biē jiǎ* (Carapax Trionycis). Song Hongxiang conducted an extraorgan bacteriostasis experiment with *Fu Yan Kang Tai Chong Ji* 妇炎康泰冲剂 . Results revealed its anti-bacterial effect is fairly strong against staphylococcus epidermidis, colibacillus, bacillus and staphylococcus albus. Experiments on laboratory animals revealed that this formula can reduce swelling in the toes of rats and the auricles of mice; relieve abdominal pain in mice; improve microcirculation in rabbits. This is indication that the mechanism of action of this medicine is to improve the absorption and dissipation of inflammation by eliminating bacteria, alleviating pain and improving microcirculation. [50]

f) *Fu Fang Mao Dong Qing Ye* 复方毛冬青液

Contains *máo dōng qīng* (Radix Ilicis Pubescentis), *é zhú* (Rhizoma Curcumae), *huáng qí* (Radix Astragali) and *dān shēn* (Radix et Rhizoma Salviae Miltiorrhizae). Liu Xiaoyu conducted an orthogonality T test using rat granuloma as a pharmacodynamic index and analyzed the optimal dose combination of *Fu Fang Mao Dong Qing Ye* 复方毛冬青液 . Results of treating rat granuloma revealed the pharmacodynamic significance of the ingredients in order is *máo dōng qīng* (Radix Ilicis Pubescentis), *é zhú* (Rhizoma Curcumae), *huáng qí* (Radix Astragali) and *dān shēn* (Radix et Rhizoma Salviae Miltiorrhizae). The optimal dose combination is *máo dōng qīng* (Radix Ilicis Pubescentis) 40g, *é zhú* (Rhizoma Curcumae) 12g, *huáng qí* (Radix Astragali) 30g and *dān shēn* (Radix et Rhizoma Salviae Miltiorrhizae) 20g. The experiment also revealed that this formula can activate the reticuloendothelial system and improve microcirculation, which implies that the formula can inhibit the hyperplasia of inflammation and promote the absorption of inflammation by improving microcirculation and increasing the immune function of the body. [51]

g) *Fu Ke Qian Jin Jiao Nang* 妇科千金软胶囊

The chief ingredients are *chuān xīn lián* (Herba Andrographis), *jī xuè téng* (Caulis Spatholobi) and *dāng guī* (Radix Angelicae Sinensis). Jia Lina conducted a study on the main pharmacodynamic actions of *Fu Ke Qian Jin Jiao Nang* 妇科千金软胶囊 (Women's Precious Capsule). She built the inflammatory models by chemical empyrosis, bacteria, and non-specificity inflammation. Results show that the capsule can significantly decrease blood viscosity in lab rats, decrease left and right uterine weight variations, and heal histologic lesions in the uteruses of rats. It can inhibit the hyperblastosis of granulation tissue caused by cotton ball in rats, and relieve the swelling of the auricles of rats caused by xylene. This capsule has anti-inflammatory and anti-bacterial effects, and improves the blood rheological index. [52]

h) *Yan Ke Ning Chong Ji* 炎克宁冲剂

The main constituents are *huáng qín* (Radix Scutellariae), *chái hú* (Radix Bupleuri), *é zhú* (Rhizoma Curcumae), *jīn yín huā* (Flos Lonicerae Japonicae), *mǔ dān pí* (Cortex Moutan) and *chì sháo* (Radix Paeoniae Rubra). Wang Ying conducted a clinical trial with the following conclusion: *Yan Ke Ning Chong Ji* 炎克宁冲剂 is an effective formula for the prevention and treatment of chronic PID. [53]

i) *Dang Gui Shao Yao San* 当归芍药散 (Proportion of ingredients: *bái sháo* (Radix Paeoniae Alba): *dāng guī* (Radix Angelicae Sinensis): *bái zhú* (Rhizoma Atractylodis Macrocephalae): *fú líng* (Poria): *zé xiè* (Rhizoma Alismatis): *chuān xiōng* (Rhizoma Chuanxiong) is 8:1.6:1:1:1:1) Wang Zhiguo treated 2 groups of chronic PID patients with *Dan Gui Shao Yao San*. Results showed a significant difference between the treatment group and the control group. The clinical trial revealed that *Dan Gui Shao Yao San* has an effect on the regulation of immune function. [54]

j) *Dan Shao Huo Xue Xing Qi Tang* 丹芍活血行气汤

Chief ingredients are *dān shēn* (Radix et Rhizoma Salviae Miltiorrhizae) 20g, *chì sháo* (Radix Paeoniae Rubra) 15g, *wū yào* (Radix Linderae) 15g, *táo rén* (Semen Persicae) 15g, *mǔ dān pí* (Cortex Moutan) 10g, *chuān liàn zǐ* (Fructus Toosendan) 10g, *xiāng fù* (Rhizoma Cyperi) 9g, *dāng guī* (Radix Angelicae Sinensis) 9g, *yán hú suǒ* (Rhizoma Corydalis) 12g and *bài jiàng cǎo* (Herba Patriniae) 30g. Conclusion: Treating pelvic hemostasis syndrome with *Dan Shao Huo Xue Xing Qi Tang* 丹芍活血行气汤 produced good results. The mechanism of action may involve the improvement of blood circulation, facilitation of the relief of inflammation, and regulation of the body's immune functions. [55]

REFERENCES

[1] Gao Yuhua. Differentiation of Symptoms and Signs in the Treatment of Pelvic Inflammation (Pen Qiang Yan De Bian Zheng Zhi Liao) 盆腔炎的辨证治疗. *Qinghai Medical Journal*, 1998, 28（6）：32

[2] Gao Hui. Summary of Clinical and Laboratory Research of Chinese Medicinals in the Treatment of Chronic Pelvic Inflammation (Zhong Yi Yao Zhi Liao Man Xing Pen Qiang Yan De Lin Chuang Yu Shi Yan Yan Jiu Gai Shu) 中医药治疗慢性盆腔炎的临床与实验研究概述. *Research of Traditional Chinese Medicine*, 1996，（6）：57 – 60

[3] Zhu Aimei, Ma Baozhang. Chinese Medical Treatment of Chronic Pelvic Inflammatory Disease (Man Xing Pen Qiang Yan De Zhong Yi Zhi Liao Ti Hui)慢性盆腔炎的中医治疗体会. *Chinese Medicine Times*, 2005, 33（5）：9

[4] Zhang Fuzhen. 46 Differentiation of Symptoms and Signs in the Treatment of Pelvic Inflammation (Bian Zheng Zhi Liao Pen Qiang Yan 46 Li) 辨证治疗盆腔炎46例. *Shanxi Traditional Medicine*, 2004, 25（11）：982－983

[5] Liang Jianping. 50 Differentiation of Symptoms and Signs in the Treatment of Pelvic Inflammation with Chinese Medicine (Zhong Yi Bian Zheng Zhi Liao Pen Qiang Yan 50 Li) 中医辨证治疗盆腔炎50例. *Jiangxi Traditional Medicine*, 2004, 35（12）34－35

[6] Yao Yuchen. *Journal of Traditional Chinese Medicine.* March 1998, Vol.39, No.3：180－181

[7] Zhou Yujie. 106 Treatments of Pelvic Inflammation with Huayu Jiedu Tang and External Therapy (Hua Yu Jie Du Tang He Wai Zhi Fa Zhi Liao Pen Qiang Yan 106 Li)化瘀解毒汤合外治法治疗盆腔炎106例. *Jiamusi Medical School Times*, 1997, 20（2）：90－91

[8] Yang Ping, Lu Zhangwen. 36 Treatments of Pelvic Inflammation with Pelvic Pyema using Jiawei Guizhi Fuling Tang (Jia Wei Gui Zhi Fu Ling Tang Zhi Liao Man Xing Pen Qiang Yan Ban Pen Qiang Ji Ye 36 Li) 加味桂枝茯苓汤治疗慢性盆腔炎伴盆腔积液36例. *Zhejiang Journal of Traditional Chinese Medicine*, 1997, 32 (5) :209

[9] Wang Ruifang, Zhang Ping. The Preparation and Clinical Application of Combined Formulas in the Treatment of Pelvic Inflammation (Pen Qiang Yan He Ji De Zhi Bei Yu Lin Chuang Ying Yong) 盆腔炎合剂的制备与临床应用. *Lishizhen Research of Medicine and the Materia Medica*, 1997, 8（3）：269－270

[10] Zhao Yuqiu, Wu Zhaodi. Observation of the Healing Effect of Bochun Granules in theTreatment of Subacute Pelvic Inflammation (Bo Chun Ke Li Zhi Liao Ya Ji Xing Pen Qiang Yan Lin Chuang Liao Xiao Guan Cha) 柏椿颗粒治疗亚急性盆腔炎临床疗效观察. *Chinese Journal of Integrated Medicine* 2001, 21(10)：777－778

[11] Su Hualin, Chen Jinghui, Lin Hua et al. The Clinical Observation of Penyanqing Capsule in the Treatment of Chronic Pelvic Inflammation (Pen Yan Qing Jiao Nang Zhi Liao Man Xing Pen Qiang Yan Lin Chuang Guan Cha) 盆炎清胶囊治疗慢性盆腔炎临床观

察. *Sichuan Traditional Chinese Medicine* 2003, 21(10)：59 – 60

[12] Ye Wenzhen, Sun Liping, Cai Zhifen, et al. Kangning Tang Retention Enema in the Treatment of 50 Cases of Pelvic Inflammation (Kang Ning Tang Bao Liu Guan Chang Zhi Liao Pen Qiang Yan 50 Li) 康宁汤保留灌肠治疗盆腔炎50例. *Shanghai Journal of Traditional Chinese Medicine*, 1987, (3): 7

[13] Zheng Zhongjie, Hou Qingchang, Zhu Xiaoke, et al. Research of Pelvic Pathogens and Observation of the Therapeutic Effects of Its Treatment (Pen Qiang Yan Bing Yuan Ti Yan Jiu Ji Qi Zhi Liao Xiao Guo Guan Cha) 盆腔炎病原体研究及其治疗效果观察. *Tianjin Medicine*, 2003, 31(5)：291 - 293

[14] Ning Yan, Ning Ye, Ye Lizi, et al. Observation of the Healing Effects Danshao Huoxue Xingqi Tang in the Treatment of Pelvic Congestion Syndrome (Dan Shao Huo Xue Xing Qi Tang Zhi Liao Pen Qiang Yu Xue Zong He Zheng Liao Xiao Guan Cha) 丹芍活血行气汤治疗盆腔瘀血综合征疗效观察. *Chinese Journal of Chinese Traditional Emergency Medicine*, 2006, 15（2）：143

[15] Yang Xiaoyu, Hang Xinfei, Cui Hongliang. The Clinical Research of Compound Fengling Granules in the Treatment of Chronic Pelvic Pain Syndrome (Fu Fang Feng Ling Ke Li Zhi Liao Man Xing Pen Qiang Teng Tong Zong He Zheng Lin Chuang Yan Jiu) 复方风灵颗粒治疗慢性盆腔疼痛综合征临床研究. *Liaoning Journal of Traditional Chinese Medicine*, 2006, 33（1）：42

[16] Yuan Junyi. Acupuncture with TDP Radiation in the Treatment of 124 Cases of Chronic Pelvic Inflammation (Zhen Ci Jie He TDP Zhao She Zhi Liao Man Xing Pen Qiang Yan 124 Li).针刺结合TDP照射治疗慢性盆腔炎124例. *Chinese Acupuncture and Moxibustion*, 1992,（2）：27

[17] Han Chonghua. The Treatment of 144 Cases of Chronic Pelvic Inflammation with Electric Needling and Warming Needling (Dian Zhen Jia Wen Zhen Zhi Liao Man Xing Pen Qiang Yan 144 Li) 电针加温针治疗慢性盆腔炎144例. *Chinese Acupuncture*, 1998,（10）：594

[18] Li He, Li Jingfen. Observation of the Healing Effects of Fire Needles in the

Treatment of Chronic Pelvic Inflammation (Huo Zhen Bian Zheng Zhi Liao Man Xing Pen Qiang Yan Liao Xiao Guan Cha) 火针辨证治疗慢性盆腔炎疗效观察. *Chinese Acupuncture*, 2002, 22 (5): 295 - 296

[19] Hong Jianyun, Ou Lanfang, Li Fu, et al. The Clinical Observation of Celiac Trunk and Sacroiliac Acupuncture in the Treatment of Chronic Pelvic Inflammation (Fu Cong Ci He Di Qia Ci Zhi Liao Man Xing Pen Qiang Yan Lin Chuang Liao Xiao Guan Cha) 腹丛刺合骶髂刺治疗慢性盆腔炎临床疗效观察. *Chinese Acupuncture*, 2005, 25（7）: 471 - 472

[20] Xu Xia. 60 Clinical Observations of the Treatment of Chronic Pelvic Inflammation with Acupuncture and Medication (Zhen Yao Jie He Zhi Liao Man Xing Pen Qiang Yan 60 Li Lin Chuang Liao Xiao Guan Cha) 针药结合治疗慢性盆腔炎60例临床疗效观察. *Practical Journal of Traditional Chinese Internal Medicine*, 2006, 20（1）: 80 – 81

[21] Zhao Jianchun. The Observation of 60 Cases of Chronic Pelvic Inflammation and Their Treatment with Acupuncture and Moxibustion (Xue Wei Wen He Jiu Zhi Liao Man Xing Pen Qiang Yan 60 Li Guan Cha) 穴位温和灸治疗慢性盆腔炎60例观察. *Clinical Journal of Acupuncture*, 1995（3）: 29 – 30

[22] Du Lei. Observation of the Healing Effects of Treating 83 Cases of Chronic Pelvic Inflammation with Acupuncture and TDP (Zhen Jiu Jia TDP Zhi Liao Man Xing Pen Qiang Yan 83 Li Liao Xiao Guan Cha) 针灸加TDP治疗慢性盆腔炎83例疗效观察. *Hebei Traditional Chinese Medicine*, 2004, 26（11）: 850

[23] Wang Zhexiang. The Treatment of 30 Cases of Chronic Pelvic Inflammation with Manpen Tang Retention Enema (Man Pen Tang Bao Liu Guan Chang Zhi Liao Man Xing Pen Qiang Yan 30 Li) 慢盆汤保留灌肠治疗慢性盆腔炎30例. *Journal of Zhejiang Academy of Traditional Chinese Medicine*, 1996（1）: 19

[24] Wang Yan. The Treatment of 30 Cases of Chronic Pelvic Inflammation with Chinese Medicinal Drops (Zhong Yao Dian Di Zhi Liao Man Xing Pen Qiang Yan 30 Li)中药点滴治疗慢性盆腔炎30例. *Journal of Chinese Traditional Medicine*, 1996, (4): 213

[25] Wang Kecan. The Treatment of 47 Cases of Chronic Pelvic Inflammation with Pen Qiang Xiao Yan Tang Retention Enema (Pen Qiang Xiao Yan Tang Guan Chang Wei

Zhu Zhi Liao Man Xing Pen Qiang Yan 47 Li) 盆腔消炎汤灌肠为主治疗慢性盆腔炎47例. *Journal of Anhui Academy of Traditional Chinese Medicine*, 1995,（2）：25

[26] Wang Jin. Observation of the Healing Effects in the Treatment of Chronic Pelvic Inflammation with Hongteng Tang Retention Enema (Hong Teng Tang Guan Chang Wei Zhu Zhi Liao Man Xing Pen Qiang Yan Liao Xiao Guan Cha) 红藤汤灌肠为主治疗慢性盆腔炎疗效观察. *Modern Journal of Integrated Chinese and Western Medicine*, 2005, 14（22）：2952

[27] Zhu Zhaolian. Observation of the Healing Effects in the Treatment of Pelvic Inflammation using External Application of Chinese Medicinals (Zhong Yao Wai Fu Zhi Liao Pen Qiang Yan De Liao Xiao Guan Cha) 中药外敷治疗盆腔炎的疗效观察. *Journal of External Treatment of Chinese Medicine*, 1995,（3）：9

[28] Zhang Wen. Treatment of 100 Cases of Chronic Pelvic Inflammation using External Application of Chinese Medicinals (Zhong Yao Wai Fu Zhi Liao Man Xing Pen Qiang Yan 100 Li) 中药外敷治疗慢性盆腔炎100例. *Liaoning Journal of Traditional Chinese Medicine*, 1993,（12）：29

[29] Zheng Hongjun. Treatment of Chronic Pelvic Inflammation with Ion-leading Chinese Medicinals (Zhong Yao Li Zi Dao Ru Zhi Liao Man Xing Pen Qiang Yan) 中药离子导入治疗慢性盆腔炎. *Jiangsu Journal of Traditional Chinese Medicine*, 1996,（4）：18

[30] Meng Wen. Treatment of Chronic Pelvic Inflammation with "Audio Frequency" Chinese Medicinal Infiltration and Ultrasound Therapy ("Yin Pin Dian" Zhong Yao Tou Ru Jia Chao Sheng Zhi Liao Man Xing Pen Qiang Yan) "音频电"中药透入加超声治疗慢性盆腔炎. *Liaoning Journal of Traditional Chinese Medicine*, 1995,（2）：75

[31] Huang Yanzhen, Lin Hua, Hang Zhenrong. Treatment of 127 Cases of Pelvic Inflammation with Frequency Ion-leading Chinese Medicinals (Yin Pin Pei He Zhong Yao Li Zi Dao Ru Zhi Liao Pen Qiang Yan 127 Li) 音频配合中药离子导入治疗盆腔炎127例. *Fujian Journal of Traditional Chinese Medicine*, 1995,（2）：20

[32] Zheng Mingying. Treatment of 36 Cases of Chronic Pelvic Inflammation with helium-neon lLaser (Hai-Nai Ji Guang Zhi Liao Man Xing Pen Qiang Yan 36 Li) 氦-氖激光治疗慢性盆腔炎36例. *Fujian Journal of Traditional Chinese Medicine*, 1995,（1）：92

[33] Wang Yanjun. 30 Clinical Case Reports of the Treatment of Chronic Pelvic Inflammation with Massage (Tui Na Zhi Liao Man Xing Pen Qiang Yan 30 Li Lin Chuang Bao Dao) 推拿治疗慢性盆腔炎30例临床报道. *Jiangsu Traditional Chinese Medicine*, 1997,3：35

[34] Dong Shihua. The Clinical Observation and Pharmacological Experiment of Compound Baijiang Injection in the Treatment of Pelvic Inflammation (Fu Fang Bai Jiang Zhu She Ye Zhi Liao Pen Qiang Yan De Lin Chuang Guan Cha Yu Yao Li Xue Shi Yan) 复方败酱注射液治疗盆腔炎及临床观察于药理学实验. *Shandong Journal of Traditional Chinese Medicine*, 1990, 9（4）：14 – 15

[35] Miao Yanxia. Recent Advances in the Clinical Application of Acupuncture Point Injection in the Treatment of Pelvic Inflammation (Xue Wei Zhu She Zhi Liao Pen Qiang Yan Lin Chuang Ying Yong Jin Kuang) 穴位注射治疗盆腔炎临床应用近况. *Shanxi Correspondence Course of Traditional Chinese Medicine*, 1992,（4）：16 – 18

[36] Zhang Yuxin. The Treatment of 100 Cases of Chronic Pelvic Inflammation with Venesection and Cupping Therapies (Ci Luo Ba Guan Zong He Liao Fa Zhi Liao Man Xing Pen Qiang Yan 100 Li) 刺络拔罐综合疗法治疗慢性盆腔炎100例. *Forum of Traditional Chinese Medicine*, 1997, 12（4）：38

[37] Qiao Yin. Treatment of 184 Cases of Chronic Pelvic Inflammation with the Application of Stasis-dissolving Pastes on Acupuncture Points (Hua Yu Gao Xue Wei Tie Zhi Man Xing Pen Qiang Yan 184 Li) 化瘀膏穴位帖治慢性盆腔炎184例. *Shanxi Journal of Traditional Chinese Medicine*, 1993, 14（6）：245 – 246

[38] Zhang Xiaoli, Yang Menggeng, Qiuxuehua, et al. The Analysis of the Healing Effects of Treating 182 Cases of Chronic Pelvic Inflammation with Medical Injection into the Uterine Cavity (Gong Qiang Yao Wu Zhi Liao Man Xing Pen Qiang Yan 182 Li Liao Xiao Fen Xi) 宫腔药物治疗慢性盆腔炎182例疗效分析. *Shanxi Journal of Medicine*, 1998, 27(10)：623 – 624

[39] Yang Huaguang, Yao Yuanqing, Qiu Zhenqin, et al. The Clinical Observation of Treating Chronic Pelvic Inflammation with Pelvic Retention Intubation (Pen Qiang Liu

Zhi Cha Guan Zhi Liao Man Xing Pen Qiang Yan De Lin Chuang Guan Cha) 盆腔留置插管治疗慢性盆腔炎的临床观察. *Chinese Journal of Integrated Chinese and Western Medicine* 2002, 22（12）：937-938

[40] Zhu Jiangwen. Treatment of 102 Cases of Chronic Pelvic Inflammation with Chinese Medicated Pads (Zhong Yao Dian Zhi Liao Man Xing Pen Qiang Yan 102 Li) 中药垫治疗恢性狆腔炎102例. *Hebei Journal of Integrated Chinese and Western Medicine*, 1998, 7（1）：66

[41] Li Cuiping. The Clinical Research of Pelvic Inflammatory Embolization in the Treatment of Chronic Pelvic Inflammation (Pen Yan Shuan Zhi Liao Man Xing Pen Qiang Yan De Lin Chuang Yan Jiu) 盆炎栓治疗慢性盆腔炎的临床研究. *Henan Traditional Chinese Medicine*, 1998, 18（2）：35－36

[42] Guo Guotian, Zhang Hua. Observation of the Healing Effects in the Treatment of 56 Cases of Chronic Pelvic Inflammation with Acupuncture Point Injection (Xue Wei Zhu She Zhi Liao Man Xing Pen Qiang Yan 56 Li Liao Xiao Guan Cha) 穴位注射治疗慢性盆腔炎56例疗效观察. *Jilin Journal of Traditional Chinese Medicine*, 2005, 25（8）：34

[43] Liu Xiaoyu, Li Liyun, Zhang Shuming, et al. The Function of Ilexonin A in Experimental Obstruction of the Oviducts in Rats (Mao Dong Qing Jia Su Dui Da Shu Shi Yan Xing Shu Luan Guan Zu Sai De Zuo Yong) 毛冬青液素对大鼠实验性输卵管阻塞的作用. *Chinese Journal of Integrated Chinese and Western Medicine*，1993，13（8）478－480

[44] Cheng Jing. The Preparation and Clinical Observation of Danshen Liquid (Dan Shen Ye De Zhi Bei Yu Lin Chuang Guan Cha) 丹参液的制备与临床观察. *Lishizhen Research of Medicine and the Materia Medica*, 1998, 9（2）：144

[45] Jiang Hong, Liu Lele, Wang Hongwei, et al. The Research Progress of the Chemical Ingredient and Clinical Function of the Chinese Medicinal Hongteng (Zhong Yao Hong Teng Hua Xue Cheng Fen Ji Lin Chuang Zuo Yong De Yan Jiu Jin Zhan) 中药红藤化学成份及临床作用的研究进展. *Scientific Technology and Economy of Inner Mongolia*, 2002,（3）：120

[46] Shen Biqiong, Situ Yi, Ou Yongquan. The Main Pharmacological Research of

Penyanqing Capsule (Pen Yan Qing Jiao Nang Zhu Yao Yao Xiao Xue Yan Jiu) 盆炎清胶囊主要药效学研究. *Journal of Guangzhou Academy of Traditional Chinese Medicine* 2001, 18(2)：159 – 162

[47] Yao Shian, Yao Yuchen, Shao Zhengyi. The Clinical and Experimental Research of Fuyou Powder in the Treatment of Chronic Pelvic Inflammation 妇友冲剂治疗慢性盆腔炎的临床与实验研究. *China Academy of Traditional Chinese Medicine Times*, 1994, 9（5）：12 – 14

[48] Ge Xin, He Xiaoying, Xie Jingwen, et al. The Effect of Penyan Tablets on the Immune System of Mice and on the Blood Rheology of Rats and Experimental Research on Its Effect on the Uterine Inflammation in Rats (Pen Qiang Yan Pian Dui Xiao Shu Mian Yi Gong Neng, Xue Yu Da Shu Xue Ye Liu Bian Xue De Ying Xiang Ji Kang Da Shu Zi Gong Yan Zheng De Shi Yan Yan Jiu) 盆腔炎片对小鼠免疫功能, 血瘀大鼠血液流变学的影响及抗大鼠子宫炎症的实验研究. *Chinese Scientific Technology of Traditional Chinese Medicine* 2000, 7(5)：291 - 292

[49] Zhang Qin, He Jialin, Zhu XiaoLing, et al. The Experimental Research of Qijie Granules in the Treatment of Chronic Pelvic Inflammation (Qi Jie Ke Li Zhi Liao Man Xing Pen Qiang Yan De Shi Yan Yan Jiu)芪竭颗粒治疗慢性盆腔炎的实验研究. *Chinese Scientific Technology of Traditional Chinese Medicine* 2002, 9(6)：337 - 338

[50] Song Hongjiang, Qing Hui, Li Shumin, et al. The Experimental Research of Fuyankangtai Granules in the Treatment of Chronic Pelvic Inflammation (Fu Yan Kang Tai Chong Ji Zhi Liao Man Xing Pen Qiang Yan De Shi Yan Yan Jiu) 妇炎康泰冲剂治疗慢性盆腔炎的实验研究. *Chinese Scientific Technology of Traditional Chinese Medicine*, 1998，5（5）：290 – 291

[51] Liu Xiaoyu, Li Liyun, Mo Lili, et al. The Component Method Principle and Dose Analysis of Compound Ilexonin orthogonality t value $L_8(2^7)$ 复方毛冬青液的正交t值法 $L_8(2^7)$的组方原则及剂量分析. *Journal of Guangzhou Academy of Traditional Chinese Medicine*, 1996, 13 (3, 4)：66 – 67

[52] Jia Lina, Zhao Shiping, Yan Jing, et al. The Pharmacological Research of Fukeqianjin Capsules in the Treatment of Pelvic Inflammation (Fu Ke Qian Jin Ruan Jiao

Nang Zhi Liao Pen Qiang Yan Yao Xiao Xue Yan Jiu) 妇科千金软胶囊治疗盆腔炎药效学研究. *New Traditional Chinese Medicine and Clinical Pharmacology*, 2006, 17（1）：18

[53] Wang Ying, Sun Kefeng, Ma Wenguang, et al. The Effects of Yankening Granules on the Cell Apoptosis of Rats with Chronic PID (Yan Ke Ning Chong Ji Dui Man Xing Pen Qiang Yan Da Shu Xi Bao Diao Wang De Ying Xiang) 炎克宁冲剂对慢性盆腔炎大鼠细胞凋亡的影响. *Chinese Scientific Technology of Traditional Chinese Medicine*, 2005, 12（6）：363

Miscarriage
by Liang Xue-fang, He Cheng-qun & Si Tu-yi

OVERVIEW

Miscarriage is defined as a pregnancy that terminates (on its own, without artificial induction) before the 28th completed week of gestation with a fetal weight of less than 1000g. Miscarriage can be categorized as early miscarriage and late miscarriage, according its time of onset. The former occurs before 12 weeks and the latter after 12 weeks. Miscarriage can also be divided into spontaneous abortion and induced miscarriage. Induced miscarriage, which is not covered in this chapter, refers to the voluntary or involuntary termination of pregnancy by artificial means. Generally speaking, though there are various categories and different clinical manifestations of miscarriage, the common symptoms are post-menstrual vaginal bleeding and abdominal pain of varying intensity. Miscarriage is the natural elimination of the products of human conception with about 75% of fertilized ova, of which only approximately 15% can be recognized because of detectable miscarriage symptoms. Other symptoms include dysfunctional uterine bleeding, and delayed menstruation. The fertilized egg may be eliminated naturally and silently in the early stage of development, which is a natural selective phenomenon of reproduction. Though there are still 3% of all neonates with birth defects, miscarriage plays a role in the process of natural selection.

Miscarriage can be classified as threatened miscarriage, habitual miscarriage, inevitable miscarriage, incomplete miscarriage, complete miscarriage and retention of dead fetus (missed abortion) according to its main symptoms and the different stages of pregnancy in which they occur. Threatened miscarriage is the appearance of these signs and symptoms before the 28th completed week of gestation - vaginal bleeding and/or lower abdominal pain without dilation of the cervix, the fetal membrane is still intact, the products of conception has not yet been expelled, and there is still hope of continuing with the pregnancy.

Habitual miscarriage is defined as spontaneous abortion occurring 3 or more times consecutively. Inevitable miscarriage refers to miscarriage that cannot be avoided, and is a development of threatened miscarriage under general circumstances. Incomplete miscarriage, which is a progression of inevitable miscarriage, is the partial expulsion of conceptive products. Complete miscarriage is the expulsion of all of the products of conception and gradual cessation of vaginal bleeding, followed by the disappearance of abdominal pain. Missed abortion is when the embryo or fetus dies in utero without the expulsion of conceptive products. All of the above fall under the categories of "threatened miscarriage", "restless fetus", "abdominal pain during pregnancy", "habitual miscarriage", "spontaneous abortion", "miscarriage", "gloomy delivery", "fallen embryo that is difficult to save", and "retention of dead fetus" in Chinese medicine.

In biomedicine, miscarriage is considered to have many causes, especially habitual miscarriage, which makes up 1% of all miscarriages; but the true cause still remains unclear. Recent advancements have been made in the identification of some definite factors (such as cytogenetic abnormalities, malformation and dysfunction of the uterus, and immune-genetic factors), yet they still have not been completely solved. The same goes for other uncertain factors, such as recurrent intrauterine infection, dysfunction of the corpus luteum, abnormal functioning of the thyroid gland, and pathological changes of collagen-blood vessels.

1) Chromosomal Abnormalities

Chromosomal abnormalities can be classified as quantitative chromosomal abnormalities and structural chromosomal abnormalities. The former includes aneuploid and polyploid abnormalities; the latter contains deletion, translocation, inversion and overlapping, of which inversion and overlapping are most commonly seen. Generally speaking, balanced translocation does not affect the growth of the embryo, because it does not result in the loss of genetic material; imbalanced translocation induces partial trisomies or monomies, and can easily cause death of the embryo or miscarriage.

2) Uterine Factors

Uterine malformation is one of the causes of miscarriage, mainly because of limited uterine cavity space, insufficient blood supply or an unhealthy internal environment of the uterine cavity. Uterine factors are various, such as malformation, adhesion within the cavity, and cervical incompetence (which is defined as a weak cervix that dilates gradually during pregnancy; a major cause of miscarriage in the second trimester).

3) Immunological Factors

The causes of some miscarriages can be found, such as cytogenetic abnormality, anatomical abnormality, hormonal imbalance or microbe infection; the causes of other miscarriages are not clear. Modern research points out the possibility that the immunological factor is the key in determining whether or not pregnancy will be successful. In the past, abnormal immune reactions in the mother were a cause of miscarriage that could not be explained. Reproductive immunity is a special protective mechanism: on one hand it can protect the mother from microbe invasions; on the other hand, when it is functioning normally, it will not reject the fetus and placenta as a foreign antigen. However, if there is immunological incompatibility between the mother and the fetus, the mother's immune system will reject the fetus, causing miscarriage.

4) Endocrine Factors

The implantation and further development of the embryo is dependent upon the mutual coordination of the ever so complicated endocrine system. A disorder of any of its components can cause miscarriage, of which the dysfunction of the corpus luteum is the most

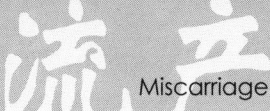

common. Less frequently encountered disorders are the abnormal functioning of the thyroid gland and diabetes.

5) Genital Tract Infection

Genital tract infection is considered as one of the causes of early miscarriage. Endometrial infection results in the failure of the ovum to implant or malformation of the gametic chromosome. The pathogens that contribute to habitual miscarriage will inevitably produce persistent infection with few maternal symptoms, and they can directly or indirectly cause fetal death by inflammatory reaction. Generally speaking, the upward infection of the lower genital tract occurs before the 12th completed week of gestation, after which the fetal membrane and decidual membrane will create a barrier by fusing together and sealing the passage. This results in the resistance infection of the amniotic fluid, which will gradually worsen throughout the course of the pregnancy.

6) Environmental Factors

In our living and working environments, it is inevitable that we encounter harmful factors that can produce adverse effects in the human body and may even impair reproductive functions if severe. The known environmental causes of miscarriage are multiple. Examples are physical factors such as x-rays, microwaves, and noise; metals such as lead, aluminum, mercury and zinc; pharmaceutical chemicals like chloroquine, antineoplastic, anesthetic gas, oral antidiabetics, polychlorinated biphenyl, carbon bisulfide and dibromochloropropane. Other causes include cigarette smoking, alcohol, coffee and harsh medicinals. All of the above can cause miscarriage.

7) Other Parental Factors

Maternal systemic disease is often one of the causes of infertility as well as miscarriage. These include severe anemia, malnutrition, septicemia, all kinds of malignant tumors, acute infectious hepatitis, chronic nephritis, hemolytic disease, food poisoning and allergies, all of which can increase the risk of miscarriage. An example of a paternal factor is bacteriospermia, which is often asymptomatic. If the bacteria existing in the sperm reaches a certain amount, this can interfere with the implantation of the ovum or cause an early miscarriage. In addition, the father's sperm can be damaged from occupational health hazards such as heat, radiation, chemical substances and harmful metals.

The clinical diagnosis of miscarriage should be made by analyzing the case history, menstrual history, basal body temperature, presence or absence of abdominal pain, vaginal bleeding, typical signs, physical examination and pelvioscopy in particular. For patients who do not present with typical clinical symptoms or those with possible miscarriage, it is necessary to use HCG, E2 and P testing; microscopic examination of vaginal discharge; B-mode ultrasound; and other auxiliary examinations make a definite diagnosis.

Once miscarriage occurs, proper treatment should be administered according to pattern differentiation. If it has been confirmed that the fetus has congenital defects, imminent post-natal functional abnormalities, and possible deformities, the expectant mother should be persuaded into terminating the pregnancy. In severe and emergency cases of missed abortion and inevitable miscarriage, biomedical treatment should be given first. Chinese medicinals are very effective for general threatened miscarriage and habitual miscarriage, so they can be given with or without biomedical treatment; integrative treatment can be considered if there is profuse vaginal bleeding and severe abdominal pain.

1. Threatened Miscarriage

a. Patient should rest in bed, refrain from sexual activities and avoid vaginal examinations. Medical personnel should give patients sympathy and comfort in order to eliminate tension and anxiety. Mild sedatives that

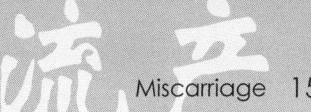

do not harm the fetus can be taken if necessary.

b. Take vitamin E and folic acid. For patients with luteal phase defects, an intramuscular injection of 20mg of progesterone can be given once or twice a day. Progesterone levels increase throughout the course of the pregnancy. However, progesterone deficiency is very likely to occur in threatened abortion patients, or during the period when progesterone dependence is shifting over to placental dependence. Early administration of HCG can promote the synthesis of progesterone.

c. If, after two weeks of treatment, there is no sign of improvement, or on the contrary the symptoms are worse, this indicates abnormal development of the embryo. In this case, discontinue the treatment and allow the miscarriage to occur. Or, use ultrasound and HCG to determine the embryo's condition, and administer the appropriate treatment, which may include termination of the pregnancy.

2. Inevitable Miscarriage

The treatment principle for inevitable miscarriage is the complete expulsion of the fetus and the placental tissues as quickly as possible to prevent continuous bleeding and infection. For early miscarriage, dilation and curettage (D&C) should be performed immediately, followed by careful inspection and examination of the removed substances for pathological clues. For late miscarriages in which D&C is rather difficult because of a large uterus, an intravenous drip of 500ml of glucose mixed with 10 units of oxytocin can be administered to promote uterine contraction. Check to see if the expulsion of the fetus and placenta are complete, and if necessary, use D&C to clear the remains of the conceptive products. For patients with severe anemia, consider blood transfusion before or during surgery, and give antibiotics to prevent post-surgical infection. For incomplete miscarriage, clear the remaining tissues of the fetus and prevent continuous bleeding. D&C is also an option for incomplete miscarriage, but the patient must be given antibiotics in order to prevent post-surgical infection.

3. Complete Miscarriage

For patients with a final diagnosis of complete miscarriage, there is no treatment. Distinguishing incomplete miscarriage from other conditions is crucial. For instance, if there is still continuous bleeding, it may be an incomplete miscarriage with retention of chorionic villi, for which D&C can be considered.

4. Missed Abortion

The treatment for missed abortion is more difficult. Performing D&C would be difficult because of the possibility of the embryonic tissues adhering tightly to the uterine wall; if the length of time since the occurrence of the miscarriage is too long, it may cause a disturbance in the body's clotting mechanism, which can lead to DIC (disseminated intravascular coagulation – severe bleeding due to the formation of blood clots throughout the body). Before treatment, it is necessary to make preparations for a blood transfusion in case it is needed. If the uterus is smaller than that of 12 gestational weeks, D&C is appropriate, along with an injection of a uterine-contracting solution during the surgery to reduce bleeding. Special caution should be given to prevent perforation during the operation if the placenta has adhered tightly to the uterine wall. If the product of conception cannot be removed all at once, attempt the surgery again within the next 5-7 days. If the uterus is larger than that of 12 gestational weeks, an intravenous injection of oxytocin can be administered, as well as an induced abortion using prostaglandin (PG) or ethacridine.

5. Habitual Miscarriage

For women with histories of habitual miscarriage, it is necessary

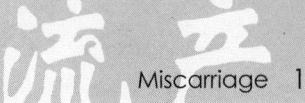

for them to undergo examination and treatment before attempting to conceive and receive early preventative treatment after conception.

a. Treatment of uterine abnormalities:

Horizontal excision of the septum can be considered for complete or incomplete uterine septa. Hysteroscopy is applicable for small submucosal myomas; horizontal excision is an option for large submucosal myomas or intramural myomas that protrude into the uterine cavity. If there are adhesions in the uterine cavity, separate them with the aid of a hysteroscope. For stubborn adhesions, cut them with a micro scissor. Place a contraceptive ring in the uterine cavity for 3 months or use an F01EY catheter until the next menstrual period to prevent the reformation of adhesions. Estrogen and antibiotics may also be given.

b. Patients who show positive signs on microbe tests of the uterine cavity and the cervix should be treated before pregnancy. During pregnancy, medicines that cause no harm to the fetus can be considered.

c. Treatment for dysfunction of the corpus luteum:

Since dysfunction of the corpus luteum can manifest as progesterone deficiency, the most sensible treatment is progesterone supplementation, which also happens to be the only feasible option during pregnancy.

d. Immunological treatment:

After ruling out genetic factors, anatomical factors, infectious factors and endocrine factors, habitual miscarriages of unknown causes are usually found to be caused by immunological factors. Immunotherapy is available for patients with defects due to blocking factors (diagnosed by immunological testing).

e. Women with histories of habitual miscarriages of unknown causes can be treated on the basis of insufficiency of the corpus luteum and given daily intramuscular injections of 10-20mg of progesterone. Continue with the treatment until the 10th week of pregnancy or beyond the month that the previous miscarriages often occur in, or with the intramuscular injections of 2000u of HCG every other day. Advise patients to stay in bed, to get plenty of rest, and to refrain from intercourse. Recommend vitamin supplements and provide psychological counseling to relieve mental and emotional stress.

CHINESE MEDICAL ETIOLOGY AND PATHOMECHANISM

In Chinese medicine, it is considered that the etiology and pathogenesis of miscarriage involves both the fetus and the mother, as stated in *Treatise on the Causes and Symptoms of All Diseases* (*Zhu Bing Yuan Hou Lun* 诸病源候论): "the mother's disease influences her fetus" and "the instability of the fetus affects the mother."

1) Fetal Aspect
Fetal instability from fetal diseases is caused by parental insufficiency of congenital essence. Even though the sperm and ovum were able to fuse, the embryo lacks stability; or the embryo is unable to grow because of defects, which may cause abnormal vaginal bleeding during pregnancy and restless movement of the fetus. If the embryo itself has defects, medication is usually inappropriate and will eventually lead to spontaneous abortion or miscarriage.

2) Maternal Aspect
The major maternal factor is the deficiency of the penetrating and conception vessels, rendering them unable to carry and support the embryo, which leads to the instability of the embryo and eventually causes miscarriage. The penetrating vessel is the sea of blood, and the conception vessel controls the placenta and the embryo. If the qi and blood of penetrating and conception vessels are sufficient, the embryo will be held by the qi and nourished by the blood, and the fetus can develop normally. If the penetrating and conception vessels are deficient, they are unable to control blood to nourish embryo or control qi to secure

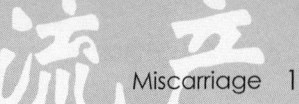

and hold the embryo. The unstable embryo can cause vaginal bleeding during pregnancy, excessive fetal movement, or possibly spontaneous abortion or miscarriage.

The causes of deficiency of the penetrating and conception vessels are kidney deficiency, qi and blood deficiency, blood heat, blood stasis and external injury. All of above can damage the penetrating and conception vessels and make the fetus unstable enough to be spontaneously aborted.

a. Kidney Deficiency

Includes insufficiency of congenital constitution or congenital kidney deficiency; early marriage (in this case it refers to an early sex life), frequent childbirth, exhaustion from excessive sexual intercourse, excessive sexual activity during pregnancy, consumption and exhaustion of kidney qi, and deficiency of the penetrating and conception vessels due to kidney deficiency causing instability of the fetus. All of the above can cause vaginal bleeding during pregnancy, restless movement of the fetus, spontaneous abortion, miscarriage and habitual miscarriage.

b. Qi and Blood Deficiency

The growth and development of the embryo requires nourishment from maternal qi and blood. If qi and blood is constitutionally deficient, or if the spleen and stomach are weak or damaged by long-term morning sickness and an unhealthy diet after pregnancy, there will be an inadequate source for the qi and blood. Qi and blood deficiency can also be caused by insufficient right qi after long-term severe disease and lack of healthcare. Deficient qi has no strength to carry the fetus and deficient blood is unable to nourish the fetus, resulting in vaginal bleeding during pregnancy, restless movement of the fetus, spontaneous abortion, miscarriage and habitual miscarriage. Or, the unsuccessful expulsion of a dead fetus due to deficiency of qi and blood can result in retention of dead fetus (missed abortion).

c. Blood Heat

Blood heat can arise from constitutional excess of yang qi, exogenous heat pathogens, excessive consumption of acrid food after pregnancy, internal damage of the seven emotions (such as long-term depression) transforming into fire, or internal heat from yin deficiency disturbing the penetrating and conception vessels and causing instability of the two vessels, or exogenous toxic heat injuring the embryo. All of the above can cause vaginal bleeding during pregnancy (threatened miscarriage), restless movement of the fetus, spontaneous abortion and miscarriage.

d. Liver Constraint

Frequent liver constraint, postpartum depression, binding constraint of liver qi, impaired qi dynamic, or the impairment of the ascending and descending of the qi dynamic by the growing fetus can all lead to abdominal pain during pregnancy or restless movement of the fetus.

e. Blood Stasis

Liver constraint and qi stagnation is a common cause of blood stasis. When qi and blood are unable to flow smoothly because of stubborn illness and the obstruction of static blood, this may lead to further deficiency of blood in the penetrating and conception vessels, hindering fetal nourishment and stability. This gives rise to abdominal pain during pregnancy, restless movement of the fetus, spontaneous abortion, miscarriage and habitual miscarriage. The internal obstruction of static blood prohibits the fetus from being expelled normally, resulting in retention of dead fetus.

f. External Trauma

External injuries such as tumbles, falls, sudden sprains and contusions during pregnancy can cause the disharmony of qi and blood. The chaotic qi is unable to carry the fetus and the disorderly blood is unable to nourish the fetus. Also, external injuries can directly damage the penetrating and conception vessels, disturb fetal qi, harm the embryo and cause vaginal bleeding during pregnancy, restless movement of the fetus and spontaneous abortion.

CHINESE MEDICAL TREATMENT

There are different treatment approaches for miscarriage because of its complexity. To prevent miscarriage is the primary goal in the treatment of threatened miscarriage and habitual miscarriage. For inevitable miscarriage, missed abortion and incomplete miscarriage, it is essential to expel the products of conception and treat the mother as soon as possible. Routine monitoring and differential diagnoses of incomplete miscarriage is important for complete miscarriage, and nursing the mother back to health after miscarriage should be emphasized if a complete miscarriage is confirmed.

1. Pattern Differentiation and Treatment

1) The Treatment of Threatened Miscarriage:
Calming the fetus and preventing miscarriage are the main treatment principles for threatened miscarriage. Tonifying the kidney, benefiting qi and nourishing blood are the primary methods of calming the fetus. If the kidney qi is sufficient, the fetus can be secured; if the kidney qi is vigorous, the fetus is stable; if blood is abundant, the fetus can be nourished and calmed. At the same time, we should distinguish between cold and heat, and between deficiency and excess, according to the principle of "basing the treatment on pattern differentiation," and apply the method of strengthening the kidney, strengthening the spleen, benefiting qi, clearing heat, regulating qi, invigorating blood, and resolving toxins to prevent miscarriage.

For the selection of formulas, attention should be paid to warming and tonifying medicinals, making sure that the combination is not excessively acrid or drying. Heat-clearing formulas should not be too bitter or too cold, and formulas that regulate qi should not produce excessive dissipation. Stasis-removing and diuretic medicinals must be used with caution. If such medicinals are required, stop using them as soon as they have taken effect, in accordance with the principle of "cease the use of medicinals when the majority of pathogens have been eliminated."

a. Kidney Deficiency

【Syndrome Characteristics】 Mild vaginal bleeding of light or dark red color and thin texture in early or middle pregnancy. Vague pain in the lower abdomen, soreness in the lumbosacral area, dizziness, tinnitus, aversion to cold with cold limbs, frequent and clear urination, a history of miscarriage, a pale tongue with thin white coating, and a deep, slippery and weak pulse.

【Treatment Principle】 Reinforce the kidney and calm the fetus; tonify qi and nourish blood.

【Commonly Used Medicinals】 *Sāng jì shēng* (Herba Taxilli), *xù duàn* (Radix Dipsaci), *tù sī zǐ* (Semen Cuscutae), *dù zhòng* (Cortex Eucommiae), *dǎng shēn* (Radix Codonopsis), *bái zhú* (Rhizoma Atractylodis Macrocephalae), *shān yào* (Rhizoma Dioscoreae), *zhì gān cǎo* (Radix Glycyrrhizae Praeparata), *ài yè* (Folium Artemisiae Argyi), *ē jiāo* (Colla Corii Asini) and *hàn lián cǎo* (Herba Ecliptae).

【Representative Formula】 Modified *Shou Tai Wan* 寿胎丸

【Ingredients】

菟丝子	tù sī zǐ	30g		Semen Cuscutae
桑寄生	sāng jì shēng	30g		Herba Taxilli
续断	xù duàn	15g		Radix Dipsaci
阿胶	ē jiāo	10g (dissolve)		Colla Corii Asini
党参	dǎng shēn	15g		Radix Codonopsis
白术	bái zhú	10g		Rhizoma Atractylodis Macrocephalae
焦艾叶	jiāo ài yè	6g		Folium Artemisiae Argyi Praeparata
炙甘草	zhì gān cǎo	6g		Radix Glycyrrhizae Praeparata cum Melle

Decoct in 500ml of water until 200ml of the decoction is left. Take warm, 1 bag a day.

【Formula Analysis】 *Tù sī zǐ* (Semen Cuscutae) can tonify the kidney, benefit essence and stabilize the penetrating and conception vessels. When the kidney qi is flourishing, the body can conceive. *Tù sī zǐ* (Semen Cuscutae), prescribed in a large dosage, is the chief medicinal; *sāng jì shēng* (Herba Taxilli) and *xù duàn* (Radix Dipsaci) are the deputies, and can tonify and benefit the liver and kidney, nourish blood and calm fetus; *ē jiāo* (Colla Corii Asini) as both the assistant and the envoy, nourishes blood. The four medicinals used together can achieve the effects of tonifying the kidney, nourishing blood, and controlling and calming the fetus. Add *dǎng shēn* (Radix Codonopsis), *bái zhú* (Rhizoma Atractylodis Macrocephalae), *zhì gān cǎo* (Radix et Rhizoma Glycyrrhizae Praeparata cum Melle) to strengthen the spleen and benefit qi to use the acquired constitution to support the congenital constitution with, produce qi and blood to nourish the essence, reinforce congenital and acquired constitution, and enhance the pacifying of the fetus. *Jiāo ài yè* (Folium Artemisiae Argyi Praeparata) warms the channels and stop bleeding to calm the fetus.

【Modifications】

For fear of cold, cold limbs and cold pain in the lower back and abdomen, *bā jǐ tiān* (Radix Morindae Officinalis) 10g is added to warm the kidney and support yang.

For severe abdominal pain, add *bái sháo* (Radix Paeoniae Alba) 15g and *gān cǎo* (Radix et Rhizoma Glycyrrhizae) to relieve spasms and alleviate pain. For sagging sensation in the lower abdomen, *huáng qí* (Radix Astragali) 15g is added to raise yang and lift the fetus.

For kidney yin deficiency with a dry bitter mouth, a red tongue with scanty coating, and a thready rapid pulse, remove *ài yè* (Folium Artemisiae Argyi) and *dǎng shēn* (Radix Codonopsis), and add *hàn lián cǎo* (Herba Ecliptae) 15g and *nǚ zhēn zǐ* (Fructus Ligustri Lucidi) 15g to nourish kidney yin. If there are symptoms of pronounced heat, add *huáng qín* (Radix Scutellariae) 12g, *shā shēn* (Radix Glehniae Littoralis) 15g and *mài dōng* (Radix Ophiopogonis) 15g to eliminate heat and nourish yin.

For dry and hard stools, add *huǒ má rén* (Fructus Cannabis) 20g and *xuán shēn* (Radix Scrophulariae) 9g to moisten the intestines and unblock the stools.

b. Qi and Blood Deficiency

【Syndrome Characteristics】 Mild occasional vaginal bleeding of light red color and thin texture in early and middle pregnancy. Vague and sagging pain in the lower abdomen, pale or sallow complexion, spiritual lassitude, palpitations, shortness of breath, a pale tongue with white thin coating, and a thready, slippery and weak pulse.

【Treatment Principle】 Benefit qi and nourish blood; tonify the kidney and calm the fetus.

【Commonly Used Medicinals】 *Dǎng shēn* (Radix Codonopsis), *huáng qí* (Radix Astragali), *bái zhú* (Rhizoma Atractylodis Macrocephalae), *zhì gān cǎo* (Radix et Rhizoma Glycyrrhizae Praeparata cum Melle), *dāng guī* (Radix Angelicae Sinensis), *bái sháo* (Radix Paeoniae Alba), *shú dì huáng* (Radix Rehmanniae Praeparata), *ē jiāo* (Colla Corii Asini), *dù zhòng* (Cortex Eucommiae), *tù sī zǐ* (Semen Cuscutae), *sāng jì shēng* (Herba Taxilli) and *xù duàn* (Radix Dipsaci). *Bái sháo* (Radix Paeoniae Alba) paired with *gān cǎo* (Radix et Rhizoma Glycyrrhizae) can relieve spasms and alleviate pain.

【Representative Formula】 Modified *Tai Yuan Yin* 胎元饮

【Ingredients】

党参	dǎng shēn	20g	Radix Codonopsis
黄芪	huáng qí	15g	Radix Astragali
白术	bái zhú	10g	Rhizoma Atractylodis Macrocephalae

当归	dāng guī	6g	Radix Angelicae Sinensis
白芍	bái sháo	15g	Radix Paeoniae Alba
熟地黄	shú dì huáng	12g	Radix Rehmanniae Praeparata
阿胶	ē jiāo	10g (dissolve)	Colla Corii Asini
杜仲	dù zhòng	10g	Cortex Eucommiae
陈皮	chén pí	6g	Pericarpium Citri Reticulatae
炙甘草	zhì gān cǎo	6g	Radix et Rhizoma Glycyrrhizae Praeparata cum Melle

Decoct in 500ml of water until 200ml of liquid remains. Take warm, 1 bag a day.

【Formula Analysis】 *Rén shēn* (Radix et Rhizoma Ginseng), *huáng qí* (Radix Astragali), *bái zhú* (Rhizoma Atractylodis Macrocephalae) and *zhì gān cǎo* (Radix et Rhizoma Glycyrrhizae Praeparata cum Melle) are all sweet and warm. They strengthen the spleen and benefit qi to secure the fetus while supporting the source of generation and transformation. *Dāng guī* (Radix Angelicae Sinensis), *shú dì huáng* (Radix Rehmanniae Praeparata), *bái sháo* (Radix Paeoniae Alba) and *ē jiāo* (Colla Corii Asini) nourishes blood and calms the fetus. *Dù zhòng* (Cortex Eucommiae) can tonify the kidney and calm the fetus. *Chén pí* (Pericarpium Citri Reticulatae) can regulate the qi and harmonize the stomach. *Tai Yuan Yin* 胎元饮 is *Ba Zhen Tang* without *fú líng* (Poria) and *chuān xiōng* (Rhizoma Chuanxiong), and with *dù zhòng* (Cortex Eucommiae) and *chén pí* (Pericarpium Citri Reticulatae) added. This formula can tonify the qi, blood and kidney simultaneously.

【Modifications】

For vaginal bleeding, *dāng guī* (Radix Angelicae Sinensis) is removed and 10g of *jiāo ài yè* (Folium Artemisiae Argyi Praeparata) is added to stop bleeding and calm the fetus.

For history of spontaneous abortion or miscarriage, *tù sī zǐ* (Semen Cuscutae) 20g is added to enhance the effect of strengthening the kidney and securing the fetus.

For nausea, vomiting and poor appetite, *shā rén* (Fructus Amomi) 6g and *zǐ sū gěng* (Caulis Perillae) 12g are added to harmonize the stomach and calm the fetus.

c. Blood Heat
A. Excess Heat

【**Syndrome Characteristics**】 Mild vaginal bleeding of bright red color and thick texture in early and middle pregnancy, lower abdominal pain, red face and lips, dry mouth, thirst, a red tongue with white coating, and a slippery rapid pulse.

【**Treatment Principle**】 Clear heat and cool blood; stanch bleeding and calm the fetus.

【**Commonly Used Medicinals**】 *Huáng qín* (Radix Scutellariae), *huáng lián* (Rhizoma Coptidis), *cè bǎi tàn* (Cacumen Platycladi Carbonisata), *chūn gēn pí* (Cortex Ailanthi), *dì yú* (Radix Sanguisorbae), *hàn lián cǎo* (Herba Ecliptae), *ē jiāo* (Colla Corii Asini), *hé shǒu wū* (Radix Polygoni Multiflori), *shān yào* (Rhizoma Dioscoreae) and *sāng jì shēng* (Herba Taxilli).

【**Representative Formula**】 Modified *Qing Re An Tai Yin* 清热安胎饮

【**Ingredients**】

黄芩	huáng qín	10g	Radix Scutellariae
黄连	huáng lián	6g	Rhizoma Coptidis
侧柏炭	cè bǎi tàn	10g	Cacumen Platycladi Carbonisata
椿根皮	chūn gēn pí	10g	Cortex Ailanthi
阿胶	ē jiāo	10g (dissolve)	Colla Corii Asini
山药	shān yào	15g	Rhizoma Dioscoreae

Decoct in 500ml of water until 200ml of the liquid remains. Take warm, 1 bag a day.

【**Formula Analysis**】 *Huáng qín* and *huáng lián* can clear heat and drain fire; *cè bǎi tàn* and *chūn gēn pí* clear heat, cool blood and stop bleeding because of their astringent nature; *ē jiāo* nourishes blood and stops bleeding; *shān yào* can strengthen the spleen, benefit the kidney and calm the fetus.

【Modifications】

For distending fullness in the chest and hypochondria, bitter taste in the mouth and dry throat, *bái sháo* (Radix Paeoniae Alba) 15g and vinegar-fried *chái hú* (Radix Bupleuri) 10g are added to nourish blood and soothe the liver.

For dry and hard stools, *xuán shēn* (Radix Scrophulariae) 12g and *mài dōng* (Radix Ophiopogonis) 15g are added to nourish yin, enrich fluids and moisten dryness to unblock the stools.

B. Deficiency Heat

【Syndrome Characteristics】 Vaginal bleeding of small quantity, dark red color and thick texture during pregnancy, lumbar soreness and sagging pain in the lower abdomen. Other symptoms include vexing heat in the five hearts, dry mouth and throat, thirst, tidal fever, night sweats, a red tender tongue with scanty or no coating, and a thready, slippery and rapid pulse.

【Treatment Principle】 Enrich yin and clear heat; nourish blood and calm fetus.

【Commonly Used Medicinals】 *Huáng qín* (Radix Scutellariae), *huáng bǎi* (Cortex Phellodendri Chinensis), *shēng dì huáng* (Radix Rehmanniae Recens), *bái sháo* (Radix Paeoniae Alba), *shān yào* (Rhizoma Dioscoreae), *xù duàn* (Radix Dipsaci), *sāng jì shēng* (Herba Taxilli), *gān cǎo* (Radix et Rhizoma Glycyrrhizae), *zhù má gēn* (Radix Boehmeriae Ramie), *nǚ zhēn zǐ* (Fructus Ligustri Lucidi) and *hàn lián cǎo* (Herba Ecliptae).

【Representative Formula】 Modified *Bao Yin Jian* 保阴煎

【Ingredients】

黄芩	huáng qín	10g	Radix Scutellariae
黄柏	huáng bǎi	10g	Cortex Phellodendri Chinensis
生地黄	shēng dì huáng	15g	Radix Rehmanniae Recens
白芍	bái sháo	15g	Radix Paeoniae Alba

山药	shān yào	15g	Rhizoma Dioscoreae
续断	xù duàn	10g	Radix Dipsaci
桑寄生	sāng jì shēng	30g	Herba Taxilli
甘草	gān cǎo	6g	Radix et Rhizoma Glycyrrhizae
苎麻根	zhù má gēn	10g	Radix Boehmeriae Ramie
女贞子	nǚ zhēn zǐ	15g	Fructus Ligustri Lucidi
旱莲草	hàn lián cǎo	15g	Herba Ecliptae

Decoct in 500ml of water until 200ml of liquid remains. Take warm, 1 bag a day.

【Formula Analysis】 *Huáng qín* (Radix Scutellariae), *huáng bǎi* (Cortex Phellodendri Chinensis), *shēng dì huáng* (Radix Rehmanniae Recens), *hàn lián cǎo* (Herba Ecliptae) and *zhù má gēn* (Radix Boehmeriae Ramie) nourish yin, clear heat, cool blood and stop bleeding; *bái sháo* (Radix Paeoniae Alba) paired with *gān cǎo* (Radix et Rhizoma Glycyrrhizae) can relieve spasms and alleviate pain; *sāng jì shēng* (Herba Taxilli), *xù duàn* (Radix Dipsaci) and *nǚ zhēn zǐ* (Fructus Ligustri Lucidi) can secure the kidney and calm the fetus.

【Modifications】 For dry mouth and throat, add *shā shēn* (Radix Glehniae Littoralis) 15g and *shí hú* (Caulis Dendrobii) 10g to nourish yin and promote the generation of fluids to quench thirst.

d. Liver Constraint

【Syndrome Characteristics】 Lower abdominal pain or mild vaginal bleeding during pregnancy. Accompanying symptoms include depression, frequent sighing, distending pain in the chest and hypochondria, belching, poor appetite, occasional nausea and vomiting of sour or bitter fluid, a normal tongue body, and a wiry slippery pulse.

【Treatment Principle】 Soothe the liver to relieve constraint; regulate qi to calm the fetus.

【Commonly Used Medicinals】 *Zǐ sū gěng* (Caulis Perillae), *chén pí* (Pericarpium Citri Reticulatae), *dà fù pí* (Pericarpium Arecae), *dāng guī*

(Radix Angelicae Sinensis), *bái sháo* (Radix Paeoniae Alba), vinegar-fried *chái hú* (Radix Bupleuri), *dǎng shēn* (Radix Codonopsis), *gān cǎo* (Radix et Rhizoma Glycyrrhizae), *sāng jì shēng* (Herba Taxilli), *tù sī zǐ* (Semen Cuscutae) and *xù duàn* (Radix Dipsaci).

【**Representative Formula**】 Modified *Zi Su Yin* 紫苏饮

【**Ingredients**】

苏梗	sū gěng	10g	Caulis Perillae
陈皮	chén pí	10g	Pericarpium Citri Reticulatae
大腹皮	dà fù pí	10g	Pericarpium Arecae
当归	dāng guī	6g	Radix Angelicae Sinensis
白芍	bái sháo	10g	Radix Paeoniae Alba
党参	dǎng shēn	15g	Radix Codonopsis
甘草	gān cǎo	6g	Radix et Rhizoma Glycyrrhizae
醋柴胡	cù chái hú	10g	Radix Bupleuri, vinegar-fried
桑寄生	sāng jì shēng	15g	Herba Taxilli
菟丝子	tù sī zǐ	15g	Semen Cuscutae

Decoct in 500ml of water until 200ml of liquid is left. Take warm, 1 bag a day.

【**Formula Analysis**】 *Zǐ sū gěng* (Caulis Perillae), *chén pí* (Pericarpium Citri Reticulatae) and *dà fù pí* (Pericarpium Arecae) have the ability to regulate qi and relieve epigastric distention; *dāng guī* (Radix Angelicae Sinensis), *bái sháo* (Radix Paeoniae Alba) and vinegar-fried *chái hú* (Radix Bupleuri) can nourish blood, soften and soothe the liver, resolve constraint and calm the fetus; *dǎng shēn* (Radix Codonopsis) and *gān cǎo* (Radix et Rhizoma Glycyrrhizae) can strengthen the spleen and benefit qi; *sāng jì shēng* (Herba Taxilli), *tù sī zǐ* (Semen Cuscutae) and *xù duàn* (Radix Dipsaci) can enrich and nourish the liver and kidney to calm the fetus.

【**Modifications**】

For nausea and vomiting of sour or bitter gastric fluid, add *huáng qín* (Radix Scutellariae) 10g, *dàn zhú rú* (Caulis Bambusae in Taenia) 10g and *zǐ sū gěng* (Caulis Perillae) 12g to clear heat, downbear counterflow and relieve vomiting.

e. Blood Stasis

【Syndrome Characteristics】 Vaginal bleeding of dark color or with mild clots, pain in the lesser abdomen, or a history of stubborn illness; a dusky tongue with possible stasis spots and maculae, and a wiry slippery pulse.

【Treatment Principle】 Invigorate blood to disperse concretions; tonify the kidney to calm the fetus.

【Commonly Used Medicinals】 *Guì zhī* (Ramulus Cinnamomi), *fú ling* (Poria), *táo rén* (Semen Persicae), *chì sháo* (Radix Paeoniae Rubra), *mǔ dān pí* (Cortex Moutan), *sāng jì shēng* (Herba Taxilli), *xù duàn* (Radix Dipsaci), *tù sī zǐ* (Semen Cuscutae) and *ē jiāo* (Colla Corii Asini).

【Representative Formula】 Modified *Gui Zhi Fu Ling Wan* 桂枝茯苓丸 and *Shou Tai Wan* 寿胎丸

【Ingredients】

桂枝	guì zhī	10g	Ramulus Cinnamomi
茯苓	fú líng	15g	Poria
桃仁	táo rén	10g	Semen Persicae
赤芍	chì sháo	10g	Radix Paeoniae Rubra
牡丹皮	mǔ dān pí	10g	Cortex Moutan
桑寄生	sāng jì shēng	15g	Herba Taxilli
续断	xù duàn	15g	Radix Dipsaci
菟丝子	tù sī zǐ	15g	Semen Cuscutae
阿胶	ē jiāo	10g (dissolve)	Colla Corii Asini

Decoct in 500ml of water until 200ml of liquid remains. Take the decoction when warm, 1 bag a day.

【Formula Analysis】 *Guì zhī* (Ramulus Cinnamomi) can warm the channels to dispel cold, unblock the collaterals and move stasis; *fú ling* (Poria) can strengthen the spleen and transform dampness; *táo rén* (Semen Persicae) can invigorate blood and dissipate nodules; *chì sháo* (Radix Paeoniae Rubra) moves the stagnation in the blood; *mǔ dān pí* (Cortex

Moutan) cools blood and transforms stasis; *sāng jì shēng* (Herba Taxilli), *xù duàn* (Radix Dipsaci), *tù sī zǐ* (Semen Cuscutae) and *ē jiāo* (Colla Corii Asini) can strengthen the kidney, nourish blood and calm the fetus. This formula has the effects of invigorating blood to transform stasis, dispersing concretions, alleviating pain, and strengthening the kidney to calm the fetus. When static blood has been removed, fresh blood can flow within the vessels to nourish the embryo.

f. External Trauma

【**Syndrome Characteristics**】 Post-traumatic lower abdominal pain, lumbar soreness and vaginal bleeding of small quality and red color during pregnancy, a normal tongue body, and a slippery or slippery weak pulse.

【**Treatment Principle**】 Benefit qi and harmonize blood; Strengthen the kidney and calm the fetus.

【**Commonly Used Medicinals**】 *Dǎng shēn* (Radix Codonopsis), *huáng qí* (Radix Astragali), *dāng guī* (Radix Angelicae Sinensis), *chuān xiōng* (Rhizoma Chuanxiong), *bái sháo* (Radix Paeoniae Alba) and *shú dì huáng* (Radix Rehmanniae Praeparata).

【**Representative Formula**】 Modified *Sheng Yu Tang* 圣愈汤 and *Shou Tai Wan* 寿胎丸

【**Ingredients**】

党参	dǎng shēn	15g	Radix Codonopsis
黄芪	huáng qí	15g	Radix Astragali
当归	dāng guī	6g	Radix Angelicae Sinensis
川芎	chuān xiōng	6g	Rhizoma Chuanxiong
白芍	bái sháo	15g	Radix Paeoniae Alba
熟地黄	shú dì huáng	10g	Radix Rehmanniae Praeparata
桑寄生	sāng jì shēng	30g	Herba Taxilli
续断	xù duàn	10g	Radix Dipsaci
菟丝子	tù sī zǐ	15g	Semen Cuscutae
阿胶	ē jiāo	10g (dissolve)	Colla Corii Asini

Decoct the medicinals in 500ml of water until 200ml of liquid remains. Take warm, 1 bag a day.

【Formula Analysis】 *Sāng jì shēng* (Herba Taxilli), *xù duàn* (Radix Dipsaci) and *tù sī zǐ* (Semen Cuscutae) can secure the kidney to calm the fetus; *dǎng shēn* (Radix Codonopsis) and *huáng qí* (Radix Astragali) can strengthen the spleen and benefit qi; *dāng guī* (Radix Angelicae Sinensis), *chuān xiōng* (Rhizoma Chuanxiong), *bái sháo* (Radix Paeoniae Alba) and *shú dì huáng* (Radix Rehmanniae Praeparata) can nourish and harmonize blood; *ē jiāo* (Colla Corii Asini), *hàn lián cǎo* (Herba Ecliptae) can nourish blood, stop bleeding and calm the fetus.

【Modifications】

For an increased volume of vaginal bleeding, remove *dāng guī* (Radix Angelicae Sinensis) and *chuān xiōng* (Rhizoma Chuanxiong), and add *zhù má gēn* (Radix Boehmeriae Ramie)10g and *zhì gān cǎo* (Radix et Rhizoma Glycyrrhizae Praeparata cum Melle) 10g to stop bleeding and calm the fetus.

For sharp lower abdominal pain due to static blood from trauma, take 2g of powdered *sān qī* (Radix et Rhizoma Notoginseng) stirred in water to transform stasis, stop bleeding and relieve pain.

2) The Treatment of Inevitable Miscarriage and Incomplete Miscarriage:
The Chinese medical approach for the treatment of inevitable miscarriage and incomplete miscarriage is "expelling the fetus to benefit the mother." These two conditions can be divided into two categories according to their clinical manifestations – obstruction of static blood, and blood deficiency with qi desertion.

a. Obstruction of Static Blood
【Syndrome Characteristics】 During early pregnancy, there is exacerbation of sagging and distending pain in the lower abdomen, profuse dark vaginal bleeding with clots, or with partial expulsion of

conceptive products. During middle pregnancy, there are aggravating labor pains, lower back soreness with sagging sensation, distension and weighed down sensation in the perineum, possible discharge of amniotic fluid or vaginal bleeding, possible retention of the placenta and fetal membrane in the uterus, a normal tongue, and a slippery or slippery thready pulse.

【Treatment Principle】 Invigorate blood and transform stasis; expel the fetus and stop bleeding.

【Commonly Used Medicinals】 *Dāng guī* (Radix Angelicae Sinensis), *chuān xiōng* (Rhizoma Chuanxiong), *hóng huā* (Flos Carthami), *táo rén* (Semen Persicae), *niú xī* (Radix Achyranthis Bidentatae), *chē qián zǐ* (Semen Plantaginis), *zhǐ qiào* (Fructus Aurantii), *yì mǔ cǎo* (Herba Leonuri) and *pú huáng* (Pollen Typhae).

【Representative Formula】 Modified *Tuo Hua Jian* 脱花煎

【Ingredients】

当归	dāng guī	20g	Radix Angelicae Sinensis
川芎	chuān xiōng	15g	Rhizoma Chuanxiong
红花	hóng huā	10g	Flos Carthami
牛膝	niú xī	15g	Radix Achyranthis Bidentatae
车前子	chē qián zǐ	10g	Semen Plantaginis
枳壳	zhǐ qiào	15g	Fructus Aurantii
益母草	yì mǔ cǎo	30g	Herba Leonuri
桃仁	táo rén	12g	Semen Persicae

Decoct the medicinals in 500ml of water until only 200ml of liquid remains. Take warm, 1 bag a day.

【Formula Analysis】 *Dāng guī* (Radix Angelicae Sinensis), *chuān xiōng* (Rhizoma Chuanxiong), *hóng huā* (Flos Carthami), *táo rén* (Semen Persicae) and *niú xī* (Radix Achyranthis Bidentatae) can nourish blood, promote blood circulation and expel the fetus; *chē qián zǐ* (Semen Plantaginis) lubricates to facilitate expulsion of the fetus; *zhǐ qiào* (Fructus

Aurantii), *yì mǔ cǎo* (Herba Leonuri) and *pú huáng* (Pollen Typhae) can promote qi flow, dispel stasis, expel the fetus and stop bleeding.

【Modifications】

For incomplete expulsion of the productions of conception, or profuse bleeding due to the retention of the placenta and fetal membrane, add *pú huáng* (Pollen Typhae) 10g, *wǔ líng zhī* (Faeces Togopteri) 10g and *sān qī* (Radix et Rhizoma Notoginseng) 3g to expel stasis and stop bleeding.

For lassitude and shortness of breath, *dǎng shēn* (Radix Codonopsis) 15g, *huáng qí* (Radix Astragali) 15g are added to benefit qi and expel the fetus.

b. Blood Deficiency and Qi Desertion

【Syndrome Characteristics】 Sudden profuse incessant vaginal bleeding during spontaneous abortion or miscarriage, pale complexion, profuse sweating, short and hasty breathing, pale lips and tongue, a faint pulse that is verging on expiry, and unconsciousness (in severe cases).

【Treatment Principle】 Benefit qi and stem desertion; restore yang and rescue counterflow.

【Commonly Used Medicinals】 *Rén shēn* (Radix et Rhizoma Ginseng) and *shú fù zǐ* (Radix Aconiti Lateralis Praeparata).

【Representative Formula】 *Shen Fu Tang* 参附汤

【Ingredients】

| 人参 | rén shēn | 30g | Radix et Rhizoma Ginseng |
| 熟附子 | shú fù zǐ | 10g | Radix Aconiti Lateralis Praeparata |

Decoct in 500ml of water until 200ml of liquid remains. Take the decoction when warm, 1 bag a day.

【Formula Analysis】 *Rén shēn* (Radix et Rhizoma Ginseng) strongly tonifies original qi; *shú fù zǐ* (Radix Aconiti Lateralis Praeparata) strengthens original yang. The two medicinals used together have the

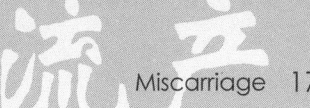

effects of benefiting qi and secures desertion, restoring yang and rescuing from counterflow.

In inevitable miscarriage and incomplete miscarriage, profuse incessant bleeding can be life-threatening, because it can lead to qi desertion with bleeding and separation of yin and yang due to the sudden blood loss, causing yang to lose its anchorage. This not only has a negative impact on the mother's health, but can also be fatal. Integrative treatment should be adopted. The uterine contents should be removed immediately, and the patient should be given a blood transfusion. For mild bleeding with partial retention of the conceptive products in the uterus, use the methods of invigorating blood, transforming stasis and contracting the uterus to facilitate complete expulsion of the fetus. D&C treatment is applicable if bleeding is profuse.

3) The Treatment of Complete Miscarriage:

If there is complete expulsion of the conceptive products (or fetus) with mild vaginal bleeding, doctors can treat this as they would a normal delivery. However, since a miscarriage is much more detrimental to the body than a normal delivery, special attention should be paid to post-miscarriage healthcare.

If there is qi and blood insufficiency (as a result of excessive bleeding consuming qi and blood) during the course of spontaneous abortion or miscarriage, the patient may present with a sallow yellow facial complexion, mental lassitude, weak limbs, soreness and weakness of the lower back and knees, palpitation, shortness of breath, a small quantity of lochia of light color and thin consistency, a pale tongue and a thready weak pulse.

【Treatment Principle】 The primary treatment principle is to benefit qi and nourish blood; the secondary treatment principle is to promote the contraction the uterus and stop bleeding.

【Commonly Used Medicinals】 *Rén shēn* (Radix et Rhizoma Ginseng), *dāng guī* (Radix Angelicae Sinensis), *páo jiāng* (Rhizoma Zingiberis Praeparatum), *chuān xiōng* (Rhizoma Chuanxiong), *yì mǔ cǎo* (Herba Leonuri), *zhì gān cǎo* (Radix et Rhizoma Glycyrrhizae Praeparata cum Melle), 6 pieces of *dà zǎo* (Fructus Jujubae), *huáng qí* (Radix Astragali) and *zhǐ qiào* (Fructus Aurantii).

【Representative Formula】 Modified *Ren Shen Sheng Hua Tang* 人参生化汤

【Ingredients】

人参	rén shēn	10g (decoct separately first)	Radix et Rhizoma Ginseng
当归	dāng guī	10g	Radix Angelicae Sinensis
炮姜	páo jiāng	6g	Rhizoma Zingiberis Praeparatum
川芎	chuān xiōng	6g	Rhizoma Chuanxiong
益母草	yì mǔ cǎo	30g	Herba Leonuri
炙甘草	zhì gān cǎo	6g	Radix et Rhizoma Glycyrrhizae Praeparata cum Melle
大枣	dà zǎo	6 pieces	Fructus Jujubae
黄芪	huáng qí	15g	Radix Astragali
枳壳	zhǐ qiào	15g	Fructus Aurantii

Decoct in 500ml of water until 200ml of liquid remains. Take warm, 1 bag a day.

【Formula Analysis】 *Rén shēn* (Radix et Rhizoma Ginseng) powerfully tonifies original qi; *huáng qí* (Radix Astragali) benefits qi and strengthens the spleen; *dāng guī* (Radix Angelicae Sinensis) and *chuān xiōng* (Rhizoma Chuanxiong) nourishes blood and promotes blood circulation; *páo jiāng* (Rhizoma Zingiberis Praeparatum) warms channel and dissipates cold; *zhì gān cǎo* (Radix et Rhizoma Glycyrrhizae Praeparata cum Melle) and *dà zǎo* warm the middle to tonify deficiency; *yì mǔ cǎo* (Herba Leonuri) dispels stasis and engenders fresh blood; *zhǐ qiào* (Fructus Aurantii) regulates qi and promotes uterine contraction. The formula has the effects of tonifying qi, containing blood, dispelling stasis and promoting the production of fresh blood.

4) The Treatment of Missed Abortion:

If the fetus dies in utero and is not expelled naturally, this is a missed abortion, which falls under the patterns of deficiency and excess. The deficiency pattern consists of deficiency of both qi and blood resulting in the lack of force needed to expel the fetus out of the body. The excess pattern is the obstruction of static blood impairing the expulsion of the fetus. To facilitate the expulsion of the fetus is the main focus of the treatment; however, the mother's constitution (deficiency or excess) should be taken into consideration, so as to avoid the careless use of drastic methods.

a. Qi and Blood Deficiency

【Syndrome Characteristics】 Prolonged retention of dead fetus, lower abdominal pain, light red vaginal discharge, pale complexion, mental lassitude, shortness of breath, disinclination to speak, foul breath, a pale tongue body with white greasy coating, and a deficient, large and rough pulse.

【Treatment Principle】 Benefit qi and nourish blood; invigorate blood to expel the fetus.

【Commonly Used Medicinals】 *Dǎng shēn* (Radix Codonopsis), *dāng guī* (Radix Angelicae Sinensis), *chuān xiōng* (Rhizoma Chuanxiong), *yì mǔ cǎo* (Herba Leonuri) and *chuān niú xī* (Radix Cyathulae).

【Representative Formula】 Modified *Jiu Mu Dan* 救母丹

【Ingredients】

党参	dǎng shēn	20g	Radix Codonopsis
当归	dāng guī	15g	Radix Angelicae Sinensis
川芎	chuān xiōng	10g	Rhizoma Chuanxiong
益母草	yì mǔ cǎo	30g	Herba Leonuri
赤石脂	chì shí zhī	30g	Halloysitum Rubrum
炒芥穗	chǎo jiè suì	10g	Spica Schizonepetae (stir-fried)
川牛膝	chuān niú xī	10g	Radix Cyathulae

Decoct the medicinals in 500ml of water until there is 200ml of liquid is left. Take warm, 1 bag a day.

【Formula Analysis】 *Dǎng shēn* (Radix Codonopsis) tonifies qi. *Dāng guī* (Radix Angelicae Sinensis) and *chuān xiōng* (Rhizoma Chuanxiong) tonifies blood; when qi and blood are both flourishing, the qi is able to propel the blood and blood is able to move. *Yì mǔ cǎo* (Herba Leonuri) invigorates blood and facilitates the expulsion of the dead fetus. *Chì shí zhī* (Halloysitum Rubrum) transforms malign blood; once the malign blood is removed, the dead fetus can be expelled. *Chǎo jiè suì* (Spica Schizonepetae, stir-fried) guides the blood into the channels and allows the fetus to be expelled without causing excessive bleeding in the process. *Chuān niú xī* (Radix Cyathulae) invigorates blood and guides the blood downward. The formula has the effects of tonifying qi and blood and discharging the dead fetus.

【Modifications】

For cold pain in lower abdomen and cold limbs with fear of cold, *ròu guì* (Cortex Cinnamomi) 6g and *wū yào* (Radix Linderae) 10g are added to warm the uterus, dissipate cold and stop bleeding;

For extreme deficiency of qi and blood, *huáng qí* (Radix Astragali) and *dān shēn* (Radix et Rhizoma Salviae Miltiorrhizae) can be added to regulate and nourish qi and blood.

b. Blood Stasis

【Syndrome Characteristics】 Retention of dead fetus, lower abdominal pain, vaginal bleeding of dark purplish color or with blood clots, blue and dark facial complexion, blue lips, foul breath, a dark purplish tongue with or without stasis spots, and a deep, rough pulse.

【Treatment Principle】 Invigorate blood and remove stagnation; dispel stasis to expel the fetus.

【Commonly Used Medicinals】 *Dāng guī* (Radix Angelicae Sinensis), *chuān xiōng* (Rhizoma Chuanxiong), *hóng huā* (Flos Carthami), *é zhú* (Rhizoma Curcumae), *yì mǔ cǎo* (Herba Leonuri), *chuān niú xī* (Radix Cyathulae), *chē qián zǐ* (Semen Plantaginis) and *máng xiāo* (Natrii Sulfas).

【Representative Formula】Modified *Tuo Hua Jian* 脱花煎

【Ingredients】

当归	dāng guī	15g	Radix Angelicae Sinensis
川芎	chuān xiōng	10g	Rhizoma Chuanxiong
肉桂	ròu guì	6g	Cortex Cinnamomi
车前子	chē qián zǐ	10g	Semen Plantaginis
川牛膝	chuān niú xī	15g	Radix Cyathulae
红花	hóng huā	10g	Flos Carthami
莪术	é zhú	10g	Rhizoma Curcumae
芒硝	máng xiāo	3g (dissolve)	Natrii Sulfas
益母草	yì mǔ cǎo	30g	Herba Leonuri

Decoct in 500ml of water until there is 200ml of liquid left. Take warm, 1 bag a day.

【Formula Analysis】*Dāng guī* (Radix Angelicae Sinensis) and *chuān xiōng* (Rhizoma Chuanxiong) nourish and invigorate blood; *hóng huā* (Flos Carthami), *é zhú* (Rhizoma Curcumae) and *yì mǔ cǎo* (Herba Leonuri) dispel stasis and break static blood; chuān *niú xī* (Radix Cyathulae) guides blood downward to discharge the fetus; *chē qián zǐ* (Semen Plantaginis) and *máng xiāo* (Natrii Sulfas) promote water flow and drains downward to facilitate expulsion of the fetus; *ròu guì* (Cortex Cinnamomi) warms and unblocks the channels. All of these medicinals, when used together, can remove static blood and discharge the dead fetus.

【Modifications】

For profuse bleeding, add *chǎo pú huáng* (Pollen Typhae, stir-fried) 10g and powdered *sān qī* (Radix et Rhizoma Notoginseng) 3g to transform stasis and stop bleeding;

For fullness and distension in the chest and abdomen, *zhǐ qiào* (Fructus Aurantii) 15g and *chuān liàn zǐ* (Fructus Toosendan) 10g are added to regulate qi and remove stagnation;

In cases of missed abortions where the fetus has been dead for a long period of time, this can easily induce a hemorrhage or a secondary infection. Therefore, it is necessary to closely monitor vaginal bleeding and abdominal pain. When removing the fetus, carefully inspect to see if the fetus, placenta and fetal membrane have been discharged completely. Integrative treatment should be adopted immediately if there is profuse bleeding or other complications.

5) The Treatment of Habitual Miscarriage:

Multiple miscarriages damage the penetrating and conception vessels, thus deficiency is a common result. The basic therapeutic principle of habitual miscarriage is tonification. Understanding that "the primary focus is prevention, in conjunction with treatment" is an important step in the treatment process. Before pregnancy, it is necessary to tonify the kidney, strengthen the spleen, benefit qi, nourish blood, regulate and stabilize the penetrating and conception vessels. After the patient is pregnant, preventing miscarriage should be the main focus of treatment.

a. Insufficiency of Kidney Qi

【Syndrome Characteristics】 Frequent miscarriages, occurring more than 3 times consecutively, listlessness, dizziness, tinnitus, soreness and weakness of the lower back and knees, frequent copious night urination, dark circles around the eye sockets or dark maculae on the face, a pale tongue and a deep, thready pulse.

【Treatment Principle】 Tonify the kidney and calm the fetus.

【Commonly Used Medicinals】 *Tù sī zǐ* (Semen Cuscutae), *xù duàn* (Radix Dipsaci), *bā jǐ tiān* (Radix Morindae Officinalis), *dù zhòng* (Cortex

Eucommiae), *lù jiǎo shuāng* (Cornu Cervi Degelatinatum), *shú dì huáng* (Radix Rehmanniae Praeparata), *gǒu qǐ zǐ* (Fructus Lycii), *ē jiāo* (Colla Corii Asini), *dǎng shēn* (Radix Codonopsis), *huáng qí* (Radix Astragali), *shā rén* (Fructus Amomi), *bái zhú* (Rhizoma Atractylodis Macrocephalae) and *shān yào* (Rhizoma Dioscoreae).

【**Representative Formula**】 Modified *Bu Shen Gu Chong Wan* 补肾固冲丸

【**Ingredients**】

菟丝子	tù sī zǐ	30g	Semen Cuscutae
续断	xù duàn	15g	Radix Dipsaci
巴戟天	bā jǐ tiān	15g	Radix Morindae Officinalis
杜仲	dù zhòng	15g	Cortex Eucommiae
熟地黄	shú dì huáng	20g	Radix Rehmanniae Praeparata
鹿角霜	lù jiǎo shuāng	12g	Cornu Cervi Degelatinatum
枸杞子	gǒu qǐ zǐ	12g	Fructus Lycii
阿胶	ē jiāo	12g (dissolve)	Colla Corii Asini
党参	dǎng shēn	15g	Radix Codonopsis
白术	bái zhú	12g	Rhizoma Atractylodis Macrocephalae
黄芪	huáng qí	15g	Radix Astragali
砂仁	shā rén	6g	Fructus Amomi

Decoct in 500ml of water until there is 200ml of liquid left. Take warm, 1 bag a day.

【**Formula Analysis**】 *Tù sī zǐ* (Semen Cuscutae), *xù duàn* (Radix Dipsaci), *bā jǐ tiān* (Radix Morindae Officinalis), *dù zhòng* (Cortex Eucommiae) and *lù jiǎo shuāng* (Cornu Cervi Degelatinatum) tonify the kidney, stabilize the penetrating vessel and calm the fetus; *shú dì huáng* (Radix Rehmanniae Praeparata), *gǒu qǐ zǐ* (Fructus Lycii) and *ē jiāo* (Colla Corii Asini) nourish blood and calm the fetus; *dǎng shēn* (Radix Codonopsis), *huáng qí* (Radix Astragali), *shā rén* (Fructus Amomi), *bái zhú* (Rhizoma Atractylodis Macrocephalae) and *shān yào* (Rhizoma Dioscoreae) tonify the spleen and benefit qi.

b. Qi and Blood Deficiency

【Syndrome Characteristics】 Frequent miscarriages, occurring more than 2 times consecutively, a weak body, a somber white or sallow yellow facial complexion, mental lassitude, dizziness, palpation, a pale tongue with thin white coating and a thready, weak pulse.

【Treatment Principle】 Benefit qi, tonify blood and calm the fetus.

【Commonly Used Medicinals】 *Dǎng shēn* (Radix Codonopsis), *huáng qí* (Radix Astragali), *bái zhú* (Rhizoma Atractylodis Macrocephalae), *zhì gān cǎo* (Radix et Rhizoma Glycyrrhizae Praeparata cum Melle), *bái sháo* (Radix Paeoniae Alba), *shú dì huáng* (Radix Rehmanniae Praeparata), *tù sī zǐ* (Semen Cuscutae), *xù duàn* (Radix Dipsaci), *sāng jì shēng* (Herba Taxilli) and *dù zhòng* (Cortex Eucommiae).

【Representative Formula】 Modified *Tai Shan Pan Shi Yin* 泰山磐石饮

【Ingredients】

党参	dǎng shēn	15g	Radix Codonopsis
黄芪	huáng qí	15g	Radix Astragali
白术	bái zhú	10g	Rhizoma Atractylodis Macrocephalae
熟地黄	shú dì huáng	20g	Radix Rehmanniae Praeparata
白芍	bái sháo	15g	Radix Paeoniae Alba
杜仲	dù zhòng	15g	Cortex Eucommiae
砂仁	shā rén	12g	Fructus Amomi
炙甘草	zhì gān cǎo	6g	Radix et Rhizoma Glycyrrhizae Praeparata cum Melle
菟丝子	tù sī zǐ	30g	Semen Cuscutae
续断	xù duàn	15g	Radix Dipsaci
桑寄生	sāng jì shēng	15g	Herba Taxilli

Decoct in 500ml of water until 200ml of liquid remains. Take warm.

【Formula Analysis】 *Dǎng shēn* (Radix Codonopsis), *huáng qí* (Radix Astragali), *bái zhú* (Rhizoma Atractylodis Macrocephalae), *zhì gān cǎo* (Radix et Rhizoma Glycyrrhizae Praeparata cum Melle) strengthen the spleen and benefit qi to hold the fetus; *bái sháo* (Radix Paeoniae Alba) and *shú dì huáng* (Radix Rehmanniae Praeparata) tonify and harmonize blood to nourish the fetus; *tù sī zǐ* (Semen Cuscutae), *xù duàn* (Radix Dipsaci), *sāng jì shēng* (Herba Taxilli) and *dù zhòng* (Cortex Eucommiae) tonify the kidney, strengthen the lower back and secure the fetus.

【Modifications】

For cold pain in lower abdomen with physical cold and cold limbs, add *bā jǐ tiān* (Radix Morindae Officinalis) 10g and *wū yào* (Radix Linderae) 10g to warm yang, dissipate cold and alleviate pain.

For sensations of emptiness and sagging in the lower abdomen with discomfort, add *shēng má* (Rhizoma Cimicifugae) 5g to raise yang and lift sinking.

c. Blood Heat due to Yin Deficiency

【Syndrome Characteristics】 Frequent miscarriages, occurring more than 2 times consecutively, flushed cheeks, dry mouth and throat, feverish sensation in the palms and soles, insomnia, profuse dreaming, vexation and agitation, emaciation, a red tongue with little or no coating and a thready, rapid pulse.

【Treatment Principle】 Enrich yin, clear heat, cool blood and calm the fetus.

【Commonly Used Medicinals】 *Shān yú ròu* (Fructus Corni), *shēng dì huáng* (Radix Rehmanniae Recens), *shú dì huáng* (Radix Rehmanniae Praeparata), *mài dōng* (Radix Ophiopogonis), *zhī mǔ* (Rhizoma Anemarrhenae), *dì gǔ pí* (Cortex Lycii), *nǚ zhēn zǐ* (Fructus Ligustri Lucidi), *hàn lián cǎo* (Herba Ecliptae) and *sāng jì shēng* (Herba Taxilli).

【Representative Formula】 Modified *Yi Yin Jian* 一阴煎

【Ingredients】

生地黄	shēng dì huáng	15g	Radix Rehmanniae Recens
熟地黄	shú dì huáng	15g	Radix Rehmanniae Praeparata
白芍	bái sháo	15g	Radix Paeoniae Alba
麦冬	mài dōng	10g	Radix Ophiopogonis

知母	zhī mǔ	10g	Rhizoma Anemarrhenae
地骨皮	dì gǔ pí	10g	Cortex Lycii
炙甘草	zhì gān cǎo	6g	Radix et Rhizoma Glycyrrhizae Praeparata cum Melle
山茱肉	Shān yú ròu	15g	Fructus Corni
女贞子	nǚ zhēn zǐ	15g	Fructus Ligustri Lucidi
旱莲草	hàn lián cǎo	15g	Herba Ecliptae
桑寄生	sāng jì shēng	15g	Herba Taxilli

Decoct in 500ml of water until 200ml of liquid remains. Take warm.

【**Formula Analysis**】 *Shān yú ròu* (Fructus Corni), *shēng dì huáng* (Radix Rehmanniae Recens), *shú dì huáng* (Radix Rehmanniae Praeparata) and *mài dōng* (Radix Ophiopogonis) enrich yin and nourish blood; *zhī mǔ* (Rhizoma Anemarrhenae), *dì gǔ pí* (Cortex Lycii) nourish yin and clear heat; *nǚ zhēn zǐ* (Fructus Ligustri Lucidi), *hàn lián cǎo* (Herba Ecliptae), *sāng jì shēng* (Herba Taxilli) enrich the kidney and calm the fetus.

【**Modifications**】

For heart vexation, insomnia and profuse dreaming, add *suān zǎo rén* (Semen Ziziphi Spinosae) 10g and *bǎi zǐ rén* (Semen Platycladi) 10g to calm the heart and tranquilize the mind.

For dry mouth and throat with decreased body fluid, add *shí hú* (Caulis Dendrobii) 10g and *xuán shēn* (Radix Scrophulariae) 10g to engender fluids and quench thirst.

d. Internal Obstruction of Static Blood

【**Syndrome Characteristics**】 Frequent miscarriages occurring more than 2 times consecutively, lower abdominal pain, coarse skin, lower abdominal masses, a dark tongue with stasis spots or maculae and a wiry or deep rough pulse.

【**Treatment Principle**】 Invigorate blood, transform stasis, nourish blood and calm the fetus.

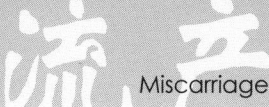

【**Commonly Used Medicinals**】 *Guì zhī* (Ramulus Cinnamomi) can be used to warm the channels, unblock the collaterals, dissipate cold and remove stasis; *chì sháo* (Radix Paeoniae Rubra), *táo rén* (Semen Persicae) and *mŭ dān pí* (Cortex Moutan) can break blood, dissipate nodules and disperse concretions; *fú líng* (Poria) can strengthen the spleen and leach out dampness; *dāng guī* (Radix Angelicae Sinensis), *bái sháo* (Radix Paeoniae Alba), *tù sī zĭ* (Semen Cuscutae) and *xù duàn* (Radix Dipsaci) can nourish blood, stabilize the kidney and calm the fetus.

【**Representative Formula**】 Modified *Gui Zhi Fu Ling Wan* 桂枝茯苓丸

【**Ingredients**】

桂枝	Guì zhī	10g	Ramulus Cinnamomi
牡丹皮	mŭ dān pí	10g	Cortex Moutan
桃仁	táo rén	15g	Semen Persicae
赤芍	chì sháo	10g	Radix Paeoniae Rubra
茯苓	fú líng	15g	Poria
当归	dāng guī	12g	Radix Angelicae Sinensis
白芍	bái sháo	15g	Radix Paeoniae Alba
菟丝子	tù sī zĭ	15g	Semen Cuscutae
续断	xù duàn	15g	Radix Dipsaci

Decoct in 500ml of water until there is 200ml of liquid left. Take warm.

【**Formula Analysis**】 *Guì zhī* (Ramulus Cinnamomi) warms the channels, unblocks the collaterals, dissipates cold and removes stasis; *chì sháo* (Radix Paeoniae Rubra), *táo rén* (Semen Persicae) and *mŭ dān pí* (Cortex Moutan) break blood, dissipate nodules and disperse concretions; *fú líng* (Poria) strengthens the spleen and leaches out dampness; *dāng guī* (Radix Angelicae Sinensis), *bái sháo* (Radix Paeoniae Alba), *tù sī zĭ* (Semen Cuscutae) and *xù duàn* (Radix Dipsaci) nourish blood, stabilize the kidney and calm the fetus.

2. Additional Treatment Modalities

A. Chinese Patent Medicine

a) *Zi Shen Yu Tai Wan* 滋肾育胎丸
Treats all types of threatened miscarriage and habitual miscarriage. Take 6 grams each time, 2 or 3 times a day.

b) *Yun Kang Kou Fu Ye* 孕康口服液
Treats all types of threatened miscarriage and habitual miscarriage. Take 1 or 2 flasks, 3 times a day.

c) *Sheng Hua Tang Wan* 生化汤丸
Invigorates blood, transforms stasis and engenders fresh blood. For incomplete miscarriage of blood deficiency and blood stasis patterns. Take 1 pill, 3 times a day.

d) *Ba Zhen Wan* 八珍丸
Regulates qi and nourishes blood. For qi and blood deficiency type complete miscarriage. Take 1 pill, 3 times a day.

e) *Yi Mu Cao Gao* 益母草膏
Nourishes and invigorates blood and transforms stasis. The formula is suitable for incomplete miscarriage or blood deficiency and blood stasis type complete miscarriage. Take 5-10ml, 15-30ml a day.

B. Acupuncture And Moxibustion

a) Acupuncture Using Filiform Needle
【Point Selection】

LI 4	hé gǔ	合谷
SP 6	sān yīn jiāo	三阴交

The prescription has the function of supplementing blood and draining qi, producing the effect of stabilizing the kidney and calming the fetus. Treats threatened miscarriage.

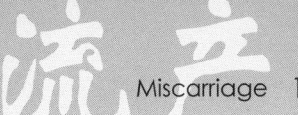
【Manipulation】 Insert the needle 1-2 cun. After obtaining the arrival of qi, retain the needle for 20 minutes and stimulate the needles intermittently. Needle LI 4 with drainage, and SP 6 with supplementation. The treatment period consists of one treatment per day, for 7 days.

b) Warming Needle Acupuncture
【Point Selection】

DU 20	bǎi huì	百会
ST 36	zú sān lǐ	足三里
SJ 5	wài guān	外关
LV 2	xíng jiān	行间
SP 6	sān yīn jiāo	三阴交
SP 10	xuè hǎi	血海
RN 4	guān yuán	关元

This point combination tonifies the kidney and calms the fetus, and is suitable for the treatment of threatened miscarriage.

【Manipulation】 DU 20 is selected with 2 or 3 other points. After needling the points and obtaining the arrival of qi, apply moxibustion and retain the needles for 15 to 30 minutes. The treatment course is once a day, for a total of 10 days.

C. Simple Prescriptions And Empirical Formulas

a) *E Jiao Ji Zi Tang* 阿胶鸡子汤

阿胶	ē jiāo	10g (dissolve)	Colla Corii Asini
鸡子	jī zǐ	2	eggs
红糖	hóng táng	30g	brown sugar

Heat *ē jiāo* (Colla Corii Asini) in 200ml of water until it boils and simmer until the *ē jiāo* has completely dissolved. Break and poach the eggs and add brown sugar after eggs are well cooked. After the brown sugar has dissolved, it is ready for consumption.

This medicinal recipe is suitable for the treatment of restless fetus and habitual miscarriage.

b) *Xiang You Mi Gao* 香油蜜膏

香油	xiāng yóu	100g	sesame oil
蜂蜜	fēng mì	200g	honey

Decoct the two ingredients over a low flame until the water boils. Turn off the flame and let the mixture cool down. When the mixture is still warm but not hot, stir it well. Take 1 tablespoon each time, 2 times a day.

This recipe is suitable for the treatment of threatened miscarriage.

c) *Gu Tai Yin* 固胎饮

莲肉	lián ròu	30g	Semen Nelumbinis
糯米	nuò mǐ	30g	glutinous rice
苎麻根	zhù má gēn	30g	Radix Boehmeriae Ramie

Decoct in 3 bowls of water until there is only 1 bowl of liquid left. This medicinal recipe is for a weak constitution with lower back pain and habitual miscarriage.

d) *Xian Shan Yao Du Zhong Tang* 鲜山药杜仲汤

鲜山药	xiān shān yào	90g	Rhizoma Dioscoreae（fresh）
杜仲	dù zhòng	6g	Cortex Eucommiae
苎麻根	zhù má gēn	15g	Radix Boehmeriae Ramie
糯米	nuò mǐ	80g	glutinous rice

Wrap *dù zhòng* (Cortex Eucommiae) and *zhù má gēn* (Radix Boehmeriae Ramie) with a gauze. Wash *nuò mǐ* thoroughly. Put the herbs together in a pot and cook them to make a porridge. This recipe can treat threatened miscarriage and habitual miscarriage.

e) *Zhu Tai Fang* 助胎方

蒸白术	bái zhú (steamed)	250g	Rhizoma Atractylodis Macrocephalae
党参	dǎng shēn	120g	Radix Codonopsis

桑寄生	sāng jì shēng	90g	Herba Taxilli
茯苓	fú líng	90g	Poria
杜仲炭	dù zhòng tàn	120g	Cortex Eucommiae Carbonisatus

Cut open some dates, decoct them and make boluses the size of dryandra seeds. Dry them in the sun and then store them away. Grind the above herbs into a powder. Every morning and night, take 9g each time, with warm water and several dates. This recipe is used for restless fetus and delayed fetal development.

f) *Du Zhong Xu Duan Tang* 杜仲续断汤

| 杜仲 | dù zhòng | 30g | Cortex Eucommiae |
| 续断 | xù duàn | 30g | Radix Dipsaci |

Decoct the above herbs in 2 bowls of water until there is half that amount of liquid left. Take it every Monday before the 5th month of pregnancy to prevent a habitual miscarriage. There are no negative side affects from taking more than the recommended dosage.

PROGNOSIS

For general threatened miscarriage, the symptoms can disappear gradually, and the patient will eventually achieve pregnancy after being treated. However, a threatened miscarriage can develop into an inevitable miscarriage or a delayed miscarriage if the embryo itself is unable to develop well, or if the matrix has irreversible pathogenic factors. For this condition, pregnancy must be terminated as soon as it is confirmed. Spontaneous abortion can become habitual miscarriage if it becomes recurrent, for which treatment must be seriously considered. Attention should be paid to treatment given before and during pregnancy; monitor the health of both the mother and the fetus, and protect the fetus when necessary. Pregnancy should be terminated in cases of fetuses with genetic defects or deformities.

PREVENTIVE HEALTHCARE

There are many causes of miscarriage. During treatment, attention must be paid to preventing miscarriage, getting enough physical exercise, strengthening the constitution, and eliminating stress and tension. We can also ensure that the mother gets sufficient nutrition by recommending a medicated diet. All of this will ensure a smooth pregnancy.

1. Lifestyle Modification

a. Avoid fatigue during the pregnancy. Let the patient rest in bed if she has bleeding.

b. Abstain from sexual intercourse. Avoid taking long walks while carrying heavy objects. Avoid climbing high hills and accidents (tumbling, falling and contusions).

c. Keep the external genitals clean.

d. Exercise caution when engaging in daily activities and avoid wind-cold invasions. Prevent catching colds and avoid touching toxic materials.

e. Do not take medicines that are harmful to the development of the fetus.

f. Make sure the bowel movement is regular. Do not strain when defecating, so as to avoid increased abdominal pressure which can cause vaginal bleeding.

g. Exercise regularly to strengthen the constitution.

2. Dietary Recommendation

Food and beverages should be light, easy-to-digest and nutritious. Avoid spicy foods and eat more vegetables and fruits instead. Tonification is the primary focus of a clinical medicated diet, particularly the strengthening of the spleen and kidney. However, transforming stasis and producing fresh blood is also necessary for missed abortion and inevitable miscarriage, in order to help expel the fetus. Refrain from eating astringent foods to avoid retention of pathogens.

A medicated diet that can strengthen the spleen and kidney: *Huáng qí* (Radix Astragali), *nuò mǐ* (glutinous rice), *dǎng shēn* (Radix Codonopsis), *ài yè* (Folium Artemisiae Argyi), eggs, sea bass, *zhù má gēn* (Radix Boehmeriae Ramie), *dù zhòng* (Cortex Eucommiae), pig's kidney, *ē jiāo* (Colla Corii Asini), *sháo yào* (Radix Paeoniae), *dāng guī* (Radix Angelicae Sinensis), *gān cǎo* (Radix et Rhizoma Glycyrrhizae), frog, *xù duàn* (Radix Dipsaci) and *huái shān yào* (Radix Dioscoreae Oppositae).

Dietary recommendation for missed abortion: *yì mǔ cǎo* (Herba Leonuri), *chuān xiōng* (Rhizoma Chuanxiong), *dāng guī* (Radix Angelicae Sinensis), *bái jiǔ* (Chinese white liquor), *yě mián huā* (wild cotton), *lián fáng* (Receptaculum Nelumbinis), *niú xī* (Radix Achyranthis Bidentatae) and *hóng huā* (Flos Carthami).

A. Threatened Miscarriage

a) *Nuo Mi Huang Qi Yin* 糯米黄芪饮

糯米	nuò mǐ	30g	glutinous rice
黄芪	huáng qí	15g	Radix Astragali
川芎	chuān xiōng	5g	Rhizoma Chuanxiong

Decoct the above medicinals in 1000g of water until 500g of liquid remains. Discard the dregs. Take the decoction warm, twice a day. This medicinal recipe nourishes qi and blood and calms the fetus.

b) *Slow-cooked Du Zhong with Pig Kidney* 杜仲煨猪肾

This recipe contains *dù zhòng* (Cortex Eucommiae), pig kidney and table salt. Cut open the pig kidney in half, and remove the tendons and membranes. Soak it in water with pepper and salt to eliminate the fishy smell. Put it in an earthenware pot together with *dù zhòng* and water. Cook slowly until ready to serve. Eat the kidney and drink the soup twice a day, for a total of 7 days (1 treatment course). This recipe tonifies deficiency, benefits the kidney and calms the fetus.

c) *Ē jiāo Wine* 胶艾酒

阿胶	ē jiāo	30g	Colla Corii Asini
艾叶	ài yè	20g	Folium Artemisiae Argyi
川芎	chuān xiōng	6g	Rhizoma Chuanxiong
芍药	sháo yào	20g	Radix Paeoniae
甘草	gān cǎo	20g	Radix et Rhizoma Glycyrrhizae
当归	dāng guī	6g	Radix Angelicae Sinensis
生地黄	shēng dì huáng	15g	Radix Rehmanniae Recens

Decoct the above medicinals with yellow rice wine and water. Divide the liquid into 3 portions, and drink 1 portion in the morning, 1 portion at noon and 1 portion at night. It is suitable for injury to fetus from accidental tumbles and falls, with the effects of nourishing blood and calming the fetus.

d) *Sāng jì shēng and Egg Tea* 桑寄生鸡蛋茶

桑寄生	*sāng jì shēng*	15g	Herba Taxilli
鸡蛋	egg	1	

Put *sāng jì shēng* (Herba Taxilli) and egg together in a pot of cold water. Bring to a boil and keep cooking until the egg is done. Crack the eggshell and continue to cook for another 30 minutes. Drink the soup and eat the egg. This recipe is suitable for threatened miscarriage.

e) *Zhu Ma Gen and Chicken Casserole* 苎麻根煲鸡

Select a 500g hen and remove the feathers, organs, head and claws. Place the dried *zhù má gēn* 30g (60-90g if fresh) inside the abdominal cavity of the hen. Boil them in a sufficient amount of water. Drink the soup and eat the chicken. This recipe is for yin deficiency with internal heat type threatened miscarriage.

B. Inevitable Miscarriage, Incomplete Miscarriage and Missed Abortion

a) *Lian Fang Wine* 莲房煮酒

Select one *lián fáng* (Receptaculum Nelumbinis) and an appropriate amount of sweet wine. Break the lián fáng into pieces and decoct it with the sweet wine. Discard the dregs and drink the decoction. This recipe has the effect of benefiting qi and nourishing blood.

b) *Hong Hua Wine* 红花煮酒

Put *hóng huā* (Flos Carthami) 6g in an earthenware pot and add a desired amount of wine. Cook them over low flame until the volume of the liquid is half the original quantity. Discard the dregs and drink 2-3 small cups. This recipe can invigorate blood and transform stasis.

C. Habitual Miscarriage

a) *Huai Shan Yao Fetus-Securing Porridge* 淮山药固胎粥

生淮山药	huái shān yào (raw)	90g	Radix Dioscoreae Oppositae
续断	xù duàn	15g	Radix Dipsaci
杜仲	dù zhòng	10g	Cortex Eucommiae
苎麻根	zhù má gēn	15g	Radix Boehmeriae Ramie
糯米	nuò mǐ	250g	glutinous rice

Wash *xù duàn* (Radix Dipsaci), *dù zhòng* (Cortex Eucommiae) and *zhù má gēn* (Radix Boehmeriae Ramie) thoroughly, and wrap them with clean gauze. Cook them together with *huái shān yào* (Radix Dioscoreae Oppositae) and *nuò mǐ* (glutinous rice). Open the gauze when the porridge is ready. Add a little oil and salt. Divide the porridge into two potions and serve warm. This recipe is suitable for liver and kidney yin deficiency. It has the effects of tonifying the liver and kidney, strengthening the spleen and calming the fetus.

b) *Chicken and Glutinous Rice Porridge* 母鸡糯米粥

Select a hen of about 750g. Wash the hen and remove its feathers and organs. Stuff its abdominal cavity with medicinal herbs. Cook a cuttlefish in water until it becomes a concentrated soup. Add *nuò mǐ* (glutinous rice) and continue to cook until rice is ready. Add a little salt and serve. This recipe treats qi and blood deficiency, and has the effects of benefiting qi, nourishing blood and securing the fetus.

3. Regulation of Emotional and Mental Health

Anxiety can cause qi stagnation and blood stasis, resulting in impaired blood flow to the uterus during pregnancy. If the fetus cannot be nourished, a miscarriage is likely to occur. Patients should be kept in high spirits and avoid situations that may cause mental and emotional stress. If a miscarriage has already occurred, the patient should avoid physical and mental exertion. For threatened miscarriage, patients should get plenty of bed rest and monitor the health of the fetus. For missed abortion, patients should be given D&C immediately. Patients are also advised to actively participate in physical exercise in order to strengthen the constitution so that they can be more prepared for the next pregnancy.

CLINICAL EXPERIENCE OF RENOWNED PHYSICIANS

1. Empirical Formulas

a. Treating habitual miscarriage with *Zi Sheng Yu Tai Wan* 滋肾育胎丸

【Ingredients】

菟丝子	tù sī zǐ	240g	Radix Codonopsis
续断	xù duàn	90g	Radix Dipsaci
巴戟天	bā jǐ tiān	90g	Radix Morindae Officinalis
杜仲	dù zhòng	90g	Cortex Eucommiae
熟地黄	shú dì huáng	150g	Radix Rehmanniae Praeparata

鹿角霜	lù jiǎo shuāng	90g	Cornu Cervi Degelatinatum
枸杞子	gǒu qǐ zǐ	90g	Fructus Lycii
阿胶	ē jiāo	120g	Colla Corii Asini
党参	dǎng shēn	120g	Radix Codonopsis
白术	bái zhú	90g	Rhizoma Atractylodis Macrocephala
无核大枣	wú hé dà zǎo	50g	Fructus Jujubae (with pits removed)
砂仁	shā rén	15g	Fructus Amomi

Grind the above medicinals into powder, except for *shú dì huáng* (Radix Rehmanniae Praeparata), *ē jiāo* (Colla Corii Asini), *gǒu qǐ zǐ* (Fructus Lycii) and *dà zǎo* (Fructus Jujubae). Decoct *shú dì huáng* (Radix Rehmanniae Praeparata) and *gǒu qǐ zǐ* (Fructus Lycii) several times, and dissolve *ē jiāo* (Colla Corii Asini) into the decoction to give it a porridge-like consistency. Crush the dates, and mix them with the porridge-like decoction and the powdered medicinals. Add a desired amount of refined honey, and stir well to make small pills. Take 6g, 3 times a day.

【Indications】 Various patterns of habitual miscarriage and threatened miscarriage.

【Formula Analysis】 Enriching kidney yin and tonifying kidney yang are the main focuses of the formula, assisted by tonifying qi, strengthening the spleen and nourishing blood. *Tù sī zǐ* (Semen Cuscutae), the chief herb, is acrid, sweet and neutral, and enters the liver and kidney channels. *Records of Renowned Physicians* <*Ming Yi Bie Lu*> 名医别录 mentions: "To treat deficiency cold in men and women, replenish essence and benefit marrow to alleviate lumbar pain and cold knees; this will tonify the kidney, benefit essence and secure the fetus." *Dǎng shēn* (Radix Codonopsis) strengthens the spleen and tonifies qi; *lù jiǎo shuāng* (Cornu Cervi Degelatinatum) reinforces original yang and produces essence and marrow; *bā jǐ tiān* (Radix Morindae Officinalis), *dù zhòng* (Cortex Eucommiae) and *xù duàn* (Radix Dipsaci), tonify the kidney and stabilize the penetrating vessel; *gǒu qǐ zǐ* (Fructus Lycii), *shú dì huáng* (Radix Rehmanniae Praeparata) and *ē jiāo* (Colla Corii Asini) nourish the liver and enrich blood; *bái zhú* (Rhizoma Atractylodis Macrocephalae) and *dà zǎo* (Fructus Jujubae) tonify qi and strengthen the spleen; *shā rén* (Fructus Amomi) regulates qi and harmonizes the middle. This formula concurrently treats the kidney, liver, spleen, qi and blood to benefit the root of the penetrating and conception vessels. Experiments on lab animals confirm that this formula improves blood flow to the ovaries and uterus, and thus promotes the growth and development of the ovaries, uterus, and corpus luteum.

(Hu Xuming: Editor-in-chief. *Compendium of Secret Chinese Medical Formulas* 中国中医秘方大全. Shanghai: Wenhui Publishing House, 1989.9)

b. Treating Habitual Miscarriage with *An Tai Fang Lou Tang* 安胎防漏汤

【Ingredients】

菟丝子	tù sī zǐ	20g	Radix Codonopsis
覆盆子	fù pén zǐ	10g	Fructus Rubi
川杜仲	chuān dù zhòng	10g	Cortex Eucommiae
白芍	bái sháo	6g	Radix Paeoniae Alba
熟地黄	shú dì huáng	15g	Radix Rehmanniae Praeparata
党参	dǎng shēn	15g	Radix Codonopsis
炒白术	chǎo bái zhú	10g	Rhizoma Atractylodis Macrocephala Praeparata
棉花根	mián huā gēn	10g	Radix Gossypii
炙甘草	zhì gān cǎo	5g	Radix Glycyrrhizae Praeparata

【Indications】 Habitual miscarriage of the following patterns: qi and blood deficiency, and instability due to kidney deficiency.

【Formula Analysis】 *Tù sī zǐ* (Semen Cuscutae) is acrid, sweet and neutral; *fù pén zǐ* (Fructus Rubi) is sweet, sour and slightly warm. When used together, they have the functions of tonifying the kidney, producing essence, strengthening the lower back and securing the fetus. *Dù zhòng* (Cortex Eucommiae), because of its sweet and warm nature, is tonifying but not cloying and warming but not drying, therefore it is an important herb for the liver and kidney. *Dāng guī* (Radix Angelicae Sinensis), *bái sháo* (Radix Paeoniae Alba) and *shú dì huáng* (Radix Rehmanniae Praeparata) all possess the ability to tonify blood and nourish the liver; sufficient liver blood can promote fetal development. *Dǎng shēn* (Radix Codonopsis), *bái zhú* (Rhizoma Atractylodis Macrocephalae) and *mián huā gēn* (Radix Gossypii) are sweet, warm and slightly bitter; they can strengthen the spleen, benefit qi, raise yang and transform dampness, facilitating the production of qi and blood and promoting the lifting, strengthening and calming of the fetus. *Gān cǎo* is sweet and neutral, which can not only harmonize all the medicinals, but also nourish qi, regulate the middle jiao, relieve spasms and alleviate pain. The whole formula has the effects of warming and nourishing qi and blood, strengthening the kidney, benefiting essence, securing the fetus and preventing a threatened miscarriage.

【Modifications】

For distention and sagging pain in the lower back and the lesser and lower abdomens, add *sāng jì shēng* (Herba Taxilli) 12g, *xù duàn* (Radix Dipsaci) 10g, *shā rén qiào* (husk of Fructus Amomi) 3g and *zǐ sū gěng* (Caulis Perillae) 5g.

For vaginal bleeding of scanty quantity and red color, and a thready rapid pulse, add *hé yè dì* (calyx of Folium Nelumbinis) 12g, *zhù má gēn* (Radix Boehmeriae Ramie) 15g, *huáng qín* (Radix Scutellariae) 10g and *ē jiāo* (Colla Corii Asini) 10g (to be melted in the decoction); if vaginal bleeding is profuse and red, remove acrid and warm *dāng guī* (Radix Angelicae Sinensis), and add *jī xuè téng* (Caulis Spatholobi) 20g, *hàn lián cǎo* (Herba Ecliptae) 20g and *dà yè zǐ zhū* (Callicarpae Macrophyllae Folium) 10g; for prolonged scanty uterine bleeding of light color without abdominal pain, add *sāng piāo xiāo* (Ootheca Mantidis) 10g, *lù jiǎo shuāng* (Cornu Cervi Degelatinatum) 20g and *huā shēng yī* (Testa Arachidis Hypogaeae) 30g, and increase the dosage of *dǎng shēn* (Radix

Codonopsis) to 15g.

Take this formula before pregnancy for 3 to 6 months to cultivate the root (*běn*); and take it again after getting pregnant. Complete expulsion can be achieved as long as the treatment adheres to the principle of tonifying qi and blood, stabilizing the kidney and strengthening the lower back.

(Zhang Fengqiang, et al. *A Selection of Effective Empirical Formulas of the First Group of National Renowned Physicians*首批国家级名老中医效验秘方精选. Beijing: International Culture Publishing Company, 1995. 305-306)

c. Treating Habitual Miscarriage with *Gu Tai Tang* 固胎汤

【**Ingredients**】

党参	dǎng shēn	30g	Radix Codonopsis
白术	bái zhú	30g	Rhizoma Atractylodis Macrocephalae
炒扁豆	chǎo biǎn dòu	9g	Semen Dolichoris Lablab
淮山药	huái shān yào	15g	Rhizoma Dioscoreae Oppositae
熟地黄	shú dì huáng	30g	Radix Rehmanniae Praeparata
山茱萸	shān zhū yú	9g	Fructus Corni
杜仲	dù zhòng	9g	Cortex Eucommiae
续断	xù duàn	9g	Radix Dipsaci
桑寄生	sāng jì shēng	15g	Herba Taxilli
白芍	bái sháo	18g	Radix Paeoniae Alba
炙甘草	zhì gān cǎo	3g	Radix Glycyrrhizae Praeparata
枸杞子	gǒu qǐ zǐ	9g	Fructus Lycii

【**Indications**】 Spleen and kidney deficiency type habitual miscarriage manifesting as dull abdominal pain, lower back pain, sagging pain in the lower abdomen, a deep, weak and forceless pulse, and a pale or tooth-marked tongue with thin coating.

【**Formula Analysis**】 Most habitual miscarriages are caused by dual deficiency of the spleen and kidney. *Dǎng shēn* (Radix Codonopsis), *bái zhú* (Rhizoma Atractylodis Macrocephalae), *biǎn dòu* (Semen Dolichoris Lablab), *huái shān yào* (Rhizoma Dioscoreae Oppositae) and *gān cǎo* (Radix

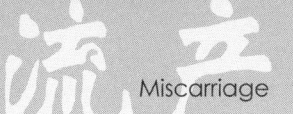

et Rhizoma Glycyrrhizae) strengthen the spleen and benefit qi to tonify the acquired constitution; *shú dì huáng* (Radix Rehmanniae Praeparata), *shān zhū yú* (Fructus Corni), *dù zhòng* (Cortex Eucommiae) and *gǒu qǐ zǐ* (Fructus Lycii) nourish blood and benefit essence to tonify the congenital constitution; *xù duàn* (Radix Dipsaci) and *sāng jì shēng* (Herba Taxilli) tonify the kidney and calm the fetus to relieve abdominal pain; *bái sháo* (Radix Paeoniae Alba) preserves yin, nourishes blood, relieves spasms, and alleviates abdominal pain. The formula is characterized by large doses of the primary medicinals, such as *bái zhú* (Rhizoma Atractylodis Macrocephalae) and *shú dì huáng* (Radix Rehmanniae Praeparata), which are required to achieve the desired specialized effects.

【Modifications】

For sagging sensation in the lower abdomen, add *shēng má* (Rhizoma Cimicifugae) 9g and *chái hú* (Radix Bupleuri) 9g to raise yang and lift sinking.

For pulling pain in lower abdomen that is sometimes severe, increase the dosages of *bái sháo* (Radix Paeoniae Alba) to 30g and *gān cǎo* (Radix et Rhizoma Glycyrrhizae) 15g to relieve spasms and alleviate pain.

For distending pain in the lower abdomen, add *zhǐ shí* (Fructus Aurantii Immaturus) 9g to regulate qi and alleviate pain.

For restless fetus and vaginal bleeding, add *ē jiāo* (Colla Corii Asini) 12g, *hàn lián cǎo* (Herba Ecliptae) 15g and *zōng lǘ tàn* (carbonized Petiolus Trachycarpi) 9g to stabilize the penetrating vessel and stanch bleeding.

For dry mouth and throat with a red tongue and yellow coating, remove *dǎng shēn* (Radix Codonopsis) and add *tài zǐ shēn* (Radix Pseudostellariae) 15g, or add *huáng qín* (Radix Scutellariae) 9g, *mài dōng* (Radix Ophiopogonis) 12g, *shí hú* (Caulis Dendrobii) 12g and *xuán shēn* (Radix Scrophulariae) 12g to nourish yin, clear heat and calm the fetus.

For chest oppression and poor appetite, add *shā rén* (Fructus Amomi) 9g and *chén pí* (Pericarpium Citri Reticulatae) 9g to aromatically harmonize the stomach.

For nausea and vomiting, add *zhú rú* (Caulis Bambusae in Taenia) 9g and *shēng jiāng* (Rhizoma Zingiberis Recens) 9g to harmonize the stomach and relieve vomiting.

For fear of cold with cold limbs and lesser abdomen, add *ròu guì* (Cortex Cinnamomi) 6g and *zhì fù piàn* (Radix Aconiti Lateralis Praeparata) 9g to warm yang and the uterus.

(Beijing Hospital of Chinese Medicine. *Clinical Gynecological Experience of Liu Fengwu.* Beijing Chinese Medicine School. Beijing: People's Medical Publishing House, 1977.286)

d. Treating threatened miscarriage with *Gu Shen An Tai Yin* 固肾安胎饮

【**Ingredients**】

桑寄生	sāng jì shēng	9g	Herba Taxilli
当归	dāng guī	9g	Radix Angelicae Sinensis
白芍	bái sháo	9g	Radix Paeoniae Alba
续断	xù duàn	9g	Radix Dipsaci
苎麻根	zhù má gēn	12g	Radix Boehmeriae Ramie
杜仲	dù zhòng	9g	Cortex Eucommiae
阿胶	ē jiāo	9g (dissolve)	Colla Corii Asini
炒艾叶	chǎo ài yè	3g	Folium Artemisiae Argyi (stir-fried)
菟丝子	tù sī zǐ	9g	Semen Cuscutae
甘草	gān cǎo	4.5g	Radix et Rhizoma Glycyrrhizae
生地黄	shēng dì huáng	12g	Radix Rehmanniae Recens
生黄芪	shēng huáng qí	12g	Radix Astragali (raw)
西党参	xī dǎng shēn	12g	Radix Codonopsis

To be decocted with water.

【**Indications**】 Threatened miscarriage due to either qi and blood deficiency or spleen and kidney insufficiency.

【**Formula Analysis**】 The primary cause of this disorder is qi and blood deficiency and spleen and kidney insufficiency, leading to instability of the penetrating and conception vessels and inability to contain blood and nourish the fetus. *Dān shēn* (Radix et Rhizoma Salviae Miltiorrhizae) and *huáng qí* (Radix Astragali) tonify the spleen and benefit qi; *dāng guī* (Radix Angelicae Sinensis), *bái sháo* (Radix Paeoniae Alba) and *shēng dì huáng* (Radix Rehmanniae Recens) nourish blood and harmonize nutritive qi; *ē jiāo* (Colla Corii Asini) and *ài yè* (Folium Artemisiae Argyi) calm the fetus and stop bleeding; *gān cǎo* (Radix et Rhizoma Glycyrrhizae) and *bái sháo* (Radix Paeoniae Alba) relieve spasms and alleviate pain; the fetus is connected to the kidney, so *dù zhòng* (Cortex Eucommiae), *xù duàn* (Radix Dipsaci), *sāng jì shēng* (Herba Taxilli) and *tù sī zǐ* (Semen Cuscutae) are used to stabilize the kidney and strengthen the lower back to calm the fetus; *zhù má gēn* (Radix Boehmeriae Ramie) nourishes yin, calms the fetus, clears heat and stops bleeding. Some consider that the function of the kidney - *tiān guǐ* - penetrating and conception vessels-uterus system in Chinese medicine is similar to that of the hypothalamus-pituitary-ovary-uterus system in biomedicine, which shows that the kidney has a close relationship with the reproductive and endocrine systems. This formula places emphasis on tonifying and benefiting kidney qi; when kidney qi is sufficient, the fetus is calm.

【Modifications】

For blood heat due to yin deficiency, remove *ài yè* (Folium Artemisiae Argyi) and add *hàn lián cǎo* (Herba Ecliptae) 9g.

For problems caused by external injury, add *shā rén* (Fructus Amomi) 3g.

(Hu Xuming: Editor-in-chief. *Compendium of Secret Chinese Medical Formulas* 中国中医秘方大全. Shanghai: Wenhui Publishing House, 1989.7)

e. Treating threatened miscarriage with *Qing Re An Tai Yin* 清热安胎饮

【Ingredients】

淮山药	huái shān yào	15g	Radix Dioscoreae Oppositae
石莲肉	shí lián ròu	9g	Semen Nelumbinis
黄芩	huáng qín	9g	Radix Scutellariae
川连	chuān lián	3g	Fructus Forsythiae
椿根皮	chūn gēn pí	9g	Cortex Ailanthi
侧柏炭	cè bǎi tàn	9g	Cacumen Platycladi (carbonized)
阿胶	ē jiāo	15g (dissolve)	Colla Corii Asini

【Indications】 Vaginal bleeding during early pregnancy (threatened miscarriage) with aching pain in the lower back due to fetal heat.

【Formula Analysis】 In early pregnancy, the blood gathers to nourish the fetus. Vaginal bleeding during pregnancy is commonly seen in yin deficiency with predominant yang causing heat that disturbs the sea of blood and forces the blood to move recklessly. This leads to vaginal bleeding during pregnancy, lower back soreness, and abdominal pain. It was mentioned in *Essentials of Materia Medica <Ben Cao Bei Yao>* 本草备要 that *bái zhú* (Rhizoma Atractylodis Macrocephalae) and *huáng qín* (Radix Scutellariae) are sacred herbs for calming the fetus. *Bái zhú* (Rhizoma Atractylodis Macrocephalae) can strengthen the spleen to replenish blood; *huáng qín* (Radix Scutellariae) can clear fetal heat because of its bitter and cold nature. It was considered by the renowned physician Liu Fengwu that *bái zhú* (Rhizoma Atractylodis Macrocephalae) is predominantly warm and dry, and since most pregnancies are characterized by blood heat due to yin deficiency, *bái zhú* (Rhizoma Atractylodis Macrocephalae) should be replaced with *huái shān yào* (Radix Dioscoreae Oppositae). *Huái shān yào* is sweet and neutral, and therefore nourishes without inducing heat. *Shí lián* (Semen Nelumbinis), which is slightly bitter and cold, can strengthen the spleen and tonify the kidney. *Huáng qín* (Radix Scutellariae) and *chuān lián* (Fructus Forsythiae) clears heat and calm the fetus; *chūn gēn pí* (Cortex Ailanthi), which is bitter, astringent and cold, stops bleeding. *Cè bǎi yè* (Cacumen Platycladi) is bitter and astringent and has the ability to cool blood and stop bleeding. When it is stir-fried until carbonized (chǎo tàn), its hemostatic function is enhanced. *Ē jiāo* (Colla Corii Asini) is sweet and neutral, and has the original function of clearing heat, cooling blood, benefiting yin and calming the fetus. Its sticky and greasy nature can also coagulate and stabilize the blood collaterals to stop bleeding. The ancients have used *Jiao Ai Tang* 胶艾汤 to treat vaginal bleeding during pregnancy. However, since *ài yè* (Folium Artemisiae Argyi) is predominantly warm, it should be replaced by *huáng qí* (Radix Astragali) and *huáng lián* (Rhizoma Coptidis) to clear heat and calm the fetus. This formula strengthens the spleen and tonifies the kidney, nourishes without producing heat, clears heat without damaging healthy qi, stops bleeding and calms the fetus.

【**Modifications**】

For profuse bleeding, add *guàn zhòng tàn* (Rhizoma Guanzhong, carbonized), *chén zōng tàn* (Petiolus Trachycarpi, carbonized), *shēng dì huáng* (Radix Rehmanniae Recens) and *hàn lián cǎo* (Herba Ecliptae).

For spleen and kidney deficiency with restless fetus, add *tù sī zǐ* (Semen Cuscutae), *xù duàn* (Radix Dipsaci) and *sāng jì shēng* (Herba Taxilli).

For qi deficiency, add *dǎng shēn* (Radix Codonopsis), *huáng qí* (Radix Astragali) and *bái zhú* (Rhizoma Atractylodis Macrocephalae).

For sagging sensation in the lower abdomen, add *shēng má tàn* (Rhizoma Cimicifugae, carbonized).

For blood heat due to yin deficiency resulting in restless fetus or lower abdominal pain, add *bái sháo* (Radix Paeoniae Alba) and zhì *gān cǎo* (Radix et Rhizoma Glycyrrhizae Praeparata cum Melle).

(Hu Xuming: Editor-in-chief. *Compendium of Secret Chinese Medical Formulas* 中国中医秘方大全. Shanghai: Wenhui Publishing House, 1989.6)

f. Treating Threatened Miscarriage with Modified *Er Zhi Wan* 二至丸 and *Shou Tai Wan* 寿胎丸

【Ingredients】

旱莲草	hàn lián cǎo	15g	Herba Ecliptae
女贞子	nǚ zhēn zǐ	15g	Fructus Ligustri Lucidi
黄芩	huáng qín	9g	Radix Scutellariae
桑寄生	sāng jì shēng	12g	Herba Taxilli
菟丝子	tù sī zǐ	12g	Semen Cuscutae
干地	gān dì (alternate name for shēng dì)	15g	Radix Rehmanniae Recens
白芍	bái sháo	8g	Radix Paeoniae Alba
麦冬	mài dōng	9g	Radix Ophiopogonis
玄参	xuán shēn	15g	Radix Scrophulariae
阿胶	ē jiāo	10g (dissolve)	Colla Corii Asini

【Indications】 Threatened miscarriage due to kidney yin deficiency.

【Formula Analysis】 *Er Zhi Wan* 二至丸 nourishes kidney yin, stops bleeding and calms the fetus; *sāng jì shēng* (Herba Taxilli) and *tù sī zǐ* (Semen Cuscutae) strengthen the penetrating and conception vessels to calm the fetus; *huáng qín* (Radix Scutellariae), *gān dì* (Radix Rehmanniae Recens), *xuán shēn* (Radix Scrophulariae) and *mài dōng* (Radix Ophiopogonis) nourish yin, clear heat and cool blood.

【Modifications】

For dry and hard stools, add *huǒ má rén* (Fructus Cannabis) to moisten the intestines and unblock the stools.

(Li Liyun: Editor-in-chief. *Chinese Medical Clinical Symptoms and Treatment in Gynecology* 中医妇科临证证治. Guangdong: People's Publishing House of Guangdong, 1999.223-224)

g. Treating Incomplete Miscarriage with *Suo Gong Zhu Yu Tang* 缩宫逐瘀汤

【Ingredients】

当归	dāng guī	10g	Radix Angelicae Sinensis
川芎	chuān xiōng	10g	Rhizoma Chuanxiong
生蒲黄	shēng pú huáng	10g	Pollen Typhae (raw)

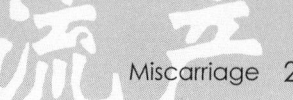

生五灵脂	shēng wǔ líng zhī	10g	Faeces Togopteri (raw)
党参	dǎng shēn	20g	Radix Codonopsis
枳壳	zhǐ qiào	10g	Fructus Aurantii
益母草	yì mǔ cǎo	15g	Herba Leonuri

【Indications】 All types of incomplete miscarriage and inevitable miscarriage.

【Formula Analysis】 *Dāng guī* (Radix Angelicae Sinensis) and *chuān xiōng* (Rhizoma Chuanxiong) nourish and invigorate blood. *Pú huáng* (Pollen Typhae) and *wǔ líng zhī* (Faeces Togopteri) expel stasis and stop bleeding, assisted by *zhǐ qiào* (Fructus Aurantii) which regulates qi; static blood can be expelled if qi and blood flow smoothly. Add *yì mǔ cǎo* (Herba Leonuri) to invigorate blood, transform stasis and produce new blood. Add *dǎng shēn* (Radix Codonopsis) to tonify qi and strengthen uterine contraction; although it is incompatible with *wǔ líng zhī* (Faeces Togopteri), it can enhance the effect of transforming stasis when used together (because they are complementary opposites).

【Modifications】

For pronounced blood deficiency, increase the dosage of *dǎng shēn* (Radix Codonopsis) to 50g.

For profuse bleeding, increase the dosage of *dǎng shēn* (Radix Codonopsis) to 100g.

For severe abdominal pain, increase the dosage of *wǔ líng zhī* (Faeces Togopteri) to 15g.

For profuse blood clots, add powdered *sān qī* (Radix et Rhizoma Notoginseng) 3g.

For prolonged bleeding, add *sāng yè* (Folium Mori) 20g.

For foul-smelling blood, add *huáng bǎi* (Cortex Phellodendri Chinensis) 10g.

For edema, add raw *huáng qí* (Radix Astragali) 50g.

For poor appetite, add raw *shān zhā* (Fructus Crataegi) 15g.

(Xu Chengji: Editor-in-chief. *Selected Famous Formulas of Renowned Physicans in Contemporary China* 中国当代名医名方精选. Jilin: Yanbian People's Publishing House, 1991. 256-257)

2. Selected Case Studies

(1) Li Shoushan's Case Studies—Instability of the Penetrating and Conception Vessels; Blood Stasis Due to Cold Uterus

Zhu, female, 29 years old, pediatrician. Initial visit: January 15th, 1958.

The patient experienced sagging distention and cold pains in the lower abdomen for 2 weeks after a miscarriage. She has had a total of 3 habitual miscarriages. The most recent miscarriage occurred during the 3rd to 4th month of pregnancy, and did not respond to any Chinese medical or biomedical measures to prevent miscarriage. During the 2nd week of the 3rd (most recent) miscarriage, the patient had symptoms of mild bleeding with clots and abdominal pain. Even after the bleeding stopped (today), there is still distention, sagging sensation, and cold pain in the lower abdomen. She also had mental lassitude, a dark and lusterless complexion, a dusky red tongue with thin white coating and a deep and wiry pulse. There is hard pain in the lower abdomen when pressed. There are no other abnormalities.

【Diagnosis】 Habitual miscarriage

【Pattern Differentiation】 Instability of the penetrating and conception vessels, and blood stasis due to a cold womb.

【Treatment Principle】 Warm the channels, dispel cold, invigorate blood and transform stasis.

【Prescription】

| 当归 | dāng guī | 15g | Radix Angelicae Sinensis |
| 川芎 | chuān xiōng | 10g | Rhizoma Chuanxiong |

赤芍	chì sháo	15g	Radix Paeoniae Rubra
炒小茴香	chǎo xiǎo huí xiāng	7.5g	Fructus Foeniculi (stir-fried)
炮姜	páo jiāng	5g	Rhizoma Zingiberis Praeparatum
肉桂	ròu guì	5g	Cortex Cinnamomi
延胡索	yán hú suǒ	15	Rhizoma Corydalis
五灵脂	wǔ líng zhī	15g	Faeces Togopteri
蒲黄	pú huáng	10g (to be wrapped for decoction)	Pollen Typhae
益母草	yì mǔ cǎo	15g	Herba Leonuri

The patient was given the following instructions: Decoct with water; use yellow rice wine as a guide.

The second visit was on January 20th. She reported having cold pain in the lower abdomen, which was alleviated after taking 3 doses of the above formula. There was cold pain and a sagging sensation in the lower abdomen with clots during menstruation, which was caused by incomplete elimination of cold in the uterus and static blood. All the symptoms disappeared immediately after taking another 3 doses of the same formula, and she got pregnant in April. During the 2nd month of pregnancy, she experienced lower back soreness and a sagging sensation in the lower abdomen, so she came to see the doctor for fear of another possible miscarriage.

The third visit was on July 6th. The patient had lower back soreness, sluggishness and a sagging sensation in the lower abdomen. She had no other complaints. She presented with a pale red tongue without coating and a deep thready pulse that is weak over chi region, which indicates a deficiency of right qi as a result of the stasis elimination. To prevent another miscarriage, the treatment plan should include benefiting qi, nourishing blood, regulating and tonifying the liver and kidney to stabilize the penetrating and conception vessels as well as the fetus. The patient was given modified *Tai Shan Pan Shi San* 泰山磐石散, which contains *huáng qí* (Radix Astragali) 15g, *dǎng shēn* (Radix Codonopsis)

15g, *bái zhú* (Rhizoma Atractylodis Macrocephalae) 15g, *dāng guī* (Radix Angelicae Sinensis) 15g, *chuān xiōng* (Rhizoma Chuanxiong) 5g, *bái sháo* (Radix Paeoniae Alba) 15g, *shú dì huáng* (Radix Rehmanniae Praeparata) 15g, *huái shān yào* (Radix Dioscoreae Oppositae) 20g, *tù sī zǐ* (Semen Cuscutae) 15g, *xù duàn* (Radix Dipsaci) 15g, *ē jiāo* (Colla Corii Asini) 10g (dissolve in decoction) and *huáng qín* (Radix Scutellariae) 10g, decocted in water for oral intake.

The patient did well on the formula, and took it as prescribed (4 - 5 doses every month until the 7th month of pregnancy). The woman carried the pregnancy full-term and gave birth to a baby boy in the winter of that year. The patient conceived again 2 years later and was treated with the same method. She had a smooth pregnancy and delivered the baby. The follow-up visit 3 years later revealed that the patient was living a happy, normal life.

Comments:

The usual method of calming the fetus is to regulate and tonify the liver and kidney, and stabilize and control the penetrating and conception vessels. If a disease results in the instability of the penetrating and conception vessels, and causes injury to the fetus, we should treat the disease first, and then calm the fetus. When treating this type of disease, treat the root; the fetus will naturally be calmed once the disease has been eliminated.

The chosen formula for this case was *Shao Fu Zhu Yu Tang* 少腹逐瘀汤, which employs the method of treating the root and calming the fetus. The pulse shows signs of stasis and stagnation, and since this is the period of time immediately following the miscarriage, it is the most opportune time to invigorate blood and transform stasis. *Shao Fu Zhu Yu Tang* warms the channels and dispels; discontinue the formula as soon as the disease has been resolved. Afterwards, if there are still symptoms of stasis and stagnation during the onset of menstruation, continue to invigorate blood and transform stasis, in accordance with the principle of treating the root. When the static blood has been removed, fresh new blood can be in a state of tranquility, and the obstacle hindering the protection of the fetus will be eliminated. This is the first step – treating disease and calming the fetus.

After the patient gets pregnant and stasis and stagnation has already been removed, we can then focus on tonifying and nourishing the liver and kidney, and regulating qi and blood to stabilize and secure the fetus. Use modified *Tai Shan Pan Shi San* 泰山磐石散 to strengthen and control the penetrating and conception vessels, calm the fetus and protect delivery, which is the second step – strengthening the root and calming the fetus. If this sequential treatment method is followed, one can achieve the effects of calming the fetus and ensuring a smooth delivery.

After a detailed inquiry, it was discovered that the patient was admitted to a hospital and given Western pharmaceuticals to prevent miscarriage, but the treatment was ineffective; she was then given Chinese medicinals to enrich and tonify the liver and kidney, stabilize and control the penetrating and conception vessels, but still to no avail. The cause of all this was stasis and stagnation. It is a known fact that just tonifying qi and nourishing the liver and kidney without first invigorating blood and transforming stasis will not achieve the desired results. After taking modified *Tai Shan Pan Shi San* 泰山磐石散, the patient had a smooth pregnancy and delivery because the "pathogen has been eliminated, and the right qi is calm." Two years later, the patient was able to conceive and carry another baby to full term. Both the mother and the baby are in good health.

(Chen Dianjun: Editor-in-chief. *The Selected Cases of Renowned Physician in Contemporary China* 中医当代名医医案话选. Changchun: Jilin Science and Technology Publishing House, 1995. 161-162)

(2) Pu Fuzhou's Case Studies—Spleen and Kidney Deficiency

Yao, female, 35 years old. Initial visit: May 30th, 1958.

The patient has had 5 miscarriages or premature deliveries during the 12 years since she has been married, one of which occurred in the 4th month of pregnancy. The rest all occurred in the 5th or 6th month. During the 1st month of each pregnancy, she experienced bleeding that lasted over ten days with low blood pressure and dizziness after. in the 3rd or 4th month, she had pain in left leg and lower back. Termination of pregnancy was inevitable even though measures to prevent miscarriage were taken. During her 4th pregnancy, she took *Tai Chan Jin Dan* 胎产金丹, which was ineffective. This time, she has been pregnant for more than 2 months. For the past 20 days, she has been experiencing nausea and vomiting, selective appetite, scanty dry stool, normal urination and low spirits. She has been sleeping well. Her pulse is deep, wiry and short in the left guan region, and deep and slippery in the right guan region. There is no coating in the center of her tongue. According to the case history, the biomedical diagnosis is habitual miscarriage, and the Chinese medical diagnosis is "slippery fetus" (habitual miscarriage). The patient is presently suffering from pernicious vomiting associated with pregnancy (morning sickness).

【Pattern Differentiation】 Liver and kidney insufficiency; spleen and stomach deficiency; instability of the penetrating and conception vessels.

【Treatment Principle】 First, regulate spleen and stomach, then stabilize the liver and kidney. When the spleen and stomach are healthy and strong, continue to tonify the liver and kidney to stabilize the fetus, while strengthening the middle qi to nourish the fetus.

【Prescription】

台党参	tái dǎng shēn	6g	Radix Codonopsis (wild)
白木	bái zhú	6g	Rhizoma Atractylodis Macrocephalae
茯苓	fú líng	6g	Poria

炙甘草	zhì gān cǎo	3g	Radix Glycyrrhizae Praeparata
广陈皮	guǎng chén pí	4.5g	Pericarpium Citri Reticulatae
砂仁	shā rén	3g (crush)	Fructus Amomi
藿香	huò xiāng	6g	Agastache Seu-Pogostemon
淮山药	huái shān yào	9g	Radix Dioscoreae Oppositae
生姜	shēng jiāng	3 pieces	Rhizoma Zingiberis Recens
大枣	dà zǎo	3 pieces	Fructus Jujubae

The patient was given the following instructions: Take 3 doses of the formula. Sip slowly. Switch to the formula below once pernicious vomiting (morning sickness) has been relieved. The formula is a modified combination of *Tai Shan Pan Shi San* 泰山磐石散 and *An Tai Yin Zhu Jiu* 安胎银苎酒.

【Prescription】

熟地黄	shú dì huáng	12g	Radix Rehmanniae Praeparata
白术	bái zhú	6g	Rhizoma Atractylodis Macrocephalae
制黑川附子	zhì hēi chuān fù zǐ	3g	Radix Aconiti Lateralis Praeparata
别直参	bié zhí shēn	3g	Radix et Rhizoma Ginseng
杜仲	dù zhòng	9g	Cortex Eucommiae
当归	dāng guī	3g	Radix Angelicae Sinensis
桑寄生	sāng jì shēng	9g	Herba Taxilli
杭巴戟	háng bā jǐ	9g	Radix Morindae Officinalis
肉苁蓉	ròu cōng róng	9g	Herba Cistanches
川续断	chuān xù duàn	6g	Radix Dipsaci (from Sichuan province)
苎麻根	zhù má gēn	9g	Radix Boehmeriae Ramie

The patient was given the following instructions: Decoct the medicinals twice (for 1 hour each time) to get 400ml of liquid, which is divided into two portions. Take one portion warm, twice a day. 1 dose (two portions) of the decoction is taken throughout 1 week. Abstain from sexual activity to avoid disturbing the fetus.

The patient took the decoction as prescribed until full term and had a smooth delivery.

Comments:

After 5 miscarriages, the patient was said to have the slippery fetus syndrome (habitual miscarriage). After the first month of every pregnancy, she would bleed for over 10 days, while also exhibiting signs and symptoms of a threatened miscarriage. There were 2 causes: one was that the spleen and stomach was too weak to nourish fetal qi, the other was insufficiency of the liver and kidney causing the root of fetus to be unstable. That is known as habitual miscarriage. The treatment method was to first regulate the spleen and stomach, and then strengthen the liver and kidney, so that the fetus can be adequately nourished and its root consolidated. All this was assisted by *zhù má gēn* (Radix Boehmeriae Ramie), which addressed the threatened miscarriage and ensured that the patient delivered another full term baby in her 6th pregnancy.

(*Pu Fuzhou's Case Studies* 蒲辅周医案, compiled by Gao Huiyuan. Beijing: People's Medical Publishing House, 1973. 137-138)

(3) Cheng Menma's Case Studies — Qi and Blood Deficiency

Tong, female, adult. Initial visit: June 16th, 1935.

The patient was pregnant and had pain and a sagging sensation in the abdomen, palpitation, lassitude, nausea, vomiting and a poor appetite. She had to avoid physical exertion to prevent injuring the fetus.

【Pattern Differentiation】 Restless fetus due to qi deficiency; liver and stomach disharmony.

【Treatment Principle】 Benefit qi and calm the stomach; harmonize the liver and spleen.

【Prescription】

炙绵芪	zhì mián qí (alternate name for zhì huáng qí)	6g	Radix Astragali Praeparata cum Melle
生白术	shēng bái zhú	6g	Rhizoma Atractylodis Macrocephalae (raw)
大白芍	dà bái sháo	6g	Radix Paeoniae Alba

云茯苓	yún fú líng	9g	Sclerotium Poriae Cocos (from Yunnan province) ·
制半夏	zhì bàn xià	4.5g	Rhizoma Pinelliae Praeparata (prepared)
炒竹茹	chǎo zhú rú	4.5g	Caulis Bambusae in Taenia (stir-fried)
浮小麦	fú xiǎo mài	12g	Fructus Tritici Levis
炒酸枣仁	chǎo suān zǎo rén	9g	Semen Ziziphi Spinosae (stir-fried)
炒黄芩	chǎo huáng qín	2.4g	Radix Scutellariae (stir-fried)
厚杜仲	hòu dù zhòng	6g	Cortex Eucommiae
桑寄生	sāng jì shēng	9g	Herba Taxilli

The patient was given 2 bags of this formula.

【Second Visit】 Pain and sagging sensation in the abdomen was alleviated. The patient had severe palpitations, lassitude, shortness of breath upon exertion, and a dry mouth and throat. The patient was given the same formula, modified by the addition of medicinals that benefit qi and nourish yin.

The ingredients of the modified formula are as follows: *Zhì huáng qí* (Radix Astragali Praeparata cum Melle) 6g, *shēng bái zhú* (Rhizoma Atractylodis Macrocephalae) 6g, *yuán shí hú* (Caulis Dendrobii, stir-fried with rice) 4.5g, *dà bái sháo* (Radix Paeoniae Alba) 6g, *fú shén* (Sclerotium Poriae Cocos Paradicis) 9g, *chǎo suān zǎo rén* (Semen Ziziphi Spinosae, stir-fried) 9g, *fú xiǎo mài* (Fructus Tritici Levis) 12g, *chǎo huáng qín* (Radix Scutellariae, stir-fried) 2.4g, *hēi dòu* (Semen Glycines Atrum) 12g, *shā yuàn jí lí* (Semen Astragali Complanati) 4.5g, *hòu dù zhòng* (Cortex Eucommiae) 6g and *sāng jì shēng* (Herba Taxilli) 9g. The patient was instructed to take 6 doses.

【Third Visit】 After benefiting qi and harmonizing the liver and spleen to protect the fetus and prevent miscarriage, all the symptoms were alleviated; the nausea and vomiting had vanished, but there was still palpitations and dry mouth. The formula was modified again, according to the same treatment method.

The newly modified formula contained: *Zhì huáng qí* (Radix

Astragali Praeparata cum Melle) 9g, *shēng bái zhú* (Rhizoma Atractylodis Macrocephalae) 6g, *shí hú* (Caulis Dendrobii) 9g, *dà bái sháo* (Radix Paeoniae Alba) 6g, *chǎo suān zǎo rén* (Semen Ziziphi Spinosae) 9g, *fú xiǎo mài* (Fructus Tritici Levis) 12g, baked *huáng qín* (Radix Scutellariae) 2.4g, *hòu dù zhòng* (Cortex Eucommiae) 6g, *hēi dòu* (Semen Glycines Atrum) 12g and *sāng jì shēng* (Herba Taxilli) 9g. The patient was instructed to take 6 doses.

Comments:

Cheng's usual method of calming the fetus method: *Bái zhú* (Rhizoma Atractylodis Macrocephalae), *bái sháo* (Radix Paeoniae Alba) and *huáng qín* (Radix Scutellariae) are selected as the main medicinals. *Bái zhú* (Rhizoma Atractylodis Macrocephalae) combined with *bái sháo* (Radix Paeoniae Alba) harmonizes the liver and spleen. When the liver is in harmony, it will not cause unrestrained ascent and disturbance to produce unremitting dizziness and nausea. When the spleen is harmonious, distention and fullness can be alleviated, and the appetite and thirst are normal.

Huáng qín (Radix Scutellariae) combined with *bái zhú* (Rhizoma Atractylodis Macrocephalae) harmonizes the spleen and downbears turbidity; *huáng qín* (Radix Scutellariae) paired with *bái sháo* (Radix Paeoniae Alba) soften the liver and clear heat. Our predecessors observed that "it is appropriate to use cooling method before the arrival of the fetus." Although this law is not set in stone, after conception the turbid qi descends and the heat from constraint either rises or sinks down to harass the fetal origin, which can definitely aggravate the prenatal disease. Heat cannot disturb the fetus after being subjected to the bitter flavor and the clearing and draining functions of *huáng qín* (Radix Scutellariae), which also has the ability to calm the fetus, which ties in to the statement above. Hence, it is one of the ingredients in a gynecological formula known as *Zi Qin Wan* 子芩丸. Zhu Danxi preferred using *huáng lián* (Rhizoma Coptidis) – also a bitter and draining herb – to

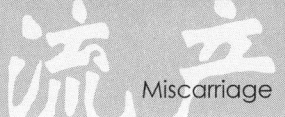

treat prenatal diseases, and would sometimes use *huáng lián* (Rhizoma Coptidis) as a single herb by itself, called *Yi Qing San* 抑青散.

If the lower back pain and downbearing sensation in the abdomen are severe, this can easily lead to a miscarriage. Cheng often uses *huáng qí* (Radix Astragali) to benefit qi and lift the fetus, and *dù zhòng* (Cortex Eucommiae) and *sāng jì shēng* (Herba Taxilli) to tonify the kidney and stabilize the fetus.

If the heart is restless, the spirit is unsettled, causing instability in the lower origin. Hence, nourishing the heart is also one approach to calming the fetus.

(*Cheng Menma's Case Studies* 程门马医案. Edited by Shanghai College of TCM. Shanghai: Shanghai Science and Technology Publishing House, 1980. 224-225)

(4) Luo Yuancai's Case Studies—Kidney Yin Insufficiency Accompanied by Deficient Heat of the Liver Channel

【Chief Complaint】 The patient did not menstruate for over 2 months. When her menstruation was delayed for more than 20 days, she was given a urine frog test (injecting a pregnant woman's urine into the dorsal lymph sac of a frog, which will either lay eggs if it is female, or produce sperm if it is male), which came back positive. On the day of her visit, she had been experiencing mild vaginal bleeding of bright red color for 5 days, accompanied by dull pain and downbearing sensation in the abdomen and slight soreness in the lower back. A year ago, the patient had already had a spontaneous abortion during the 2nd month of pregnancy. She has no children.

The patient was emaciated and often suffered dizziness and lower back soreness. She had mild pregnancy reactions and fatigue. The patient had not been getting adequate rest in the recent days. Her tongue was slightly pale with slightly red tip and margins, and her pulse was thready, slippery and slightly wiry.

【Pattern Differentiation】 Kidney yin insufficiency accompanied by deficiency heat of the liver channel and heat disturbing the penetrating and conception vessels.

【Treatment Principle】 Enrich the kidney, nourish the liver, benefit qi and calm the fetus.

【Prescription】

菟丝子	tù sī zǐ	24g	Semen Cuscutae
续断	xù duàn	12g	Radix Dipsaci
桑寄生	sāng jì shēng	12g	Herba Taxilli
阿胶	ē jiāo	12g(to be melted for decocting)	Colla Corii Asini
旱莲草	hàn lián cǎo	15g	Herba Ecliptae
女贞子	nǚ zhēn zǐ	15g	Fructus Ligustri Lucidi
白芍	bái sháo	9g	Radix Paeoniae Alba
甘草	gān cǎo	6g	Radix et Rhizoma Glycyrrhizae
荆芥炭	jīng jiè tàn	9g	Herba Schizonepetae Carbonisatum

4 bags of the formula were prescribed and the patient was given 1 bag a day. (The cooked medicinals were saved and decocted a second time.) The patient was instructed to rest in bed.

The vaginal bleeding and abdominal pain gradually disappeared after taking 3 doses of the prescription, but the lower back soreness and dry stools still remained. Then *jīng jiè tàn* (Herba Schizonepetae Carbonisatum) and *bái sháo* (Radix Paeoniae Alba) were removed from the formula, and *sāng shèn* (Fructus Mori) and *ròu cōng róng* (Herba Cistanches) were added. After taking 4 doses of the modified formula, most of the patient's symptoms disappeared, and the tongue and pulse returned to normal. *Hàn lián cǎo* (Herba Ecliptae) was then subtracted, and *huái shān yào* (Radix Dioscoreae Oppositae) added. The patient took 6 doses of the formula and continued to take 3 doses each week thereafter to consolidate the effect. The formula was discontinued in 5th month of pregnancy, and the patient eventually delivered a full-term baby boy.

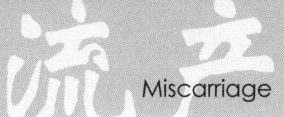

Comments:

This was a case of threatened miscarriage with restless fetus, pain and downbearing sensation in the abdomen and vaginal bleeding. The miscarriage was of the liver and kidney insufficiency pattern, manifesting as instability of the fetus, red tongue, emaciation, and a thready, slippery and slightly wiry pulse, which are all symptoms of liver and kidney yin deficiency.

It is necessary to enrich and nourish the liver and kidney yin, benefit qi and calm the fetus. Modified *Shou Tai Wan* 寿胎丸 [*tù sī zǐ* (Semen Cuscutae), *xù duàn* (Radix Dipsaci), *sāng jì shēng* (Herba Taxilli) and *ē jiāo* (Colla Corii Asini)] was used, in which *hàn lián cǎo* (Herba Ecliptae) and *nǔ zhēn zǐ* (Fructus Ligustri Lucidi) were added to benefit the liver and kidney, cool blood and stop bleeding. *Bái sháo* (Radix Paeoniae Alba) and *gān cǎo* (Radix et Rhizoma Glycyrrhizae) were added to soften and astringe the liver; *jīng jiè tàn* (Herba Schizonepetae Carbonisatum) was added to calm the fetus and stop bleeding, which alleviated the bloody stools in just one visit. However, on the second visit, her stools were still dry and hard, which required the removal of *jīng jiè tàn* (Herba Schizonepetae Carbonisatum) and *bái sháo* (Radix Paeoniae Alba) and the addition of *sāng shèn* (Fructus Mori) and *ròu cōng róng* (Herba Cistanches) to benefit kidney yin and moisten the intestines, which facilitated the recovery of right qi and the calming of the fetus. At last, the patient delivered a full-term baby.

(Tao Guangzheng: Editor-in-chief. *Selected Case Translations of Ancient and Modern Renowned Physicians* 古今名医医案选译, Beijing, Chinese Medical Publishing House of China, 1997.333)

(5) Qian Bo's Case Studies—Liver and Kidney Yin Deficiency

Gong, 28 years old. Initial visit: April 10th, 1959.

The patient had been pregnant for 6 months and had already had 3 habitual miscarriages. In the last 2 months, the patient had been experiencing irregular and remote vaginal hemorrhage of dark purplish color and moderate quantity, lumbar soreness, pain and downbearing sensation in the abdomen, normal appetite, and normal urination and bowel movement. Her tongue was pale with yellow and greasy coating which was peeled in the middle. The left pulse was thready, soft and slightly slippery; the right pulse was wiry, slippery and rapid.

【Pattern Differentiation】 Liver and kidney yin deficiency, instability of the fetus, and accumulation of heat in the stomach and intestines.

【Treatment Principle】 Nourish yin and clear heat using modified *Jiao Ai Si Wu Tang* 胶艾四物汤.

【Prescription】

干地黄	gān dì huáng	12g	Radix Rehmanniae Recens
当归	dāng guī	9g	Radix Angelicae Sinensis
白芍	bái sháo	9g	Radix Paeoniae Alba
川芎	chuān xiōng	3g	Rhizoma Chuanxiong
艾叶	ài yè	3g	Folium Artemisiae Argyi
阿胶	ē jiāo	12g (dissolve)	Colla Corii Asini
生甘草	shēng gān cǎo	3g	Radix et Rhizoma Glycyrrhizae (raw)
黄芩	huáng qín	6g	Radix Scutellariae
知母	zhī mǔ	9g	Rhizoma Anemarrhenae
藕节	ǒu jié	12g	Nodus Nelumbinis Rhizomatis

The patient was instructed to decoct and take 4 bags.

【Second Visit】 April 17th. After taking the prescribed formula, her vaginal bleeding stopped for 3 days, but she still had lumbar soreness, thin and yellow tongue coating, a slightly red tongue tip, and a thready, slippery and rapid pulse that was weak over chi position. Treatment required nourishing the liver and tonifying the kidney to stabilize the fetus.

【Prescriptiont】 *Gān dì huáng* (Radix Rehmanniae Recens) 12g, *dāng guī* (Radix Angelicae Sinensis) 9g, *bái sháo* (Radix Paeoniae Alba) 9g, *ē jiāo* (Colla Corii Asini) 12g, *shēng guī jiǎ* (Carapax et Plastrum Testudinis, raw) 15g, *xù duàn* (Radix Dipsaci) 12g, *dù zhòng* (Cortex Eucommiae)

12g, *huái shān yào* (Radix Dioscoreae Oppositae) 9g, *sāng jì shēng* (Herba Taxilli) 12g and *jú pí* (Pericarpium Citri Reticulatae) 3g. The patient was given 3 bags.

【Third Visit】 April 20th. The bleeding had stopped and the lumbar soreness was relieved. The patient had not been getting much sleep at night. She had a thin white tongue coating, and a wiry slippery pulse that was weak in the left chi position. The treatment involved nourishing and benefiting the liver and kidney to stabilize the fetus.

【Prescription】 *Gān dì huáng* (Radix Rehmanniae Recens) 12g, *dāng guī* (Radix Angelicae Sinensis) 6g, *bái sháo* (Radix Paeoniae Alba) 9g, *ē jiāo zhū* (Colla Corii Asini pearls)12g, *shēng guī jiǎ* (Carapax et Plastrum Testudinis, raw)15g, *xù duàn* (Radix Dipsaci) 12g, *dù zhòng* (Cortex Eucommiae) 9g, *huái shān yào* (Radix Dioscoreae Oppositae) 9g, *sāng jì shēng* (Herba Taxilli) 12g and *yuǎn zhì* (Radix Polygalae) 6g. The patient was given 4 bags.

Comments:

This was, without a doubt, a case of habitual miscarriage of the liver and kidney insufficiency type with instability of the fetus. During her 4th pregnancy she once again experienced dark purplish vaginal bleeding. Her tongue coating was light yellow and greasy, and her right pulse was wiry, slippery and rapid, which are symptoms of internal accumulation of heat from deficiency. The appropriate treatment principle for this case should be to enrich yin, clear heat, tonify the kidney and calm the fetus. *Jiao Ai Tang* 胶艾汤 was used to nourish blood, pacify the fetus and stop leakage (vaginal bleeding). *Huáng qín* (Radix Scutellariae) was added to clear stomach heat; *zhī mǔ* (Rhizoma Anemarrhenae) was added to clear the ministerial fire in the lower jiao; *ǒu jié* (Nodus Nelumbinis Rhizomatis) was added to cool blood and stop bleeding. After taking 4 doses the bleeding stopped. *Shou Tai Wan* 寿胎丸 and *Jiao Ai Tang* 胶艾汤 were then used together to tonify and nourish the kidney and liver, nourish blood and stabilize the fetus, which resulted in a smooth pregnancy and a full-term delivery.

(Tao Guangzheng: Editor-in-chief. *Selected Case Translations of Ancient and Modern Renowned Physicians* 古今名医医案选译, Beijing, Chinese Medical Publishing House of China, 1997.333-334)

(6) Lu Zhizheng's Case Studies—Threatened Miscarriage Due To Qi Obstruction and Phlegm Heat

Huang, female, 27 years old. Profession: doctor in a big hospital in Beijing.

Initial visit: Jan 26th, 1992.

【Chief Complaint】 The patient was pregnancy for more than 6 months until she started having lumbar soreness and dull abdominal pain, which lasted 2 months. She had not been resting well because of her busy work schedule and daily house chores. During the 4th month of pregnancy, she began having restless movement of the fetus which gave her insomnia and sometimes would wake her up with a startle in the middle of the night, accompanied by night sweats, vexation and irascibility, an upset stomach, poor appetite, sticky sensation and bland taste in the mouth, dizziness, and fatigue. In the 5th month, she started experiencing irregular uterine contractions that would last 10 seconds each time, and occurred in intervals of 10 minutes to several hours. The symptoms were alleviated after taking phenobarbital and salbutamol, but reoccurred after discontinuing the medication. This was what prompted the patient to come in for treatment. Besides the symptoms above, the patient had a superficially red face, a pale red tongue with thin greasy coating, and a slippery rapid pulse. All the symptoms were caused by heat from blood deficiency, an inability to nourish the fetus, liver constraint transforming into fire (which in turn, harasses the heart sovereign), and a disturbance of the gall bladder. Treatment therefore should include clearing heart fire, eliminating vexation, nourishing blood and calming the fetus.

【Prescription】 *Zhú rú* (Caulis Bambusae in Taenia) 15g, *zǐ sū gěng* (Caulis Perillae) 10g [add towards the end – e.g., last 10 minutes], *huáng qín* (Radix Scutellariae) 9g, *chǎo bái zhú* (Rhizoma Atractylodis Macrocephalae, stir-fried) 10g, *huáng lián* (Rhizoma Coptidis) 1.5g, *shā rén* (Fructus Amomi) 3g [add towards the end], *dān shēn* (Radix et Rhizoma Salviae Miltiorrhizae) 12g, *bái sháo* (Radix Paeoniae Alba) 15g, *chǎo zhǐ qiào* (Fructus Aurantii, stir-fried) 12g, *chǎo zǎo rén* (Semen Ziziphi Spinosae, stir-fried) 10g, *yīn chén* (Herba Artemisiae Scopariae) 10g, *yù hú dié* (Semen Oroxyli) 6g and *gān cǎo* (Radix et Rhizoma Glycyrrhizae) 3g. The patient was given 4 bags. The medicinals decocted with water for oral intake.

【Feb. 1ˢᵗ】 After taking the prescribed medicinal formula, the patient no longer had vexation, her sleep had improved, the uterine contractions were less frequent, and the superficially-red facial complexion had receded. Her tongue was pale red with a thin greasy coating, and her pulse was still slippery and rapid. Since the formula was effective, it was prescribed again with some modifications.

【Prescription】 *Zǐ sū yè* (Folium Perillae) 6g [add towards the end], *huáng lián* (Rhizoma Coptidis) 1.5g, *zhú rú* (Caulis Bambusae in Taenia) 12g, *fó shǒu* (Fructus Citri Sarcodactylis) 9g, *chǎo bái zhú* (Rhizoma Atractylodis Macrocephalae, stir-fried) 12g, *shān yào* (Rhizoma Dioscoreae) 15g, *dān shēn* (Radix et Rhizoma Salviae Miltiorrhizae) 15g, *chǎo zhǐ qiào* (Fructus Aurantii, stir-fried) 10g, *chǎo zǎo rén* (Semen Ziziphi Spinosae, stir-fried) 10g, *bái sháo* (Radix Paeoniae Alba) 15g, *shā rén* (Fructus Amomi) 4g [add towards the end], *huáng qín* (Radix Scutellariae) 9g, *gān cǎo* (Radix et Rhizoma Glycyrrhizae) 3g. The patient was given 6 bags.

【Third visit on Feb. 7ᵗʰ】 Restless movement of the fetus and uterine contractions decreased significantly after taking the prescribed formula.

The patient was advised to temporarily cease taking the formula, and to participate in outdoor activities to strengthen her constitution.

【Fourth visit on Feb. 23ʳᵈ】 In the 7ᵗʰ month of pregnancy, the patient presented with the following symptoms: fatigued limbs and mental lassitude; restless insomnia; gradual worsening of restless movement of the fetus; uterine contractions that are accompanied by abdominal pain; vexation and irascibility, nasal obstruction and itchiness of the throat; belching and acid reflux. It was diagnosed as a breech position of the fetus with signs of premature delivery. The patient was advised to stay in the hospital and receive treatment to prevent miscarriage. She had more faith in Chinese medicine after being treated with Chinese medicinals, and would like to study Chinese medicine instead of working in the hospital.

In her next visit, the patient had a red tongue with thin white coating, and a wiry slippery pulse, which were caused by insufficiency of qi and yin that resulted in an inability to nourish blood. Treatment should involve benefiting qi, nourishing yin, tonifying blood, harmonizing the ying (nutritive level), strengthening the spleen, unblocking the middle, clearing heat and calming the fetus. Also, moxibusiton should be applied at BL 67 (zhì yīn) to rectify the fetal position.

【Prescription】 *Shā rén* (Fructus Amomi) 1.5g [add near the end], *bái sháo* (Radix Paeoniae Alba) 15g, *chǎo bái zhú* (Rhizoma Atractylodis Macrocephalae, stir-fried) 12g, *huáng qín* (Radix Scutellariae) 10g, *zǐ sū gěng* (Caulis Perillae) 9g [add near the end], *zhú rú* (Caulis Bambusae in Taenia) 12g, *chǎo zhǐ qiào* (Fructus Aurantii, stir-fried) 12g, *gān cǎo* (Radix et Rhizoma Glycyrrhizae) 6g, *tài zǐ shēn* (Radix Pseudostellariae) 10g, *shā shēn* (Radix Glehniae Littoralis) 12g, *mài dōng* (Radix Ophiopogonis) 10g and *dān shēn* (Radix et Rhizoma Salviae Miltiorrhizae) 15g. The patient was prescribed 5 bags, to be decocted with water for oral intake.

【Fifth visit on Mar 15ᵗʰ】 All the discomforts were significantly alleviated after taking the above formula. The fetal movements were milder, and she experienced only occasional uterine contractions. Her breathing was smoother and she no longer had vexation and insomnia. Her appetite and energy level were improved. She had a red tongue with thin white coating, and a wiry and slightly slippery pulse. She was prescribed another 10 bags of the previous formula.

【Sixth visit on Mar 28th】: After taking 10 bags of the formula and receiving moxibusiton at BL 67 (zhì yīn), all of the symptoms improved. She slept well, and had a good appetite and unobstructed bowel movement and urination. Obstetric examination revealed that the fetus had returned to a normal position. The treatment principle for this visit was to benefit qi, nourish blood, clear heat, calm the fetus, regulate the penetrating and conception vessels, strengthen the spleen and harmonize the middle.

【Prescription】 *Tài zǐ shēn* (Radix Pseudostellariae) 12g, *mài dōng* (Radix Ophiopogonis) 10g, *dān shēn* (Radix et Rhizoma Salviae Miltiorrhizae) 15g, *chǎo bái zhú* (Rhizoma Atractylodis Macrocephalae, stir-fried) 12g, *chǎo bái sháo* (Radix Paeoniae Alba, stir-fried) 15g, *dāng guī* (Radix Angelicae Sinensis) 9g, *huáng qín* (Radix Scutellariae) 10g, *shā rén* (Fructus Amomi) 2g [add near the end], *chǎo zhǐ shí* (Fructus Aurantii Immaturus, stir-fried) 12g, *chǎo zǎo rén* (Semen Ziziphi Spinosae, stir-fried) 10g, *gān cǎo* (Radix et Rhizoma Glycyrrhizae) 6g, *zǐ sū yè* (Folium Perillae) 6g [add near the end]. 6 bags were prescribed.

The patient delivered a full term baby boy, and both the mother and the baby were in good health. The baby weighed 3kg at birth, with a strong cry and good appetite. He weighed 4.2kg when he was 30 days old, and 9.5kg at 6 months with good reflexes and a strong constitution.

Comments:

The patient was pregnant at the age of nearly 28 (when kidney qi is abundant). During the pregnancy, the patient had symptoms of qi and blood disharmony, qi obstruction and blood heat, reckless movement of hot blood, and threatened miscarriage (vaginal bleeding). Interior excess of yang qi, and liver constraint transforming into fire and harassing the heart spirit (mind) can cause vexation, insomnia and waking in the middle of the night from fright. Heat scorches the yin fluids and leads to the internal generation of deficiency heat, which causes deficiency vexation and night sweats. Qi obstruction and blood heat causes blockages in the channels and impaired flow of water and fluids. The heat accumulates and generates phlegm, which leads to uncontrolled ascending and descending. As a result, there may be poor appetite, stomach upset, stickiness and bland taste in the mouth, dizziness and fatigue. The greasy tongue coating and slippery rapid pulse were symptoms of qi obstruction and phlegm heat in the middle jiao, which was treated using the methods of clearing heat, transforming phlegm, nourishing blood and calming the fetus.

The formula used was a modified combination of *Zhi Qiao Tang* 枳壳汤, *Zhu Ru Wen Dan Tang* 竹茹温胆汤 and *Qin Zhu Tang* 芩术汤. The chief medicinals of this formula include *zhú rú* (Caulis Bambusae in Taenia), *yīn chén* (Herba Artemisiae Scopariae), *huáng lián* (Rhizoma Coptidis) and *huáng qín* (Radix Scutellariae), which clear heat, transform phlegm, warm the gall bladder and calm the heart. The deputies appointed are *bái zhú* (Rhizoma Atractylodis Macrocephalae) and *shā rén* (Fructus Amomi) to strengthen the spleen and harmonize the stomach, *zhǐ qiào* (Fructus Aurantii) to promote qi flow and free stagnation, and *yù hú dié* (Semen Oroxyli) to course the liver and remove constraint. The assistants, *dān shēn* (Radix et Rhizoma Salviae Miltiorrhizae), *bái sháo* (Radix Paeoniae Alba) and *chǎo zǎo rén* (Semen Ziziphi Spinosae, stir-fried), nourish blood, harmonize ying, calm the spirit and eliminated vexation. *Gān cǎo* (Radix et Rhizoma Glycyrrhizae), as the envoy, harmonizes all the medicinals.

The formula was created on the basis of Hejian and Danxi's theory that "it is suitable to clear heat before delivery", but it is not confined to medicinals such as *huáng qín* (Radix Scutellariae) and *bái zhú* (Rhizoma Atractylodis Macrocephalae). The effects of regulating qi without injuring yin and nourishing without causing obstruction can be achieved by transforming phlegm and clearing heat, assisted by regulating qi and nourishing blood. One can also use a small dosage of *shā rén* (Fructus Amomi), which is acrid and warm, as an opposing assistant to promote qi flow and awaken the spleen to eliminate obstruction, calm the fetus and alleviate pain. Danxi said: "pregnancy is like a bell hung on a beam; the bell will fall down if the beam is soft." *Bái zhú* (Rhizoma Atractylodis Macrocephalae) can be likened to a mother who supports and fosters, *huáng qín* (Radix Scutellariae) stabilizes the middle qi to drain fire, and nourishes yin to control ministerial fire. The fetus is naturally calmed when its harmful factors are removed.

All the symptoms were alleviated on the 2nd visit, which is attributed to the removal of gall bladder heat, thus *yīn chén* (Herba Artemisiae Scopariae) was removed from the formula. The fire from constraint had been eliminated, so *yù hú dié* (Semen Oroxyli) was also removed. The qi dynamic was no longer obstructed, hence *zǐ sū gěng* (Caulis Perillae) was replaced with *Su Ye Huang Lian Tang* 苏叶黄连汤 to stop vomiting and eliminate vexation. *Bái zhú* (Rhizoma Atractylodis Macrocephalae) strengthens the spleen to stabilize the penetrating vessel; *shān yào* (Rhizoma Dioscoreae) enriches spleen yin to harmonize ying; *fó shǒu* (Fructus Citri Sarcodactylis) courses stagnation and protects yin to prevent obstruction and stagnation. *Bái sháo* (Radix Paeoniae Alba) and *gān cǎo* (Radix et Rhizoma Glycyrrhizae) can be used together in large dosages (*Shao Yao Gan Cao Tang* 芍药甘草汤) to retain yin, harmonize ying, relieve spasms, alleviate pain and calm the fetus.

The patient was pregnant for more than 7 months during her 3rd to

5th visits. The fetus was gradually growing and developing, consuming the mother's qi for nourishment; this resulted in fetal excess and maternal deficiency, giving rise to restless stirring of the fetus, abnormal fetal position and the tendency for premature delivery. *Mai Men Dong Tang* 麦门冬汤 was selected, based on Wu Zhiwang's <*Ji Yin Gang Mu*> 济阴纲目 (written in the Ming Dynasty), which recorded its usage to treat " restless fetus that starts in the 6th month of pregnancy … panic, sudden vaginal bleeding and pains similar to labor." *Tài zǐ shēn* (Radix Pseudostellariae), *shā shēn* (Radix Glehniae Littoralis), *mài dōng* (Radix Ophiopogonis) and *dān shēn* (Radix et Rhizoma Salviae Miltiorrhizae) benefit qi and nourish yin to clear deficiency heat, accompanied by *shā rén* (Fructus Amomi) to stabilize the penetrating vessel, and *zǐ sū yè* (Folium Perillae) and *zhǐ shí* (Fructus Aurantii Immaturus) to regulate qi, calm fetus and alleviate pain. Once the bleeding stopped, the fetus was able to be nourished. Both the mother and the fetus were safe and sound after the treatment.

By the 6th visit, all the symptoms were improved, and the fetus returned to its normal position. The next treatment step included benefiting qi, nourishing blood, regulating the penetrating and conception vessels to consolidate the therapeutic effect. The mother eventually carried the pregnancy to full term and gave birth to a healthy baby.

(Deng Tietao. *The Fifth Set of Stone Collection* <*Bian Shi Ji Di Wu Ji*> 碥石集 第五集. Guangzhou: People's Publishing House of Guangdong, 2003. 67-70).

3. Discussions

(1) Li Dingming's Pattern Differentiation and Treatment of Threatened Miscarriage:

A. Etiology

Threatened miscarriage is a biomedical disease name. However, in ancient Chinese medical classics, it was referred to as "restless fetus", "fetal bleeding", "fetal spotting", "fetal obstruction", "bleeding during pregnancy", and "abdominal pain during pregnancy", which all belong to the category of threatened miscarriage. Chinese medicine divides the pathogenesis into maternal causes and fetal causes, as recorded in Jiu Yin's <Jing Xiao Chan Bao> 经效产宝 (Tang Dynasty): "There are two methods for calming the fetus: for restless fetus due to maternal disease, just treat the disease of the mother and the fetus will naturally be at peace; if the mother's health is affected by a restless and unsubstantial fetus, just treat the disease of the fetus and the mother's ailment will be alleviated. This principle is too effective to disobey." The concrete cause of miscarriage may be spleen and kidney insufficiency, depletion of qi and blood, deficiency and impairment of the penetrating and conception vessels, or injury due to the seven emotions. Clinical experience concludes that Chinese medical treatment is highly effective for threatened miscarriage due to maternal disease; but treatment of threatened miscarriage due to fetal disease (e.g., undeveloped fetus) with Chinese medicine has not been very successful.

B. Pathomechanism

The causes of threatened miscarriage are mentioned a lot in Chinese medicine, but the major ones are qi and blood deficiency, spleen and kidney insufficiency, liver constraint and qi stagnation, blood heat due to yin deficiency, and injuries due to accidents. It can be understood from clinical experience that insufficiency of the spleen and kidney plays an important role, since the spleen is the root of acquired constitution and the source of transformation. If spleen qi is deficient, the spleen is unable to transport and transform the essence of water and grain to produce blood, which causes deficiency of the penetrating and conception vessels, and fetal malnourishment during pregnancy. The kidney is the root of congenital constitution, and is connected to the uterus. Its function includes the storing of essence. Also, since the kidney channel is interconnected with the penetrating and conception vessels, kidney qi will lack the strength to stabilize the uterus if it is exhausted by immoderate sexual intercourse and excessive and indulgent emotions. The transformation and transportation of the spleen and kidney directly influences the waxing and waning of the body's essential qi and vessels, and its reproductive function. Therefore, insufficiency of the spleen and kidney is considered as one of the basic causes of threatened miscarriage.

Another factor of threatened miscarriage is blood heat due to yin deficiency, and heat disturbing the penetrating and conception vessels, causing the blood to move sporadically and the fetus to be malnourished. Fire can easily burn out of control if the source of water is insufficient; it is easy for blood to flow recklessly if there is excessive heat. These conditions are what cause restless fetus and threatened miscarriage. Blood heat due to yin deficiency has a negative effect on the development of the fetus. When we encounter pregnant women in clinical practice, always advise them not to eat acrid, hot and dry foods, especially those who normally have yin deficiency and fire excess constitutions, or those that prefer acrid and hot food in their diet. Abstinence of sexual intercourse is also very important, since miscarriage is more likely to occur if kidney qi is exhausted, which is often the case with sexual intercourse during pregnancy or excessive sexual activity.

C. Clinical Pulse and Syndrome

Although there are various causes of threatened miscarriage, and symptoms vary from person to person, it usually manifests as mild, paroxysmal and sagging pain in the lower abdomen, soreness in the lower back and knees, mild or severe vaginal bleeding that aggravates the pain in the lower back and knees, and daily worsening of the condition. Most cases are accompanied by nausea, vomiting, no appetite, mental lassitude and fatigued limbs. The pulse is usually thready, slippery and rapid or thready and wiry, which is especially pronounced over both chi regions. The slippery pulse indicates pregnancy; the thready and rapid pulse is the manifestation of water depletion and blood insufficiency; the rapid pulse represents the stirring of fire; the slippery and rapid pulse over both chi regions represents heat accumulation in the lower burner.

D. Treatment

Three principles of the usage of medicinals:

a) Aside from adopting different measures according to different pathogeneses, the key to treatment is clearing heat, nourishing yin, strengthening the spleen and benefiting the kidney.

b) Adopt the principle of treating the root and branch simultaneously. Generally speaking, if threatened miscarriage can be treated on time, the prognosis can be quite positive. However, due to the urgency of this condition, excellent results can be achieved by the simultaneous application of medicinals that stopping bleeding, relieve spasms, alleviate pain, strengthen the spleen, benefit the kidney, nourish yin, and clear heat.

c) In the past, some physicians concluded 3 principles of the use of medicinals during the prenatal period, namely clearing heat, nourishing yin, regulating the spleen and coursing qi, assisted by other medicines according to specific conditions. There are a variety of medicinals that clear heat with strong or weak functions, hence selecting the proper medicinals and making effective combinations are very important. *Huáng qín* (Radix Scutellariae), which is considered one of the best herbs to clear fetal heat and protect the fetus, also anchors liver yang to pacify the fetus. This herb was honored as the "sacred herb for calming the fetus" by Zhu Danxi. Modern medical analysis concludes that *huáng qín* (Radix Scutellariae) sedates the excitatory effect of the central nervous system on the cerebral cortex, and successfully prevent miscarriage. In clinical practice, we have encountered patients who voluntarily take *Bao Tai Wan* 保胎丸 or prevent miscarriage during the prenatal period. Although they took these preventative measures on their own, they often end up coming to see the doctor for incessant vaginal bleeding and unremitting lumbar and abdominal pain. Miscarriage can be prevented by taking *huáng qín* (Radix Scutellariae) and other medicinals that nourish yin and clear heat, in combination with medicinals that smooth qi, strengthen the spleen, relieve spasms and alleviate pain. *Shān yào* (Rhizoma Dioscoreae), *bái zhú* (Rhizoma Atractylodis Macrocephalae), *chén pí* (Pericarpium Citri Reticulatae), *bǎi biǎn dòu* (Semen Lablab Album) and other Chinese medicinals that regulate the spleen and course qi allow the spleen to restore its function of transformation and transportation; if the spleen is healthy, qi is produced with ease. Smoothing qi unblocks the qi dynamic and harmonizes qi and blood. Regulating the spleen and smoothing qi is also one of the main methods of preventing miscarriage. In particular, *bái zhú* (Rhizoma Atractylodis Macrocephalae) can strengthen the spleen and disperse phlegm. *Bái zhú* (Rhizoma Atractylodis Macrocephalae) and *huáng qín* (Radix Scutellariae) are considered essential herbs for calming the fetus. Use *bái zhú* (Rhizoma Atractylodis Macrocephalae) for spleen deficiency and *huáng qín* (Radix Scutellariae) for blood heat. If the deficiency of the spleen is mild, replace *bái zhú* (Rhizoma Atractylodis Macrocephalae) with *shēng huái shān yào* (Rhizoma Dioscoreae, raw). *Shēng huái shān yào* (Rhizoma Dioscoreae, raw) can strengthen the spleen and tonify the kidney with its sweet flavor and neutral property, without the disadvantage of *bái zhú* (Rhizoma Atractylodis Macrocephalae)'s warm and drying nature.

Besides the commonly used fetus-protecting medicinals mentioned above, it is also necessary to use medicinals that relieve spasms, alleviate pain and stop bleeding. Persistent bleeding and gradual worsening of abdominal pain will affect the fetus and eventually cause a miscarriage. It is crucial that we use blood-stanching, spasm-relieving and pain-killing medicinals under these circumstances. According to the principle of "treating the branch in acute conditions", it is imperative to use hemostatic medicinals such as *ē jiāo* (Colla Corii Asini), *zhù má gēn* (Radix Boehmeriae Ramie), *dì yú tàn* (Radix Sanguisorbae Carbonisatus), *cè bǎi tàn* (Cacumen Platycladi Carbonisatus) and *zōng tàn* (Petiolus Trachycarpi Carbonisatus), and spasm-relieving analgesics such as *bái sháo* (Radix Paeoniae Alba).

Ē jiāo (Colla Corii Asini) enriches kidney yin, nourishes blood, stops bleeding and calms the fetus; *zhù má gēn* (Radix Boehmeriae Ramie) clears the heat of the anterior yin to stop bleeding. These two medicinals are the primary choices for stanching bleeding and calming the fetus.

The above summarizes the usage of medicinals that treat yin deficiency with blood heat syndrome.

For spleen deficiency and insufficiency of qi and blood, we primarily use *Gui Pi Tang* 归脾汤 to strengthen the spleen, benefit qi and calm the fetus. Since clinical manifestations may differ from patient to patient, the formula can be modified accordingly. For immoderation of the seven emotions, medicinals that smooth qi and resolve constraint are required; for traumatic injuries, blood-invigorating and stasis-transforming medicinals are added.

In short, only by mastering the principles and seizing the key points while taking all factors into account can one succeed in preventing a miscarriage.

(*The Compiled Experience of Senior Renowned Physicians of TCM* 名中医经验汇编 Compiled by a committee of editors. Beijing: Beijing Publishing House, 1994. 396-398)

(2) Wang Mengyin advocates:

- **Identifying patterns and determining treatment in the prenatal period**
    - **Treating the disease is calming the fetus**
    - **Forcing the expulsion of the dead fetus**

In *Pathogenesis of Diseases Occurring in the Prenatal Period* 胎前病源论, Shen Xiaofeng divided obstetric disease into 3 main phenomena: "The first is yin depletion. Given the fact that the human body's essence and blood are limited, and that they are required to nourish the fetus, yin depletion is inevitable. The second is qi stagnation; the presence of the fetus in the abdomen acts as a physical barrier that disrupts the ascent and descent of the qi dynamic. The third is phlegm rheum; the normal functions of the zang-fu organs are disturbed by the sudden appearance of a physical mass (the embryo) in the abdomen, giving rise to fluid stagnation (phlegm rheum)." Mengying added, "As for the pathogenesis of obstetric disease, yin deficiency and qi stagnation have already been recognized by others before, but phlegm rheum is considered a new discovery. Shen was the only one who pointed out the key reason behind postpartum delirium." As for nourishing the fetus, he advocates "monthly monitoring of the fetus and maintaining its normal healthy state.

There are the following: premature delivery, post-term birth and early or late delivery, all of which are not necessarily considered pathological conditions. Only premature babies that are not fully developed or extremely small full-term newborns, both of which are caused by maternal qi deficiency, are thought of as pathological. In these cases, patients' health should be regulated and reinforced before getting pregnant again, so that her constitution will be strong and ready." For prenatal conditions, close observation and careful diagnosis is required, and treatment should be based on pattern identification.

The dead fetus should be expelled immediately. There are different causes of fetal death in utero: blood not nourishing fetus, fever harming the fetus, stasis and stagnation, and other factors. How to tell if the fetus has died in the womb? Mengying cited that a red face with a blue tongue, lack of fetal movement, and no labor even after the due date are all signs of intrauterine death. Physicians in ancient times, such as Yu Jiayang for instance, used *Xie Bai San* 泻白散 with the addition of *huáng qín* (Radix Scutellariae) and *jié gěng* (Radix Platycodonis) to expel the dead fetus. Mengying uses a method derived from personal experience, which was oral administration of *dān shēn* (Radix et Rhizoma Salviae Miltiorrhizae) as a single herb for a period of 20 days, to discharge the dead fetus. Modified *Tiao Wei Cheng Qi Tang* 调胃承气汤 is also applicable. Overall, the usage of formulas and medicinals should be flexible, not limited to the theories and applications of a single school of thought.

Treating disease is calming the fetus: Mengying explains that "if fetal instability is caused by a deficiency of original qi, it is then appropriate to tonify right qi; if it is caused by the invasion of pathogenic qi, it is then suitable to treat the disease." As for fetus-calming medicinals, appoint *zhú rú* (Caulis Bambusae in Taenia), *sāng yè* (Folium Mori) and *sī guā luò* (Retinervus Luffae Fructus) as the chief medicinals, assisted by other medicinals according to the different syndromes, which are applicable to all patients with blood deficiency and fire excess. Also, the usage of *huáng qín* (Radix Scutellariae) is only appropriate if there is blood heat. As for the fetal sedation effect of *chuān xù duàn* (Radix Dipsaci) and *dù zhòng* (Cortex Eucommiae), Mengying proposed that "*chuān xù duàn* (Radix Dipsaci) is not applicable in cases of qi sinkage and qi weakness. If infertility is caused by kidney qi lacking warmth with coagulation and stagnation of menstrual blood, use the two medicinals to warm qi and moisten blood; then there will be no more stagnation or spotting, and the fetus will naturally be calm." In short, it has been recognized that treating disease is calming the fetus.

(Shen Xiesun. *The Essence of Wang Mengying's Medical Works* 王孟英医
著精华. Shanghai: Shanghai Science & Technology Press, 1992. 87-88.)

(3) Mao Meirong proposes that the treatment of habitual miscarriage should emphasize nourishing blood while tonifying the spleen and kidney:

Habitual miscarriage of the deficiency type is commonly seen in
clinical practice. For this, "tonifying the deficiency to consolidate and
protect the fetus" is emphasized. I have tried using *Tai Shan Pan Shi San*
泰山磐石散, which originates from *The Complete Works of Jing Yue <Jing
Yue Quan Shu>* 景岳全书 as the basic formula whenever I encountered this
pattern. Use *dǎng shēn* (Radix Codonopsis), *huáng qí* (Radix Astragali),
xù duàn (Radix Dipsaci), *huáng qín* (Radix Scutellariae), *dāng guī* (Radix
Angelicae Sinensis), *shú dì huáng* (Radix Rehmanniae Praeparata), *chuān
xiōng* (Rhizoma Chuanxiong), *bái sháo* (Radix Paeoniae Alba), *bái zhú*
(Rhizoma Atractylodis Macrocephalae), *zhì gān cǎo* (Radix et Rhizoma
Glycyrrhizae Praeparata cum Melle) and *shā rén* (Fructus Amomi) with
necessary modifications. For restless fetus with a tendency to sink and
vaginal bleeding, remove *dāng guī* (Radix Angelicae Sinensis) and *chuān
xiōng* (Rhizoma Chuanxiong), and add *ē jiāo* (Colla Corii Asini), *nǚ zhēn
zǐ* (Fructus Ligustri Lucidi) and *hàn lián cǎo* (Herba Ecliptae) to nourish
blood, stanch bleeding and calm the fetus. For lumbar soreness with a
sagging sensation in the abdomen, add *tù sī zǐ* (Semen Cuscutae), *sāng
jì shēng* (Herba Taxilli) to consolidate the kidney and calm the fetus. For
dizziness, dry mouth, bitter taste in the mouth, and a wiry slippery pulse,
replace *huáng qí* (Radix Astragali), *dǎng shēn* (Radix Codonopsis), *dāng
guī* (Radix Angelicae Sinensis) and *chuān xiōng* (Rhizoma Chuanxiong)
with *shēng dì huáng* (Radix Rehmanniae Recens), *xuán shēn* (Radix
Scrophulariae) and *mài dōng* (Radix Ophiopogonis) to nourish yin, clear
heat and calm the fetus. If prescribed for the correct pattern, this formula
and its modifications should produce quick and satisfactory results.

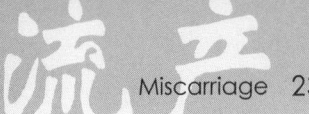

Furthermore, mastery of the key points listed below is crucial in the treatment of miscarriage.

The first is tonfiying qi and benefiting blood using *dǎng shēn* (Radix Codonopsis) *tài zǐ shēn* (Radix Pseudostellariae) and *huáng qí* (Radix Astragali) in large dosages to make the middle qi sufficient, the girdling vessel stable, and the fetus tranquil; benefiting blood allows the fetus to be adequately nourished, and this is achieved through the usage of *shú dì huáng* (Radix Rehmanniae Praeparata), *ē jiāo* (Colla Corii Asini), *bái sháo* (Radix Paeoniae Alba) and *gǒu qǐ zǐ* (Fructus Lycii).

The second key is tonifying the kidney and strengthening the spleen to consolidate the root of the fetus; the fetus can be secured if kidney qi is sufficient. The spleen is the source of production and transformation, and the nourishment of the fetus depends upon the spleen and stomach. The spleen and stomach are like the beam to which a bell is tied; the bell will fall down if the beam is soft. If spleen qi is sufficient, the source will be abundant and unobstructed, and the fetus can then be nourished. Medicinals such as *bái zhú* (Rhizoma Atractylodis Macrocephalae), *huái shān yào* (Rhizoma Dioscoreae), *tù sī zǐ* (Semen Cuscutae), *xù duàn* (Radix Dipsaci) and *dù zhòng* (Cortex Eucommiae) can be selected according to different conditions.

The third key point is that both the consumption and the stirring of blood are most feared in cases of habitual miscarriage. Therefore, herbs like *dāng guī* (Radix Angelicae Sinensis) and *chuān xiōng* (Rhizoma Chuanxiong) should be used cautiously to avoid disturbing the fetus.

The fourth point is nourishing while moving. Refrain from improper nourishment and drainage to avoid impairing the qi dynamic. The more severe the fetal distention is, the greater the chance of miscarriage. Medicinals that regulate qi and calm the fetus should be added when nourishing and benefiting qi and blood; for instance, use *shā rén* (Fructus Amomi), *zǐ sū gěng* (Caulis Perillae).

(Song Zujing. *The Pattern Differentiation and Treatment of Renowned Physicans of the Modern Era* 当代名医证治荟萃. Shijiazhuang: Hebei Science & Technology Press, 1990. 606-607)

(4) Ban Xiuwen believes that regulating the spleen and kidney before pregnancy and calming the fetus after pregnancy should be emphasized in the treatment of habitual miscarriage:

Generally speaking, there are different causes of habitual miscarriage, including spleen and kidney qi deficiency, blood heat stirring fire, and external trauma. Of these, spleen and kidney qi deficiency is the most commonly seen pattern in clinical practice.

In treatment, there are two steps that are required besides pattern differentiation and treatment: the first step is administering treatment before pregnancy, with consolidation of the kidney as the treatment focus; the second step is the prevention of miscarriage during pregnancy, and treating the disease early if it should occur.

The so-called "administering treatment before pregnancy, with consolidation of the kidney as the treatment focus" refers to emphasizing the regulation of kidney qi before the patient gets pregnant. The general pathomechanism of recurrent miscarriage is instability of the penetrating and conception vessels, or failure of the kidney to hold; therefore, attention must be paid to regulating qi and blood, warming and nourishing the penetrating and conception vessels, with focus on strengthening the kidney to stabilize and protect its root and stem. In general, rotate the use of *Ren Shen Yang Rong Tang* 人参养容汤 with the addition of *tù sī zǐ* (Semen Cuscutae), *lù jiǎo shuāng* (Cornu Cervi Degelatinatum), *fù pén zǐ* (Fructus Rubi); and *Wu Zi Yan Zong Wan* 五子衍宗丸 with *chē qián zǐ* (Semen Plantaginis) removed and medicinals like *xù duàn* (Radix Dipsaci), *dù zhòng* (Cortex Eucommiae) and *sāng jì shēng* (Herba Taxilli) added.

Pregnancy can be achieved after half a year to one year of treatment and healthcare. During pregnancy, proper medical treatment should be given according to the woman's constitution, in order to prevent miscarriage ahead of time. *Tiao Gan Tang* 调肝汤 with the addition of medicinals such as *tù sī zǐ* (Semen Cuscutae), *fù pén zǐ* (Fructus Rubi), *sāng jì shēng* (Herba Taxilli), *dù zhòng* (Cortex Eucommiae) and *xù duàn* (Radix Dipsaci) to tonify the kidney and nourish the liver is preferred; use modified *Tai Shan Pan Shi San* 泰山磐石散 to regulate qi and blood. If the congenital and acquired constitutions are nourished simultaneously, qi and blood will be harmonized and the fetus can be nourished. Most patients carry the pregnancy to full term under these conditions.

If there is restless fetus and threatened miscarriage, it is necessary to treat the branch and root concurrently, not only by regulating qi and calming the fetus, but also by strengthening the kidney and stanching bleeding. For vexing heat and dry throat due to blood heat, and threatened miscarriage with mild vaginal bleeding, use *Liang Di Tang* 两地汤 to nourish yin and clear heat, which treats the root; add medicinals like *hé yè dì* (Folium Nelumbinis Basis Hindu), *zhù má gēn* (Radix Boehmeriae Ramie) and *hàn lián cǎo* (Herba Ecliptae), which treat the branch; as a result, yin will be sufficient, the heat will be cleared, and the fetus will be pacified.

When selecting formulas for restless fetus caused by external trauma and injuries (e.g., carrying heavy loads, falls, tumbles) with blood stasis and damage to the uterine vessels, attention should be paid to nourishing qi and transforming stasis without harming the fetus. Modified *Dang Gui Bu Xue Tang* 当归补血汤 is commonly used, which not only tonifies qi and produces blood, but also promotes qi flow and invigorates blood. Add medicinals like *sāng jì shēng* (Herba Taxilli), *tù sī zǐ* (Semen Cuscutae), *xù duàn* (Radix Dipsaci), *dù zhòng* (Cortex Eucommiae) and *gǔ suì bǔ* (Rhizoma Drynariae) to relax the tendons, strengthen the lumbus, tonify the kidney; the stasis will be dispersed and the fetus will be secured.

Besides receiving medical treatment, patients should establish a balance between work and rest to keep qi and blood harmonious and maintain a pleasant state of mind. Reduce or abstain from sexual intercourse to avoid damaging the penetrating and conception vessels and causing the stirring of internal fire which can harass the fetus. Regulate and control the diet, which should include sweet, bland and nutritious foods that are not fatty, rich nor greasy; in particular, patients whose constitutions are prone to dryness or dampness should pay extra attention to their diet.

(Song Zujing. *The Pattern Differentiation and Treatment of Renowned Physicans of the Modern Era* 当代名医证治荟萃. Shijiazhuang: Hebei Science & Technology Press, 1990. 604)

(5) Luo Yuancai treats habitual miscarriage by administering treatment before delivery and strengthening the kidney after delivery:

In ancient times, recurrent miscarriage that occurs 3 or more times was referred to as repeated miscarriage; frequent pregnancy followed by frequent miscarriage is called habitual miscarriage in modern medicine. There are many causes of miscarriage: from congenital factors to acquired factors such as overstrain, immoderate sexual intercourse, frequent D&C and external trauma. The consumption and impairment of blood and qi can be caused by excessive miscarriages that lead to the instability of the penetrating and conception vessels, and inability of the kidney to hold. Therefore, most miscarriage patients have weak constitutions, which often lead to menstrual disorders accompanied by dizziness, lower back soreness, fatigue, lassitude, dark circles around the eyes, a pale enlarged tongue, and a weak thready or wiry thready pulse that is weakest over the chi position.

For the prevention and treatment of this disease, the patient's health must be built up before attempting to get pregnant again, which will strengthen the constitution and prevent another miscarriage. It is imperative that the patient does not conceive for a whole year after the last miscarriage, which gives the patient a chance to rest and recover her energy while building up her constitution with medicinals. When the patient is pregnant again, she should practice abstinence from all sexual activity and take measures to calm the fetus to ensure the therapeutic effect of treatment.

Tonification of the kidney is stressed in the treatment and prevention of miscarriage. The kidney stores essence, dominates reproduction, and is linked with the uterine collaterals; kidney qi carries the fetus. The major cause of habitual miscarriage is instability of kidney qi and failure of the kidney to hold and store, thus resulting in frequent pregnancy followed by frequent miscarriage. Because of this, there is a saying: "pregnancy can be achieved naturally if the kidney is vigorous." However, the enrichment of the kidney qi is dependant upon nourishment by essential qi which is derived from the water and grain absorbed by the spleen and stomach; therefore, tonification of the kidney must be assisted by strengthening the spleen and benefiting qi.

The health of women depends primarily on blood; menstruation, pregnancy, childbirth and breastmilk all requires blood. This explains why nourishing blood is just as important as tonifying the kidney and strengthening the spleen. If qi and blood of the spleen and kidney are abundant and the constitution is strong, the fetus will flourish and develop normally.

"*Bu Shen Gu Chong Wan* 补肾固冲丸" is composed of *tù sī zǐ* (Semen Cuscutae), *xù duàn* (Radix Dipsaci), *ē jiāo* (Colla Corii Asini), *shú dì huáng* (Radix Rehmanniae Praeparata), *lù jiǎo jiāo* (Colla Cornus Cervi), *bái zhú* (Rhizoma Atractylodis Macrocephalae), *rén shēn* (Radix et Rhizoma Ginseng), *dù zhòng* (Cortex Eucommiae), *gǒu qǐ zǐ* (Fructus Lycii), *bā jǐ tiān* (Radix Morindae Officinalis), *dāng guī* (Radix Angelicae Sinensis), *shā rén* (Fructus Amomi) and *dà zǎo* (Fructus Jujubae). It is made into small pills with honey, and taken in 6g doses, 2 times a day. 3 months is a course of treatment; it can be taken for 1-3 courses with temporary interruption during menstruation.

When the patient is pregnant again, she should rest as much as possible, avoid things and situations that bring her anxiety, and be given medicinals that calm the fetus. The pills mentioned above are still appropriate to take; however, if some pregnant women feel dry and hot, prescribe *Shou Tai Wan* 寿胎丸 combined with *Si Jun Zi Tang* 四君子汤, modified by adding *hé shǒu wū* (Radix Polygoni Multiflori). If there is no sign of threatened miscarriage, take 1 dose every other day until the 3rd month of pregnancy.

Some frequent miscarriages are caused by unhealthy embryos, as in the following cases: consanguineous marriage, if either of the couple have genetic diseases, or if the embryo has congenital defects. In these situations, the common medicinals that calm the fetus will have no effect. Consequently, when treating patients of habitual miscarriage, more examinations are required to arrive at an accurate diagnosis.

(Song Zujing. *The Pattern Differentiation and Treatment of Renowned Physicans of the Modern Era* 当代名医证治荟萃. Shijiazhuang: Hebei Science & Technology Press, 1990. 605-606)

(6) Xia Guicheng treats habitual miscarriage by restoring communication between the heart and kidney:

It is written in *Fu Qing zhu's Gynecology* <Fu Qing Zhu Nv Ke> 傅青主女科 that the uterus is the place where heart and kidney communicate, so the focal point of the disease is disharmony between heart and kidney. Kidney deficiency, in particular, is the precondition; thus tonifying the kidney is the primary focus of treatment. *Shou Tai Wan* 寿胎丸 is the established formula for tonifying the kidney and calming the fetus, of which *tù sī zǐ* (Semen Cuscutae), *sāng jì shēng* (Herba Taxilli) and *dù zhòng* (Cortex Eucommiae) are the most essential medicinals. Since habitual miscarriage possesses the characteristics of falling and sagging, it is necessary to add or use large dosages of medicinals that tonify qi and stem desertion, such as *huáng qí* (Radix Astragali), *dǎng shēn* (Radix Codonopsis), *bái zhú* (Rhizoma Atractylodis Macrocephalae) and *zhù má gēn* (Radix Boehmeriae Ramie) to reinforce the effect of tonifying the kidney and stemming desertion.

A clinical empirical formula—*Niu Bi Bao Tai Wan* 牛鼻保胎丸 – was recorded in Concise TCM Genecology <*Jian Ming Zhong Yi Fu Ke Xue*> 简明中医妇科学 for "restless movement of the fetus." However, in order to tonify the kidney, the heart must be calmed. It is said in *Careful Study of Lost Ancient Works* <*Shen Zhai Yi Shu*> 慎斋遗书 that: "If tonification of the heart is desired, it is necessary to solidify the kidney to allow its energy to ascend; if tonification of the kidney is desired, it is necessary to tranquilize the heart to allow its energy to descend." When the heart is tranquil, the kidney is solidified, the essence is sufficient, and the uterus can store and hold." The common approaches to calming the heart are clearing fire, calming the spirit, and dredging. Clearing fire and calming the heart while tonifying the kidney and stabilizing the fetus is a method often used in patients with heat in the upper region and cold in the lower region of the body. In this situation, we should warm and tonify the kidney and spleen to secure the fetus, and clear both heart and liver heat to stabilize the spirit. Use *Shou Tai Wan* 寿胎丸 or *Niu Bi Bao Tai Wan* 牛鼻保胎丸 with the addition of *gōu téng* (Ramulus Uncariae Cum Uncis), *chǎo huáng lián* (Rhizoma Coptidis, stir-fried) and *lián zǐ xīn* (Plumula Nelumbinis).

Beware of the effect that the heat-clearing and heart-calming medicinals have on the both the fetus and the deficiency cold of the spleen and kidney. For instance, in cases of cold in the lower body, it is necessary to add *shā rén* (Fructus Amomi), *ài yè* (Folium Artemisiae Argyi) and *páo jiāng* (Rhizoma Zingiberis Praeparatum). When trying to calm the spirit while tonifying the kidney, the medicinals that mainly target insomnia and poor sleep are *chǎo suān zǎo rén* (Semen Ziziphi Spinosae), *wǔ wèi zǐ* (Fructus Schisandrae Chinensis), *hé huān pí* (Cortex Albiziae), *fú shén* (Sclerotium Poriae Cocos Paradicis) and *bǎi zǐ rén* (Semen Platycladi). In severe cases, add *qīng lóng chǐ* (Dens Draconis), *mǔ lì* (Concha Ostreae) and *guī jiǎ* (Carapax et Plastrum Testudinis), which will restore the communication between the heart and the kidney. "Dredging stagnation to tranquilize the heart" refers to the use of spiritual counseling to enlighten the patient, in an attempt to eliminate mental stress and resolve psycho-emotional issues. After receiving such counseling, the patient's heart and spirit will be at ease, the essence is stabilized, and the kidney will be consolidated. For patients of habitual miscarriage - especially those who are anxiously looking forward to having a baby, or those who are emotionally weak – this is of great significance. If there is restlessness, one must follow the principle of treating the branch when there is acute disease; first calm the heart and spirit, and in addition to spiritual counseling, use *Sheng Mai San* 生脉散 with the addition of *chǎo suān zǎo rén* (Semen Ziziphi Spinosae, stir-fried), *qīng lóng chǐ* (Dens Draconis), *hé huān pí* (Cortex Albiziae), *gōu téng* (Ramulus Uncariae Cum Uncis), *bái sháo* (Radix Paeoniae Alba), *lǜ è méi* (Flos Pruni Mume) and *zhù má gēn* (Radix Boehmeriae Ramie), and advise the patient to take sleeping pills. After the spirit is calmed, switch to tonifying the kidney and stabilizing the fetus.

(Song Zujing. *The Pattern Differentiation and Treatment of Renowned Physicans of the Modern Era* 当代名医证治荟萃. Shijiazhuang: Hebei Science & Technology Press, 1990. 607-608)

(7) Shan Zhiqun selects fetus-calming medicinals based on pattern identification:

Patients of threatened miscarriage and restless fetus are often very sensitive to medicinals. Extreme caution must be exercised when prescribing formulas for these patients.

The first step in calming the fetus is to stanch bleeding. For qi deficiency, select medicinals such as *huáng qí* (Radix Astragali) and *rén shēn* (Radix et Rhizoma Ginseng) to benefit qi and control blood; for blood cold, select *ài yè tàn* (Folium Artemisiae Argyi Carbonisatus), *páo jiāng tàn* (Rhizoma Zingiberis Praeparatum, carbonized) to warm the channels and stop bleeding; for blood heat, select *dì yú* (Radix Sanguisorbae), *cè bǎi tàn* (Cacumen Platycladi Carbonisatus) and *lián fáng tàn* (Receptaculum Nelumbinis Carbonisatus) to cool blood and stop bleeding. In addition, *shēng dì huáng* (Radix Rehmanniae Recens) has the ability to tonify and move blood. Since it becomes thick and gooey when processed, use it in large dosages to take advantage of its sticky and cloying nature, which can stop bleeding rapidly in patients who are qi and blood deficient. Meanwhile, select medicinals that enter the extraordinary vessels as well. *Lù jiǎo jiāo* (Colla Cornus Cervi) tonifies the governing vessel and has an astringent property; *ē jiāo* (Colla Corii Asini) tonifies the penetrating vessel and has an anchoring effect; and *jīng jiè tàn* (Herba Schizonepetae Carbonisatum) has the effect of guiding blood to flow within the vessels. Using the medicinals together produces stronger therapeutic effects.

The ancient physicians dubbed *huáng qín* (Radix Scutellariae) and *bái zhú* (Rhizoma Atractylodis Macrocephalae) "sacred medicinals for calming the fetus", which is suspected to be an overstatement. *Huáng qín* (Radix Scutellariae) is bitter and cold, and is suitable for patients who have blood heat with restless fetus. Zhang Zhengshi, a physician who lived during the Qing Dynasty, said: "*Huáng qín* (Radix Scutellariae) is appropriate for restless fetus in emaciated patients with blood heat and overflow of nutritive blood causing ascent of the fetus; for patients who are large but have weak qi and frequent sagging of the fetus, only *rén shēn* (Radix et Rhizoma Ginseng) can lift this; for large patients with qi excess, only *mù xiāng* (Radix Aucklandiae) and *shā rén* (Fructus Amomi) can consume the excess and restore tranquility; for hyperactivity of fire due to blood deficiency with abdominal pain, only *sháo yào* (Radix Paeoniae) can nourish and restore peace; for obese patients with phlegm abundance leading to unremitting vomiting and regurgitation, only *chén pí* (Pericarpium Citri Reticulatae) can promote qi flow and resolve the problem. All of these herbs treat the imbalance of maternal qi." Zhang's comparison of *huáng qín* (Radix Scutellariae) to other medicinals shows that the application of medicinals should be direct. Wang Mengying uses *huáng qín* (Radix Scutellariae) to calm the fetus; it is also commonly used for patterns of excess heat. For deficient blood with fire, *zhú rú* (Caulis Bambusae in Taenia), *sāng yè* (Folium Mori) and *sī guā luò* (Retinervus Luffae Fructus) are the main medicinals selected. Wang adds: "All three medicinals can nourish blood and clear heat to extinguish internal wind. For instability of the fetus due to liver deficiency, this combination is better than *Si Wu E Jiao Tang* 四物阿胶汤."

Bái zhú (Rhizoma Atractylodis Macrocephalae) is sweet, bitter and warm. Its sweet flavor can strengthen the spleen and benefit qi; its bitter flavor can dry dampness. There is no damp pathogen if the spleen is fortified, and the fetus is secured if qi is sufficient. Fu Qingzhu used *bái zhú* (Rhizoma Atractylodis Macrocephalae) to calm the fetus; he believed that this herb has the effect of benefiting the qi of the waist and the navel. The girdling vessel, which is controlled by the spleen, encircles the waist; *bái zhú* (Rhizoma Atractylodis Macrocephalae) can strengthen the spleen and benefit qi to allow the qi between the waist and the navel to flow smoothly without damp pathogen, thus calming the fetus. Since *bái zhú* (Rhizoma Atractylodis Macrocephalae) is, after all, a warm and drying herb, so for patients with yin deficiency, it can be replaced with *huái Shān yào* (Rhizoma Dioscoreae Oppositae), *bǎi biǎn dòu* (Semen Lablab Album) and *shí lián* (Semen Nelumbinis). For qi deficiency that manifests as abdominal pain and sagging and dry and hard stools, use a large dose of *bái zhú* (Rhizoma Atractylodis Macrocephalae), which has the effect of benefiting qi and unblocking the stools.

Finally, the nourishment and growth of the fetus in the womb is dependant upon the stability of qi. For sinking due to qi deficiency, *shēng má* (Rhizoma Cimicifugae) and *chái hú* (Radix Bupleuri) are often used to raise and lift, but the dosage should not be excessive, so as to avoid the rising and scattering of fetal qi. Although *ài yè tàn* (Folium Artemisiae Argyi Carbonisatus) can stop bleeding, its property is warm; therefore its usage should be discontinued as soon as the bleeding has stopped. *Dāng guī* (Radix Angelicae Sinensis) is an acrid, sweet and warm herb, and is considered a yang blood-nourishing herb; it has the disadvantage of moving blood and assisting heat, so it should be used with caution. For stagnation of fetal qi, select medicinals such as *shā rén* (Fructus Amomi), *chén pí* (Pericarpium Citri Reticulatae) and *mù xiāng* (Radix Aucklandiae) to regulate qi. Pay careful attention to the dosage and the combination of medicinals to regulate qi without harming the fetus and consuming yin. When using tonics, try to use those that niether cause stagnation nor assist the transformation of heat into fire. Meanwhile, do not forget to tonify the deficiency of the spleen and stomach.

(Sun Jifen. *Medical Maxims of the Yellow River* <Huang He Yi Hua> 黄河医话. Beijing: Beijing Science & Technology Press, 1994. 374-375)

(8) Shen Jinao recorded how threatened miscarriage and restless fetus were treated by ancient physicians:

A. Restless Fetus

Chen Ziming: If healthcare during pregnancy is well-managed, qi and blood will be in harmony, the fetus will be nourished, and the delivery will be smooth; otherwise the fetus will be disturbed, qi will ascend and delivery will be difficult, which can be a very dangerous situation. If a frightened fetus is close to full-term and the spirit of the fetus is already solidified, a traumatic injury (falling, tumbling, etc.) can damage the fetus and cause the mother to have vaginal bleeding and loss of consciousness. If one wants to check whether the mother and the fetus are safe, give her *Dang Shen Tai Dong Bu An Fang* 当参胎动不安方. Select *Gou Teng Tang* 钩藤汤, *Zi Su Yin* 紫苏饮, *Gui Pi Tang* 归脾汤 and *Fo Shou San* 佛手散 according to pattern differentiation. If fetal restlessness is severe, it will inevitably lead to a miscarriage. If there is a red face with a blue tongue, this means that the fetus is dead; if there is a blue face with a red tongue, this indicates that the mother is dead; if there is a blue mouth with foaming at the sides, both the mother and the fetus are dead.

Yan Yonghe: If restless fetus occurs in the 2ⁿᵈ or 3ʳᵈ month of pregnancy, it is due to long-term deficiency of the uterus, and can easily induce a miscarriage. For this condition, take *Du Zhong Wan* 杜仲丸 in advance to nourish the fetus. If there is restless fetus with abdominal pain, this can easily turn into to a threatened miscarriage, for which *Ru Sheng Tang* 如圣汤 is indicated. He also said that if the patient has palpitations, fearful waking during sleep, hypochondriac expansion and swelling, abdominal fullness with acute pain over the umbilical region, inability to sit or lie down peacefully, short and labored breathing, this is due to qi oppression; or if there is falling and screaming which frighten the fetus, and injury of the tendons and bones which causes restlessness of the four limbs, *Da Shen San* 大圣散 should be taken immediately.

Zhu Zhengheng: If the postpartum mother has fire stirring the fetus and causing upward counterflow that results in rapid panting, immediately prescribe *huáng qín* (Radix Scutellariae) and *xiāng fù* (Rhizoma Cyperi) in powdered form. If threatened miscarriage is due to qi deficiency with heat, take *Si Wu Tang* 四物汤 in combination with *ē jiāo* (Colla Corii Asini), *bái zhú* (Rhizoma Atractylodis Macrocephalae), *huáng qín* (Radix Scutellariae), *xiāng fù* (Rhizoma Cyperi), *shā rén* (Fructus Amomi), and *nuò mǐ* (glutinous rice).

Li Chan: If restless fetus is caused by qi counterflow due to excess of

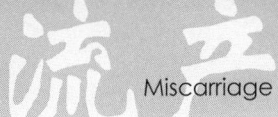

the seven emotions, take *Zi Su Yin* 紫苏饮; if there is an external invasion manifesting as headaches, vomiting, and hypochondriac distention and fullness, prescribe *An Tai Yin* 安胎饮 with the addition of *chái hú* (Radix Bupleuri) and *dà fù pí* (Pericarpium Arecae). For qi and blood deficiency, prescribe *An Tai Yin* 安胎饮 with double the dosage of *rén shēn* (Radix et Rhizoma Ginseng) and *bái zhú* (Rhizoma Atractylodis Macrocephalae).

For vaginal bleeding, take *Jiao Ai Xiong Gui Tang* 胶艾芎归汤 with *shā rén* (Fructus Amomi), *qín jiāo* (Radix Gentianae Macrophyllae), *huáng bǎi* (Cortex Phellodendri Chinensis) and *dù zhòng* (Cortex Eucommiae).

For unbearable abdominal pain with vaginal bleeding, or with yellow discharge that is like oil paint and bean milk, decoct 5 qian each of *yě zhù gēn* (Radix Boehmeriae Ramie, wild) and *jīn yín huā* (Flos Lonicerae Japonicae) with wine. For bleeding with vaginal pain, take 1 qian of *huáng lián* (Rhizoma Coptidis) powder with wine.

For restless fetus with abdominal pain due to cold, take *Li Zhong Tang* 理中汤 combined with *shā rén* (Fructus Amomi) and *xiāng fù* (Rhizoma Cyperi); for restless fetus with abdominal pain due to heat, take *Huang Qin Tang* 黄芩汤.

For abdominal pain due to blood deficiency, take *Si Wu Tang* 四物汤, or decoct *Ping Wei San* 平胃散 with salt and take it with *Er Yi Wan* 二宜丸.

For pain due to qi deficiency, take *Si Jun Zi Tang* 四君子汤 with the addition of *bái sháo* (Radix Paeoniae Alba) and *dāng guī* (Radix Angelicae Sinensis). For distending pain in the stomach and abdomen due to qi excess, take *xiāng fù* (Rhizoma Cyperi) and *zhǐ qiào* (Fructus Aurantii) in powdered form.

For restless fetus with heart pain due to cold, decoct equal dosages of *ài yè* (Folium Artemisiae Argyi), *xiǎo huí xiāng* (Fructus Foeniculi) and *chuān liàn zǐ* (Fructus Toosendan); for restless fetus with heart pain due to heat, take *Er Chen Tang* 二陈汤, replacing *bàn xià* (Rhizoma Pinelliae) with *shān zhī zǐ* (Fructus Gardeniae) and *huáng qín* (Radix Scutellariae).

The ancient formula *Qin Zhu Tang* 芩术汤 with the addition of *ē jiāo* (Colla Corii Asini) is commonly used to treat restless fetus. For wind pathogen, add *shēng jiāng* (Rhizoma Zingiberis Recens) and *dòu chǐ* (Semen Sojae Praeparatum); for cold, add *cōng bái* (Bulbus Allii Fistulosi); for heat, add *huā fěn* (Radix Trichosanthis); for alternating cold and heat, add *chái hú* (Radix Bupleuri); for neck stiffness, add *gé gēn* (Radix Puerariae Lobatae); for warmth and heat in the abdomen with pain, add *bái sháo* (Radix Paeoniae Alba); for abdominal distention, add *hòu pò* (Cortex Magnoliae Officinalis); for vaginal bleeding, add *ài yè* (Folium Artemisiae Argyi) and *dì yú* (Radix Sanguisorbae); for lower back pain, add *dù zhòng* (Cortex Eucommiae); for fright palpitations, add *huáng lián* (Rhizoma Coptidis); for vexation and thirst, add *mài dōng* (Radix Ophiopogonis) and *wū méi* (Fructus Mume); for excessive thinking and anxiety, add *fú shén* (Sclerotium Poriae Cocos Paradicis); for vomiting of phlegm, add *xuán fù huā* (Flos Inulae) and *bèi mǔ* (Bulbus Fritillaria), or consider using *bàn xià qū* (Rhizoma Pinelliae Fermentata); for exhaustion due to excessive physical labor, add *huáng qí* (Radix Astragali); for asthma, replace *bái zhú* (Rhizoma Atractylodis Macrocephalae) with *xiāng fù* (Rhizoma Cyperi); for constipation, add *huǒ má rén* (Semen Cannibis); for habitual difficult labor, add *zhǐ qiào* (Fructus Aurantii) and *zǐ sū yè* (Folium Perillae); for habitual miscarriage, add *dù zhòng* (Cortex Eucommiae); for blood deficiency, add *chuān xiōng* (Rhizoma Chuanxiong) and *dāng guī* (Radix Angelicae Sinensis); these are the most effective medicinals for calming the fetus. For extreme and urgent cases, take 3 to 5 doses a day; for mild cases, take 1 dose every 5 to 10 days. If taken regularly, this formula can calm the fetus and facilitate delivery. As a result, the newborn will be healthy and without fetal toxins.

B. Threatened Miscarriage

Li Chan: Vaginal bleeding with heart and abdominal pain indicates fetal restlessness; vaginal bleeding without heart and abdominal pain indicates a threatened miscarriage. That is the difference between the two conditions. Most threatened miscarriages are caused by heat, hence the bleeding is profuse. For internal heat with thirst, take *Si Wu Tang* 四物汤 with *huáng qín* (Radix Scutellariae), *huáng lián* (Rhizoma Coptidis), *bái zhú* (Rhizoma Atractylodis Macrocephalae) and *yì mǔ cǎo* (Herba Leonuri); for bleeding with dark clots, take *San Bu Wan* 三补丸 combined with *xiāng fù* (Rhizoma Cyperi) and *bái sháo* (Radix Paeoniae Alba); for blood deficiency with scanty bleeding, take *Jiao Ai Tang* 胶艾汤, or combined with *Si Wu Tang* 四物汤; for qi deficiency, take *Si Jun Zi Tang* 四君子汤 with the addition of *huáng qín* (Radix Scutellariae) and *ē jiāo* (Colla Corii Asini); for qi deficiency with vaginal bleeding and sagging sensation due to excessive physical labor and exposure to cold, take *Xiong Gui Bu Zhong Tang* 芎归补中汤; for monthly bleeding (like that of menstruation) that dries up the uterus and harms both the mother and the fetus, prescribe 2 qian each of *chǎo shú dì huáng* (Radix Rehmanniae Praeparata, stir-fried) and *gān jiāng* (Rhizoma Zingiberis) in powdered form, to be taken with porridge.

Vaginal bleeding only during sexual intercourse is a sign of a real threatened miscarriage; rescue the patient with *Ba Wu Tang* 八物汤 combined with *ē jiāo* (Colla Corii Asini) and *ài yè* (Folium Artemisiae Argyi).

(Shen Jinao. *Shen's Classic of Honoring Life* 沈氏尊生书. Beijing: Chinese Medical Publishing House of China, 1997 [first written in the Qing Dynasty]. 874-875)

(9) Lu Zhengzhi treats threatened miscarriage and restless fetus based on pattern differentiation:

A. Liver and Kidney Insufficiency, Instability of the Penetrating and Conception Vessels

"If there is occasional menstrual bleeding several months into the pregnancy, it is caused by deficiency of the penetrating and conception vessels which are unable to control the blood of the greater yin and the lesser yin channels." The kidney is the root of congenital constitution. In men, this refers to the storage of semen; in women, this refers to the fastening of the uterus. The liver stores blood, and therefore plays an important role in the adulthood of women. The conception vessel originates from the uterus and is attached to the liver and kidney. These two organs – the liver and the kidney – have a mother-child relationship; when the kidney is full, the liver flourishes and the penetrating and conception vessels are in harmony, which results in a healthy mother and baby. If there is insufficiency of the liver and kidney and disharmony between the penetrating and conception vessels, both the mother and the fetus will be harmed and illness will occur. As was explained in *Treatise on the Causes and Symptoms of All Diseases • Spotting During Pregnancy <Zhu Bing Yuan Hou Lun • Ren Shen Lou Bao>* 诸病源候论·妊娠漏胞候, "there will be leakage from the uterus if qi of the penetrating and conception vessels are deficient". In *The Complete Works of Jingyue <Jing Yue Quan Shu>* 景岳全书, it is said that, "if maternal qi is weak, the zang organs will not be able to cope, and there will be spotting."

B. Spleen and Stomach Weakness

The spleen and stomach are the roots of acquired constitution and the sources of production and transformation. If appetite and digestion are good, both qi and blood are vigorous, the sea of blood is full, and both the mother and baby are healthy. If the mother eats too much spicy, rich and greasy foods, or indulges in cold and raw foods, her spleen and stomach will be impaired, and she will suffer from poor appetite and slow digestion; and since production and transformation is disrupted, deficient qi is unable to carry the fetus and deficient blood cannot nourish the fetus. If the mother takes excessively warm tonics or eats foods that are harmful, her yin will be burned up and her fluids will be consumed. Yin deficiency with interior heat forces the blood to move

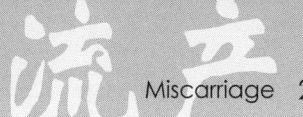

recklessly, which can cause threatened miscarriage, fetal restlessness, or spontaneous abortion.

C. Indisposition of the body and mind, emotional disharmony

In women, the liver is considered the congenital constitution. Pregnancy is the period when a woman's physiology goes through special changes. The liver as a physical organ is yin, but utilizes yang; its blood converges in the penetrating and conception vessel to nourish the fetus. As a result, not only is liver yin easily depleted in the process, but liver qi easily ascends, thus blood is easily consumed and damaged. This manifests in excessive thinking and worry, vexation and insomnia, irritability and irascibility (which can invade the spleen and stomach), nausea, dizziness, and disharmony of the mind and body. If this condition is not treated or if it is mistreated, the health of the mother and child can be affected.

Zhu Danxi said, "If qi and blood are in harmony, there is no disease; when there is anxiety, anger, sorrow and depression, and all kinds of diseases appear." Therefore, various diseases arise from constraint. For women, especially during pregnancy, more attention should be paid to cultivating the body and mind, molding one's temperament, and broadening the mind, which will not only benefit the mother, but also benefit prenatal education (as a result of the mother's good thoughts and actions).

D. Overstrain

It was mentioned in *Treatise on the Causes and Symptoms of All Diseases* <*Zhu Bing Yuan Hou Lun*> 诸病源候论 that fetal restlessness is often caused by "excessive physical labor", and that "because of damage from exhaustion, the channels are deficient and wind cold will take the opportunity to invade the body, resulting in lower back pain." It was further elaborated in <*Jing Xiao Chan Bao*> 经效产宝 that if after 8 or 9 months of pregnancy, there is restless fetus, fatigue upon physical exertion, heart and abdominal pain, blue facial complexion and eyes, cold sweat, and faint breathing that is verging on expiry, this is caused by physical overstrain frightening the fetus. Cheng Ziming of the Song Dynasty wrote in *Compendium of Effective Formulae for Gynecological Diseases* <*Fu Ren Liang Feng Da Quan*> 妇人良方大全 that, "excessive physical exertion harms the health." All of the above are in agreement that excessive physical labor during pregnancy is an important cause of fetal restlessness and premature delivery. In the Southern and Northern dynasties, Xu Zhicai pointed out in his method of "nourishing fetus in ten months" that moderate exercise combined with a proper balance between work and rest during pregnancy is beneficial for the development of the fetus, and is necessary for a smooth delivery.

Pattern differentiation and treatment summarizes that although threatened miscarriage and restless fetus are two separate diseases, their etiology and pathomechanism are basically identical. They are both caused by liver and kidney insufficiency, instability of the penetrating and conception vessels resulting in the inability to control the blood and nourish the fetus. Their treatments are similar, but there are also some slight differences. In pattern differentiation and treatment, aside from applying the four examinations and the eight principles, one should first find out how many times the patient has been pregnant. In addition, find out if the patient has ever had an abortion, if she has any long-term illnesses, the number of past threatened miscarriages with spotting and the duration of these conditions, and determine whether there is cold, heat, deficiency or excess.

If the spotting during threatened miscarriage is of darkish pale color similar to that of black bean milk, and is accompanied by lower back soreness, weakness of the knees, dizziness and tinnitus, then the condition is due to liver and kidney insufficiency; treatment involves tonifying the liver and kidney, regulating the penetrating and conception vessels, while benefiting qi and strengthening the spleen to provide a source of transformation.

If the color of the spotting is dark red, accompanied by a red face, irritability, yellow urine, constipation, and a rapid slippery pulse, then this indicates excess heat; treatment requires clearing heat, cooling blood, stanching bleeding and calming the fetus.

If the spotting is of bright red color, and is accompanied by vexing heat in the five hearts, dryness of the mouth with no desire to drink, insomnia with profuse dreaming, and a thready slippery pulse, this indicates yin deficiency with blood heat; treat by nourishing yin, clearing heat, stanching bleeding and calming the fetus.

If the patient has a yang deficiency constitution manifesting as fear of cold and lack of warmth in the uterine vessels after getting pregnant, treat with *Gui Zhi Fu Ling Wan* 桂枝茯苓丸 with the addition of *tài zǐ shēn* (Radix Pseudostellariae) and *shēng huáng qi* (Radix Astragali, raw). Use this formula with caution to avoid excessive invigoration of blood, and discontinue its usage when the majority of pathogens have been eliminated.

During middle or late pregnancy, if there is sudden profuse bleeding (similar to flooding), pale facial complexion, sweating with cold limbs and a faint pulse verging on expiry, prescribe *Du Shen Tang* 独参汤 plus *Shen Fu Tang* 参附汤 (orally or via injection) and send the patient to the hospital immediately.

For fetal restlessness that is caused by constitutional kidney deficiency, exhaustion and immoderate sexual intercourse after pregnancy, resulting in vaginal bleeding, soreness and weakness of the lower back and knees, sagging sensation in the lower abdomen, poor appetite and digestion, fatigued limbs, frequent night urination, and a deep, weak, thready and slippery pulse that is forceless over the chi region, treat this condition by benefiting qi, tonifying the kidney, and stabilizing and controlling the penetrating and conception vessels.

In patients with constitutional weakness with insufficiency of qi and blood, symptoms include vaginal bleeding; sagging sensation, distention or dull pain in the lower abdomen; mental lassitude; a pale tongue with thin coating; and a thready weak pulse that lacks force. Treatment requires strengthening the spleen and benefiting qi to provide a source of transformation to produce blood; when there is an ample supply of blood, the patient will acquire nourishment and tranquility.

If the patient has constitutional yang deficiency, she will have preference for spicy and nourishing foods during pregnancy. If the five minds (five expressions of emotions) transform into fire, sudden violent anger will impair the liver to cause intense liver fire and scorch the uterine collaterals. The excess heat from this intense liver fire combined with the excessive consumption of spicy foods can induce vaginal bleeding of bright red color and profuse quantity, accompanied by lower abdominal pain, dry mouth and tongue, reddish urine and hard stools, a red tongue with yellow coating, and a slippery and rapid pulse. This condition should be treated by clearing heat, cooling blood, stanching bleeding and calming the fetus.

Patients with restless fetus due to yin deficiency and blood heat are quite common; they should be treated by nourishing yin and blood and calming the fetus. As for patients who suffered accidental tumbles, falls, contusions and other external injuries, they need to be sent to the hospital for appropriate examination and treatment.

On the whole, "calming the fetus before delivery" and assuring the safety of both mother and infant are the most important aspects of treatment.

When calming the fetus, the first step is to "nourish blood and smooth qi", using *E Jiao San* 阿胶散, which is *Si Wu Tang* 四物汤 plus *ē jiāo* (Colla Corii Asini), *ài yè* (Folium Artemisiae Argyi), *huáng qí* (Radix Astragali) and *gān cǎo* (Radix et Rhizoma Glycyrrhizae). "Smoothing qi" refers to regulating the qi dynamic, which aims to resolve the pathological convergence of blood during pregnancy in order to nourish the fetus, and to remove the stagnation of zang qi (*see Effective Formulae of Renzhai House <Ren Zhai Zhi Zhi Fang>* 仁斋直指方: "Smoothing qi should come before calming the fetus"). The second step is to "clear heat and nourish blood during the prenatal period." Zhu Danxi said in *Discussion of the Study of Natural Phenomena, "Discussion of Spontaneous Abortion" <Ge Zhi Yu Lun, Tai Zi Duo Lun>* 格致余论, 胎自堕论 that "most miscarriages are caused by interior heat and deficiency."

Liu Wansu observed that during pregnancy, blood is deficient and nutritive and defensive qi are stagnant. Expecting mothers should often take medicinals that nourish the fluids, moisten dryness and allow blood to flourish, such as *dāng guī* (Radix Angelicae Sinensis), *chuān xiōng* (Rhizoma Chuanxiong), *shēng dì huáng* (Radix Rehmanniae Recens) and *huáng qín* (Radix Scutellariae); and medicinals that free binds and unblock stagnation, such as *bái zhú* (Rhizoma Atractylodis Macrocephalae) and *zhǐ qiào* (Fructus Aurantii). In clinical practice, I often use the observations of Danxi, Hejian and Fushan to guide me in pattern differentiation and treatment; however, there are always variations due to the uniqueness of each case, especially in the application of medicinals.

(Deng Tietao. *Bian Stone Collection, No. 5 <Bian Shi Ji Di Wu Ji>* 碥石集第五集. Guangzhou: People's Publishing House of Guangdong, 2003.67-70)

PERSPECTIVES OF INTEGRATIVE MEDICINE

1. Challenges and Solutions

Threatened miscarriage (especially habitual miscarriage) is an intractable disease, although it is recognized early and there is an abundance of clinical experience in the treatment of this disease. There are many challenges faced when treating this condition because of its recurring nature and uncertain etiology. To patients and their families, recurring miscarriages bring much despair and suffering. Therefore, problems relating to the prevention and treatment of this condition with integrative medicine become pressing challenges that are in dire need of solutions.

Challenge #1: How to Prevent Miscarriage

The causes of miscarriage are complicated, and may involve both the mother and the fetus. Maternal factors include external injury, history of other disease, medication, and other causes; hence all these possible causes should be eliminated or resolved before proceeding with treatment.

A) Eliminating the causes:

Some pregnant women have symptoms of threatened miscarriage because of poor diet and an unhealthy lifestyle. Advise patients to avoid heavy exercise and external injury during pregnancy and to abstain from sexual intercourse during the first 3 months of pregnancy. Patients of habitual miscarriage should avoid sexual intercourse throughout the entire pregnancy; do not knead or press on the lower abdomen so as to avoid inducing uterine contractions that could cause a miscarriage. Eat foods that are nutritious, and make sure the diet contains enough proteins and vitamins without abusing excessively nourishing medicinals like *rén shēn* (Radix et Rhizoma Ginseng) and *lù róng* (Cornu Cervi Pantotrichum), or drastic medicinals like *yì yǐ rén* (Semen Coicis) and *dà huáng* (Radix et Rhizoma Rhei). For women with histories of habitual miscarriage, check the following: ovarian function, the chromosomes of the couple, blood type, and the husband's sperm. Also, test to see if either of the couple has Mediterranean anemia. Women need to get a detailed examination of the genital tract (including testing for infections of special causative organisms such as chlamydia and mycoplasma) as well as examinations for uterine cancer and intrauterine adhesions. In

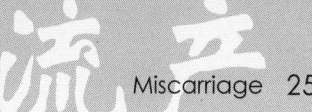

addition, a hysterosalpingography can detect whether or not there are uterine diseases or malformation, and examine the patient for dilation of the cervical os. After identifying the causes, the patient should receive treatment preferably before attempting pregnancy. For patients with corpus luteum dysfunction, hyperthyroidism, hypothyroidism, antisperm antibodies, or autoimmune HLA-related diseases, take regulatory measures in advance to prevent miscarriage.

B) Administer Treatment before Pregnancy:

Patients should not conceive for half a year to one year after a miscarriage, and should receive Chinese medicinal treatment to restore their health gradually. Whether or not the patient has received the relevant examinations mentioned above, keep track of the BBT to monitor ovarian function.

Kidney tonification with Chinese medicinals should be employed under the guidance of pattern differentiation. Tonify kidney yang or nourish kidney yin according to the patient's constitution. Use medicinals according to the appropriate stage of the menstrual cycle; during early ovulation, add *yù jīn* (Radix Curcumae) and *dān shēn* (Radix et Rhizoma Salviae Miltiorrhizae) to move qi and invigorate blood to promote ovulation; during late ovulation, use *yín yáng huò* (Herba Epimedii), *huái Shān yào* (Rhizoma Dioscoreae) and *lù jiǎo shuāng* (Cornu Cervi Degelatinatum) to regulate the function of the corpus luteum. According to Chinese medical theory, the mechanism of fastening the fetus lies primarily in the stability and control of the penetrating and conception vessels. The penetrating vessel is the sea of blood, while the conception vessel governs the uterine vessels; the root of the penetrating and conception vessels is the kidney. Maintaining the vigor of kidney qi and guaranteeing the abundance of qi and blood is an important step in ensuring normal fetal development and preventing miscarriage. Since the replenishment and nourishment of kidney cannot be achieved overnight, patients of habitual miscarriage (with the exception of those with chromosomal abnormalities, uterine malformations and other untreatable factors, or if both couples have Mediterranean anemia) should be treated for a period of time in advance before attempting to conceive, in order to ensure a smooth pregnancy.

Challenge #2: How to Ensure a Smooth Pregnancy

Repeated miscarriages can cause many problems for the patient as well as her family. Ensuring a smooth pregnancy is a common concern shared by the patient, her family members, and her healthcare providers.

A) Calm the fetus as soon as the patient has conceived: For women with histories of miscarriage, the basal body temperature (BBT) should be recorded regularly before the patient plans the next pregnancy. It's very possible that the patient is pregnant if the peak temperature phase lasts over 18 days. At this time, advise the patient to get more bed rest, to abstain from sexual intercourse, and to exercise caution while engaging in daily activities. Do not take drastic substances such as *yì yǐ rén* (Semen Coicis) and *dà huáng* (Radix et Rhizoma Rhei) to avoid a miscarriage; meanwhile, perform routine ultrasounds to monitor fetal development.

B) Provide active treatment to patients of threatened miscarriage: Vaginal bleeding, abdominal pain and lumbar soreness occurring during pregnancy are signs of a threatened miscarriage. Treatment must be provided immediately; if the situation permits, it is best for the patient to be in the hospital while receiving treatment. Tonification of the kidney is the primary treatment principle. Use large dosages of *tù sī zǐ* (Semen Cuscutae), *sāng jì shēng* (Herba Taxilli), *xù duàn* (Radix Dipsaci), *dù zhòng* (Cortex Eucommiae) and *ē jiāo* (Colla Corii Asini). For tendency towards yang deficiency, add *ài yè* (Folium Artemisiae Argyi), *lù jiǎo shuāng* (Cornu Cervi Degelatinatum), *dǎng shēn* (Radix Codonopsis) and *bái zhú*

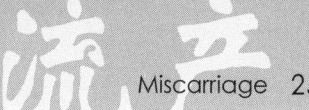

(Rhizoma Atractylodis Macrocephalae); for tendency towards heat, add *nǚ zhēn zǐ* (Fructus Ligustri Lucidi) and *huáng qín* (Radix Scutellariae). If necessary, administer intramuscular injections of 2000Iu of HCG (every other day) and 20mg of progesterone (daily). If there are paroxysmal uterine contractions, administer oral progesterone with salbutamol 2.4mg q8h to relieve them. For mental stress, give the patient phenobarbital and provide psychological counseling. In addition, routine ultrasounds are required to monitor fetal development.

Challenge #3: How to Determine Whether the Pregnancy Is Still Intact and How to Deal With a Dead Fetus

A) Judge precisely: If there is still incessant dripping of vaginal blood after treatment and the color of the blood is dark red, this means that the fetus will not develop well. Perform quantitative analysis of urine HCG and monitor HCG levels; if levels are lower than the standard norm for that week of pregnancy, this indicates that fetal development is poor. Additionally, an ultrasound may further assist in determining an accurate diagnosis, but a detailed analysis combining the patient's menstrual cycle with the time of ovulation before this pregnancy is also required. If conception occurred during late ovulation, the gestational week of the fetus can be estimated by subtracting the ovulation day from the number of weeks since her last menstrual period. If the patient is unable to provide the accurate ovulation day, the situation should be approached with caution; it is recommended that the patient receives ultrasounds regularly to monitor the growth and development of the fetus.

B) If the fetus is dead, it will drop down: Perform D&C if fetal death has been confirmed or if the patient has increased vaginal bleeding accompanied by expulsion of matter from the uterus. Most dead fetuses adhere to the uterine wall, so the operation must be performed carefully and thoroughly. The Chinese medical pattern commonly seen after operation is blood stasis obstructing the uterus. This can be treated with formulas that invigorate blood, transform stasis and engender fresh blood; modified *Sheng Hua Tang* 生化汤 is the main formula for this condition. If heat signs are pronounced, remove *páo jiāng* (Rhizoma Zingiberis Praeparatum) and *chuān xiōng* (Rhizoma Chuanxiong) to avoid excessive warming and drying. Studies show that *yì mǔ cǎo* (Herba Leonuri) and *zhǐ qiào* (Fructus Aurantii) speed up involution of the uterus (shrinking of the uterus to its pre-pregnancy size), so they can be used in large dosages to transform stasis and engender new blood. Take measures to prevent post-surgical infection.

2. Insight from Empirical Wisdom

Miscarriage is categorized as threatened miscarriage, habitual miscarriage, inevitable miscarriage, complete miscarriage and missed abortion. The fetuses of the first two patterns can be calmed; the fetuses of the latter four patterns cannot be calmed. Miscarriage occurring before the 12th completed week of gestation is called early miscarriage, and that occurring between the 12th and 28th week is called late miscarriage; early miscarriage is more commonly seen in clinical practice. Since the development of obstetric and neonatal monitoring techniques in recent years, it has been established that miscarriage is pregnancy that terminates before the 20th completed week of gestation. Some miscarriages belong to natural selection and decrease the incidence of congenital malformation. However, some fetuses are normal, and can be rescued successively by treatments that calm the fetus. Therefore, for fetuses that can be calmed, one should give immediate treatment; for the fetuses that cannot be calmed, terminate the pregnancy as soon as possible.

(1) Most Threatened Miscarriage and Habitual Miscarriages are Attributed to Kidney Deficiency

"For calming the fetus, ancient physicians and even modern

physicians advocate applying different treatments according to different patterns, as mentioned in *The Complete Works of Jingyue <Jingyue Quanshu>* 景岳全书 by Zhang Jiebin in the Ming Dynasty: "For restless fetus, give different treatments because its root and branch are different. Some of the causes of restless fetus are the same, such as deficiency or excess, cold or heat, all of which can affect fetal qi; eliminating the causes is calming the fetus." In Chinese medicine, we consider the kidney as the root of congenital constitution, which stores the essence, governs reproduction and fastens the uterine vessels. If kidney qi is vigorous, *tian gui* arrives on time, the penetrating and conception vessels are unblocked and sufficient, and menstruation is regular. If kidney qi is sufficient, the fetus can be secured; if the kidney qi is vigorous, it can carry the fetus; if blood is abundant, the fetus can be nourished and calmed. Fetal restlessness can easily occur if the patient has a weak constitution, deficient kidney qi and instability of the penetrating and conception vessels. Most modern women get married and give birth late because they are preoccupied with their professional lives in their younger years. *Basic Questions · Discussion of Nature <Su Wen · Shang Gu Tian Zhen Lun>* 素问·上古天真论 states, "at the age of 35, yang brightness channel is weakened, the complexion begins to darken, and hair begins to fall. If the woman considers having a baby after the age of 30, fetal restlessness is likely to occur."

In addition, due to the influence of modern Western culture, the modern day Chinese have more open views about sex, and as a result, many of them have histories of miscarriage or abortion. A survey was taken of 62 women with threatened miscarriage; those over 31 years old occupied 46.7%, and those with more than 1 experience of miscarriage occupied 74.2%. Frequent pregnancy followed by frequent miscarriage consumes essence and blood, impairs kidney qi, and easily leads to fetal restlessness. Professor Luo Yuankai pointed out that "the pathogenesis of threatened miscarriage is the impairment and consumption of the kidney and spleen, qi and blood, the penetrating and the conception vessels. Of these, depletion of kidney qi is the main cause."

(2) Tonifying the Kidney is the Main Treatment Principle for the Treatment of Threatened Miscarriage and Habitual Miscarriage

Based on the causes and pathogenesis above, tonification of the kidney is considered the main treatment principle for calming the fetus. Professor Luo Yuankai agrees that "tonifying the kidney to calm the fetus is an important treatment principle." Kidney yin deficiency, kidney yang deficiency and kidney deficiency are the three commonly seen patterns in clinical practice.

If the patient presents with lower back soreness and abdominal pain after the cessation of menses, accompanied by mild vaginal bleeding, bland taste in the mouth, a pale complexion, loose stools, a pale tongue with thin white coating, and a slippery thready pulse, this indicates kidney yang deficiency. Combine *tù sī zǐ* (Semen Cuscutae), *xù duàn* (Radix Dipsaci), *sāng jì shēng* (Herba Taxilli), *ē jiāo* (Colla Corii Asini), *dǎng shēn* (Radix Codonopsis), *bái zhú* (Rhizoma Atractylodis Macrocephalae), *dù zhòng* (Cortex Eucommiae), *shú dì huáng* (Radix Rehmanniae Praeparata), *bái sháo* (Radix Paeoniae Alba) *zǐ sū gěng* (Caulis Perillae) and *gān cǎo* (Radix et Rhizoma Glycyrrhizae) to tonify the kidney (congenital constitution) and strengthen the spleen (acquired constitution).

For morning sickness, add *shā rén* (Fructus Amomi) and *bàn xià* (Rhizoma Pinelliae).

If the patient has a dry mouth, dry and hard stools, red facial complexion and lips, a red tongue with thin yellow coating, and a slippery and slightly rapid pulse, this indicates kidney yin deficiency. Select *tù sī zǐ* (Semen Cuscutae), *xù duàn* (Radix Dipsaci), *sāng jì shēng* (Herba Taxilli), *ē jiāo* (Colla Corii Asini), *hàn lián cǎo* (Herba Ecliptae), *nǚ zhēn zǐ* (Fructus Ligustri Lucidi), *huáng qín* (Radix Scutellariae), *zhú rú*

(Caulis Bambusae in Taenia), *tài zǐ shēn* (Radix Pseudostellariae), *bái sháo* (Radix Paeoniae Alba) and *gān cǎo* (Radix et Rhizoma Glycyrrhizae) to nourish the liver and kidney.

For dry and hard stools, add *ròu cōng róng* (Herba Cistanches) and *huǒ má rén* (Fructus Cannabis).

If the patient presents with a dry mouth, bland taste in the mouth, a pale red tongue with thin white coating, and a slippery pulse, this indicates kidney deficiency. Select *tù sī zǐ* (Semen Cuscutae), *xù duàn* (Radix Dipsaci), *sāng jì shēng* (Herba Taxilli), *ē jiāo* (Colla Corii Asini), *hàn lián cǎo* (Herba Ecliptae), *dǎng shēn* (Radix Codonopsis), *bái zhú* (Rhizoma Atractylodis Macrocephalae), *shēng dì huáng* (Radix Rehmanniae Recens), *bái sháo* (Radix Paeoniae Alba) and *gān cǎo* (Radix et Rhizoma Glycyrrhizae) to tonify both qi and yang.

Integrative treatment is also applicable for patients with a history of habitual miscarriage or those of advanced age who have symptoms of miscarriage. Administer intramuscular injections of 2000Iu of HCG every other day until the end of the 3rd month of pregnancy. It is still controversial whether or not progesterone can cause malformation, so it is not always used, except in cases with typical luteal phase defects. For paroxysmal uterine contractions, it can be used for a short time to reduce uterine sensitivity.

(3) Treat Fetuses That Cannot Be Calmed According to Their Categories

A. If a threatened miscarriage turns into an inevitable miscarriage, expel the fetus as soon as possible:

The method of expulsion depends on the month of pregnancy and the patient's condition. For early pregnancy, perform D&C; for middle pregnancy, administer intravenous oxytocin to promote delivery (mix 10u of oxytocin with 500ml of 5% glucose solution, and gradually accelerate the speed from 20d/m until there are active uterine contractions). Another option is to insert 600ug of misoprostol into the vagina, and carefully observe the uterine contraction and expulsion, paying close attention to the condition of the placenta. D&C is necessary if the placental expulsion is difficult, or if there are partial remains of the placenta in the uterine cavity.

B. Incomplete miscarriage:

If there is profuse vaginal bleeding or shock caused by partial retention of the placenta in the uterine cavity, give antishock treatment and perform D&C as soon as possible. After the surgery, administer intravenous oxytocin to strengthen uterine involution and reduce bleeding; and take *Sheng Hua Tang* 生化汤 plus *yì mǔ cǎo* (Herba Leonuri), *zhǐ qiào* (Fructus Aurantii), *dān shēn* (Radix et Rhizoma Salviae Miltiorrhizae) and *chì sháo* (Radix Paeoniae Rubra) internally to invigorate blood, transform stasis and promote the production of fresh blood. In addition, take measures to prevent infection.

C. Eliminating the products of conception is the treatment principle of missed abortion, and the method of expelling the fetus is decided according to gestational month and relevant examinations:

Performing D&C within the first three months of gestation can cause blood coagulation disorders. Coagulation function test should be given before the operation. During and after the operation, beware of DIC, which is a life-threatening condition. At the same time, although the patient has not had menstrual bleeding for 3 months, a simple D&C can be done if the fetus is smaller than normal; if the fetus is large and the patient's cervix is tight, insert 600ug of misoprostol into the vagina 1 hour before the D&C, which dilates the cervix and strengthens uterine contractions to facilitate the operation. If the fetal biparietal diameter (BPD) is larger than 2.5cm, it may take 100mg of mifepristone every 12 hours and for a total of 3 times on an empty stomach or 2 hours after meals. On the third day, take misoprostol orally or insert it into the vagina to promote the expulsion of the fetus; repeat this every 2-3 hours. The daily dosage of misoprostol generally should not exceed 1600ug. Other options include administering oxytocin intravenously or taking

5mg of orgabolin orally before the operation, which is taken 3 times a day for a total of 3 days, to enhance the sensitivity of the uterus to oxytocin. Beware of the possibility that an incomplete miscarriage may occur during the course of taking orgabolin.

Infection may occur during or after the course of the various types of miscarriages mentioned above. If infection occurs before miscarriage, control it immediately. For a moderate amount of vaginal bleeding, first use broad-spectrum antibiotics for 5-7 days, and then perform D&C. Before giving antibiotics, it is best to use bacterial culture of the cervical secretions to clearly identify the pathogens. For profuse vaginal bleeding, perform D&C and have the patient take antibiotics until 7-10 days after the operation. Prescribe *Wu Wei Xiao Du Yin* 五味消毒饮 combined with *dà huáng* (Radix et Rhizoma Rhei). Also select *pú gōng yīng* (Herba Taraxaci), *jīn yín huā* (Flos Lonicerae Japonicae), *zǐ huā dì dīng* (Herba Violae), *dà huáng* (Radix et Rhizoma Rhei), *qīng tiān kuí* (Nervilia Fordii), *mǔ dān pí* (Cortex Moutan) and *bài jiàng cǎo* (Herba Patriniae).

(4) Chinese Medicine and Biomedicine Have Respective Advantages in the Treatment of Different Types of Miscarriages

Chinese medicine has abundant experience and success in the treatment and prevention of miscarriage; excellent curative effects have been achieved in the different stages of miscarriage with Chinese medicinal treatment. However, integrative treatment is still required in various stages of miscarriage to achieve better results.

A. Using integrative medicine to determine the cause of miscarriage:

Some cases of threatened miscarriage and habitual miscarriage are caused by unusual (but clear-cut) factors, such as uterine cavity malformation, chromosomal abnormalities and genital tract infections. Some of these patients will not present with apparent symptoms, and are therefore not aware of their condition until they receive lab tests; this often results in delayed treatment. An accurate diagnosis can be made from the start if we utilize the technology of biomedical examinations; begin treatment before pregnancy to prevent the occurrence of miscarriage.

B. Treating the primary disease with biomedicine, and using Chinese medicine as a complementary therapy:

After determining the exact cause (such as genital tract infection, dysfunctional uterine bleeding, etc.), one may use Chinese medicine in addition to biomedicine to enhance the therapeutic effect and reduce the side affects of biomedical treatment.

C. Chinese medicine and biomedicine have respective emphases on the different stages of miscarriage:

For cases of threatened miscarriage or habitual miscarriage with no evident symptoms during early pregnancy, they may be treated with Chinese medicinals according to the patient's constitution to prevent the occurrence of disease - either by tonifying the kidney or strengthening the spleen. Chinese medicinals are especially effective in the early stage of miscarriage; if treated in accordance with pattern differentiation, the patient's symptoms can be relieved. Progestogen and HCG treatment should be given in the early stage for patients with inadequate luteal function and uterine sensitivity. If the patient is entering the inevitable miscarriage stage, it is imperative to use surgery to expel the fetus. After fetal expulsion or complete miscarriage, the patient should be treated with Chinese medicinals to facilitate recovery.

3. Summary

Threatened miscarriage and habitual miscarriage are common and frequently-occurring gynecological disease. Since they can develop into inevitable miscarriage and missed abortion, they severely affect the pregnant women's physical and mental health, cause much despair and sorrow, and affect the quality of family life. In recent years, research on the pathogenesis of miscarriage has made great progress in areas of immunity, endocrinology and genetic defects. For endocrine factors, aside from inadequate luteal function, which has already been recognized, it has been established that placental hormonal insufficiency also can cause miscarriage. If HCG, HPL, and estrogen levels secreted by the placenta are decreased after the 8th gestational week, this indicates a high possibility that pregnancy will terminate and a miscarriage will occur. Biomedical treatment approaches for miscarriage are simple, which include the supplementation of progesterone, vitamin E and HCG; however, they lack the overall regulation of maternal health.

The treatment of miscarriage in Chinese medicine has a long history with several millennia of rich clinical experience, and contributes greatly to the national population of China. Chinese medical treatment of miscarriage can be administered before pregnancy, especially for patients of habitual miscarriage. Pre-pregnancy healthcare lays the groundwork for a smooth pregnancy and prevents miscarriage. The methods of tonifying the spleen and kidney, replenishing qi and blood, nourishing yin, clearing heat, invigorating blood and transforming stasis are selected according to pattern differentiation as soon as the symptoms of miscarriage appear. Treatment improves patients' symptoms, calms their minds and reinforces their confidence. In addition, Chinese medical treatment can prevent fetal malformation, making it a safe and effective therapy for miscarriage.

By comparison, Chinese medicine is slower and less effective than biomedicine in the treatment of paroxysmal uterine contractions associated with miscarriage. Integrative treatment is often required to relieve paroxysmal uterine contractions with profuse vaginal bleeding.

How to quickly and effectively reverse the process of miscarriage is an important topic for discussion. We should conduct more research to find out which formulas and dosages are the most effective, and consider integrative treatments to enhance the curative effect.

Chinese medicine has more advantages than biomedicine for pre and post-miscarriage healthcare. Chinese medical treatment can be tailored-specific to the unique constitution of each patient, such as stabilizing the kidney (congenital constitution), tonifying the spleen (acquired constitution), and regulating qi and blood to benefit the fetus.

SELECTED QUOTES FROM CLASSICAL TEXTS

Chen Suan's Interpretation of Gynecology - Category of Complicated Prenatal Syndromes <Chen Suan Fu Ke Bu Jie · Tai Qian Za Zheng Men> 陈素庵妇科补解.胎前杂证门:

"Nourishing blood to calm the fetus can cause the masses to enlarge and make the pathogens vigorous; the elimination of old pathogens can lead to blood and qi deficiency and stirring of the fetus. The therapeutic method should be chosen in accordance with the pulse condition - deficient or excess, slow or rapid, and slippery or rough. A slow, deficient and rough pulse indicates that the root of the disease is constitutional insufficiency. For this condition, the main treatment principle is to pacify the fetus, assisted by medicinals that promote qi flow. A rapid, excess and slippery pulse indicates the disease branch; treatment requires dispersion of concretions (masses) as well as nourishing blood. The fetus is the root and the concretions are the branch."

Abstracts of Obstetrics and Gynecology <Nv Ke Ji Yao> 女科辑要:
"Some fetuses are able to develop despite its atrophied condition due to the fact that they were a product of weak sperm; however, because

of the invasion of maternal disease toxins, some fetuses may die as a result. In addition, some fetuses die from traumatic injuries resulting in damage to the umbilical cord and placenta; others die because of difficult labor."

The Complete Works of Jingyue · Regulation of Women's Health <Jing Yue Quan Shu · Fu Ren Gui> 景岳全书·妇人规:

"Frequent miscarriages are caused by the depletion of qi and vessels. There are different causes of depletion, such as a weak congenital constitution; senile weakness; decreased vigor due to anxiety, anger and overstrain; and severe loss of kidney qi due to indulgence in sexual activity. In addition, factors like diet can also damage qi and vessels; however, the fetus may still be healthy despite injury to qi and vessels."

The Complete Works of Jingyue · Regulation of Women's Health <Jing Yue Quan Shu · Fu Ren Gui> 景岳全书·妇人规:

"Many fetuses die in the womb as a result of external injuries, violation of contraindications, or deficient fetal qi... If the expectant mother's abdomen is distended and her tongue is black, the fetus is already dead. If during pregnancy, the mother has cold, heaviness and downbearing sensation, nausea and vomiting, or... upward rushing of qi with a black tongue, this indicates that the fetus is dead. For this condition, the dead fetus must be expelled using a fetus-expelling formula as quickly as possible."

Complete Records of Medicine · Gynecology <Yi Bu Quan Lu · Fu Ke> 医部全录·妇科:

"Restless fetus is caused by deficiency of the penetrating and conception vessels, and insufficiency of the embryo, as well as other factors like excessive alcohol and sexual intercourse which injure and stir the fetus; careless handling and contact which can arouse the fetus;

qi constraint caused by excessive joy or anger that damage the heart and liver and affect the blood vessels; and taking warm tonics recommended by a doctor that are actually harmful. If restless fetus is caused by maternal disease, the fetus can only be calmed by treating the maternal disease; for maternal disease caused by an unstable fetus, the mother will recover by herself when the fetus is pacified."

Effective Prescriptions for Women · Discussions of Prescriptions for Pregnancy and Threatened Miscarriage with Bleeding, Number Five <Fu Ren Da Quan Liang Fang · Ren Shen Tai Luo Xia Xue Fang Lun Di Wu> 妇人大全良方. 妊娠胎漏下血方论第五:

"Threatened miscarriage is pregnancy of several months with occasional menses, which is caused by deficient penetrating and conception vessels that are unable to control the blood of hand greater yang channel and hand lesser yin channel. The penetrating and conception vessels are the reservoir of the channels and collaterals, and they originate in the uterus. The hand greater yang small intestine channel and the hand lesser yin heart channel have an exterior-interior relationship, and they provide breast milk to the upper region of the body and menses to the lower region of the body. The reason pregnant women do not menstruate is because blood is being used to nourish the fetus and produce milk. If the qi of the penetrating and conception vessels is deficient, the uterus leaks because it loses its ability to control menstrual blood; thus there is occasional spotting, which is also known as threatened miscarriage. If blood is exhausted, the patient will die. In addition, overstrain, immoderate pleasure, anger, sorrow and joy, a raw and cold diet, and exposure to pathogenic wind cold can all lead to fetal restlessness. If the mother has long-standing illness, the fetal zang organs will be easily susceptible to the invasion of wind cold, qi and blood will be in disharmony, and there will be fetal restlessness and bleeding."

Jade Ruler of Gynecology · The Prenatal Period <Fu Ke Yu Chi · Tai Qian> 妇科玉尺 • 胎前:

"Miscarriage occurs because original qi is deficient and is therefore unable to nourish the fetus. The ancients likened this to the following metaphors: the fruits fall off the branches if the branches are dried and withered, and the flowers fall if the vines are wilted. Miscarriage can also occur as a result of excessive anger causing the stirring of internal fire. This resembles the wind shaking the trees, or a person breaking a branch. …the normal delivery is like a ripe chestnut, whose shells opens naturally by itself without any damage to both the shell and the fruit. The patient needs to be nursed back to health after a miscarriage, focusing mainly on tonifying blood, engendering flesh, nourishing zang organs, removing the old (blood) and producing new (blood)."

Correction of Errors in Medical Classics · Discussion of Shao Fu Zhu Yu Tang <Yi Lin Gai Cuo · the Description of Shao Fu Zhu Yu Tang> 医林改错 • 少腹逐瘀汤说:

"The pregnant woman has a strong constitution with sufficient qi. She has a good appetite and did not suffer from any traumatic injuries. However, she is prone to having recurrent miscarriages that occur around the 3rd month of pregnancy, without any apparent causes. There are many medical books written on this topic, but most of them discuss nourishing yin and blood. There are few effective formulas in them for strengthening the spleen, nourishing the stomach, calming the fetus and preventing miscarriage. These texts fail to mention that if there is initial phlegm and blood occupying the uterus, this leaves no room for a fetus larger than that of 3 gestational months. The fetus and pathogens are squeezed together into the same small space; blood is unable enter uterus and flows down laterally instead, hence there is bleeding. Miscarriage occurs because blood is unable to enter uterus and as a result, the fetus cannot be nourished by the blood."

MODERN RESEARCH

1. Clinical Research

(1) Pattern Differentiation and Corresponding Treatment

1) Na Sumei summarized Chen Shiduo's treatment of restless fetus, and after adding this knowledge to her own comprehension and clinical experience, categorized restless fetus into the following five patterns:

A. Strengthen the acquired constitution, benefit the congenital constitution and solidify the two constitutions:

This pattern is commonly seen in kidney (yin and yang) deficiency restless fetus. Chen Shiduo emphasized that the spleen is unable to perform its function of transformation without congenital qi, and the kidney cannot govern reproduction without congenital qi. The essential qi of the kidney will not be able to continue governing reproduction if only the kidney is strengthened without reinforcing the spleen. To treat restless fetus, tonification of both the spleen and the kidney is needed to stabilize the penetrating and conception vessels. The main symptoms of the pattern are lower abdominal pain during pregnancy, and restless fetus with sagging sensation. The cause of this pattern is considered to be weakness of the girdling vessel and therefore its inability to hold the uterus; in fact, it is caused by the depletion of both the spleen and kidney. The uterus is linked to the girdling vessel, but excess of the girdling vessel is related to the spleen and kidney.

To sum up the above, Chen Shiduo proposes the principle of reinforcing acquired constitution, benefiting congenital constitution and solidifying the two constitutions by using the formula *An Dian Er Tian Tang* 安奠二天汤. Ingredients: 30g of *rén shēn* (Radix et Rhizoma Ginseng), 30g of *bái zhú* (Rhizoma Atractylodis Macrocephalae), 30g of *shú dì huáng* (Radix Rehmanniae Praeparata), 15g of *shān zhū yú* (Fructus Corni), 15g of *huái shān yào* (Rhizoma

Dioscoreae), 3g of *zhì gān cǎo* (Radix et Rhizoma Glycyrrhizae Praeparata cum Melle), 9g of *dù zhòng* (Cortex Eucommiae), 6g of *gǒu qǐ zǐ* (Fructus Lycii) and 6g of *biǎn dòu* (Semen Lablab Album). All the medicinals are decocted in water for oral intake.

B. Tonify lung metal, engender kidney water and moisten dryness to calm the fetus:

The indication of this treatment method is what is commonly known as kidney yin deficiency type restless fetus syndrome, and the usual therapeutic principle is to enrich yin and tonify the kidney. Chen Shiduo emphasizes that the original cause of kidney yin deficiency is, without a doubt, insufficiency of kidney water. Under general circumstances, kidney water cannot be produced quickly; one must first tonify the lung (metal), which in turn can engender water. Once water has a transformative source, the unrooted fire is naturally controlled. Kidney yang is comparatively more hyperactive if kidney yin is deficient, thus symptoms of hyperactive fire due to yin deficiency are commonly seen in the clinic.

The main symptoms of this disease are in the 3rd to 4th month of pregnancy, the patient present with dry mouth and tongue, mild sore throat that lacks moisture, and restless fetus. In severe cases, there may be bleeding similar to menstruation. For this condition, just clearing the ministerial fire is inadequate, simply because hyperactivity of ministerial fire is caused by kidney yin deficiency. In this case, the best therapeutic approach is to tonify lung metal, engender kidney water and moisten dryness to calm the fetus. Chen Shiduo uses *Run Zao An Tai Tang* 润燥安胎汤, which consists of *shú dì huáng* (Radix Rehmanniae Praeparata) 15g, *shān zhū yú* (Fructus Corni) 15g, *yì mǔ cǎo* (Herba Leonuri) 6g, *huáng qín* (Radix Scutellariae) 3g, *mài dōng* (Radix Ophiopogonis) 5g, *shēng dì huáng* (Radix Rehmanniae Recens) 9g, *ē jiāo* (Colla Corii Asini) 6g and *wǔ wèi zǐ* (Fructus Schisandrae Chinensis) 1g. The medicinals are decocted in water for oral intake.

C. For severe spleen and stomach deficiency, tonify the fire of the heart and kidney and support earth to stabilize the fetus:

This method is indicated for extremely deficient spleen and stomach qi which can cause restlessness of the fetus. Deficiency of the spleen and stomach usually does not cause restless fetus, but extreme deficiency may cause vomiting, diarrhea, fetal movement with a sagging sensation and unbearable pain. This condition is often considered extreme cold of the spleen and stomach, but in actuality, it is extreme deficiency of the spleen and stomach. The uterus and fetus are also weak from the spleen and stomach deficiency which is further exacerbated by vomiting and diarrhea. Under these circumstances, if a miscarriage does not occur (even though there is severe fetal restlessness), it is an indication that the kidney qi is still stable. Kidney qi can connect with the spleen, and heart qi can assist stomach qi. Chen Shiduo mentions: "If the spleen and stomach are deficient but has not yet been exhausted, the fetus will be restless but will not fall."

When treating this condition, one should tonify the spleen and kidney while boosting the heart and kidney fire at the same time. Because at this moment the spleen and stomach qi are verging on exhaustion, it is difficult to restore them by simply treating the spleen and stomach qi. Therefore, it is imperative to reinforce the fire of the heart and spleen as well as strengthen the spleen and kidney. Since fire engenders earth, this is an especially easy task to accomplish. Chen Shiduo created *Yuan Tu Gu Tai Tang* 援土固胎汤 for this purpose. The ingredients of the formula are *rén shēn* (Radix et Rhizoma Ginseng) 30g, *bái zhú* (Rhizoma Atractylodis Macrocephalae) 60g, *róu guì* (Cortex Cinnamomi) 6g, *huái shān yào* (Rhizoma Dioscoreae) 30g, *shú fù zǐ* (Radix Aconiti Lateralis Praeparata) 2g, *zhì gān cǎo* (Radix et Rhizoma Glycyrrhizae Praeparata cum Melle) 30g, *dù zhòng* (Cortex Eucommiae) 9g, *gǒu qǐ zǐ* (Fructus Lycii) 9g, *shān zhū yú* (Fructus Corni) 30g, *tù sī zǐ* (Semen Cuscutae) 9g and *shā rén* (Fructus

Amomi) 1g. All the medicinals are decocted in water for oral intake.

Chen Shiduo speculated that "80% of the formula's effect is restoring the earth of the spleen and stomach; 20% involves rescuing the fire of the heart and kidney." He concluded that at this moment, since spleen and stomach qi are extremely deficient and on the verge of exhaustion but heart and kidney yang are still intact, one should reinforce spleen and stomach qi with large dosages of medicinals.

D. If there is fullness and distention in the chest and abdomen during pregnancy due to liver constraint, course the liver to relieve these symptoms:

If there is restless fetus caused by liver constraint, accompanying symptoms may include oppression and pain in the hypochondriac region, and fullness and distention in the chest and abdomen. Chen Shiduo said: "Nourishing the fetus depends on kidney water, but kidney water must be able to generate itself without the help of liver blood." This disorder is referred to as fullness and distention in the chest and abdomen during pregnancy in *Effective Prescriptions for Women <Fu Ren Liang Fang>* 妇人良方, and is commonly known as the upward flow of fetal qi. The usual treatment method is to regulate qi and calm the fetus, using *Zi Su Yin* 紫苏饮 as the preferred formula. Chen Shiduo concluded that the main pathomechanism is obstruction of liver qi. Conception depends first on the nourishment of kidney water and then on the assistance of liver blood. If there is liver constraint, liver blood is unable to flow down to aid kidney water, and consequently the fetus will attempt to move upward to acquire the assistance of liver blood. As a result, the pregnant woman will experience oppression and pain in the hypochondriac region and the rising of fetal qi.

Treatment should involve removing liver constraint and moistening dryness of liver blood, which will alleviate the fullness and distention in the chest and abdomen. Use *Jie Xuan Tang* 解悬汤, which contains *bái sháo* (Radix Paeoniae Alba) 30g, *dāng guī* (Radix Angelicae Sinensis) 30g, *chǎo zhī zǐ* (Fructus Gardeniae, stir-fried) 9g, *zhǐ qiào* (Fructus Aurantii) 2g, *shā rén* (Fructus Amomi) 1g, *bái zhú* (Rhizoma Atractylodis Macrocephalae) 15g, *rén shēn* (Radix et Rhizoma Ginseng) 30g, *fú ling* (Poria) 9g and *bò hé* (Herba Menthae) 6g.

E. Exuberant stomach fire will consume kidney water, therefore it is necessary to drain the fire and benefit the water immediately:

This method is indicated for restless fetus caused by excess stomach fire injuring kidney water and a malnourished fetus. The main symptoms of this disorder are thirst, sweating, increased intake of cold water, vexation and agitation with possible mania, abdominal pain, lumbar soreness and restless fetus. According to Chen Shiduo, "stomach fire is the reservoir of water and grain, and it has an abundance of qi and blood to nourish all zang-fu organs." The stomach belongs to earth; earth contains fire inside it to keep it alive, but if there is no water inside the earth, it becomes scorched earth. However, exuberant stomach fire will burn and consume kidney water, causing the flaring up of fire and heat and giving rise to heart fire. The fetus is tied to the kidney and connected to the heart; heart qi communicates with the fetus. If stomach and heart fire burns fiercely, this will lead to the depletion of water, then water cannot be distributed to the fetus; how can the fetus be secure?

The treatment in this case should be to quickly drain fire and benefit water. If there is abundant water, fire will decline on its own, and the fetus will be undisturbed. Use the formula *Zi Tai Yin* 滋胎饮: *mài dōng* (Radix Ophiopogonis) 30g, *shēng dì huáng* (Radix Rehmanniae Recens) 30g, *dāng guī shēn* (Radix Angelicae Sinensis) 30g, *huáng qín* (Radix Scutellariae) 9g, *tiān huā fěn* (Radix Trichosanthis) 9g, *gān cǎo* (Radix et Rhizoma Glycyrrhizae) 3g. A large dosage of *mài dōng* (Radix Ophiopogonis) is used in the formula in combination with *shēng dì huáng* (Radix Rehmanniae Recens), *tiān huā fěn* (Radix Trichosanthis) and *gān cǎo* (Radix et Rhizoma Glycyrrhizae) to nourish yin, clear heat and drain fire from the lung and stomach channels; *dāng guī* (Radix Angelicae Sinensis) moistens dryness, nourishes blood and pacifies the fetus. [1]

2) Zhao Meifeng adopted the method of preventing miscarriage by activating blood and transforming stasis, which was inspired by Zhang Zhongjing's *Gui Zhi Fu Ling Wan* 桂枝茯苓丸:

The usage of this formula was based on the notion that "the symptom which has not been eliminated is the cause of bleeding; therefore, it should be eliminated." This statement refers to long-term accumulation of static blood. If this accumulated blood remains in the uterus during pregnancy, it will impede blood supply to the fetus. If not removed, this accumulation will eventually cause fetal death. Immediate transformation of stasis and removal of static blood is required.

If the restless fetus is caused by maternal disease, treat the disease first, and the fetus will be pacified. However, special care should be taken not to injure the fetus during the elimination of disease.

When treating restless fetus with bleeding caused by internal obstruction of static blood, first determine the correct pattern and then proceed to invigorate blood, transform stasis, dissolve masses and disperse stasis while nourishing and stabilizing the fetus. In clinical practice, the treatment can be modified according to specific circumstances; when prescribing medicinals, start from small dosages and gradually increase when necessary.

Zhao Meifeng thinks that it is fine to refer to the treatment approaches of the ancient physicians, and broadly apply them in clinical practice as long as they are closely related to the pathogenesis of the disease being treated. For instance, treating habitual miscarriage and threatened miscarriage would require activating blood and transforming stasis. Using other methods would be ineffective in some patients because of poor blood supply to the embryo due to the existence of blood stasis in the womb long before plantation of the ovum occurred. Under these conditions, the embryo cannot develop well, and it may even lead to a miscarriage.

Repeated miscarriage can injure and consume qi and blood, and damage the penetrating and conception vessels, causing impaired circulation of qi and blood, under-nourished blood, and vaginal bleeding during pregnancy. Transforming stasis and invigorating blood is needed to free the stagnation; improving the nutritional supply from mother to fetus will create a good environment for the development of the fetus.

In recent years, some practitioners in the gynecological field consider the impairment of maternal blood flow and the disturbance of placental microcirculation important causes of recurrent miscarriage. *Si Wu Tang* 四物汤 combined with *dān shēn* 丹参 (Radix et Rhizoma Salviae Miltiorrhizae) is often used, which consists of *dāng guī* (Radix Angelicae Sinensis), *chuān xiōng* (Rhizoma Chuanxiong), *sháo yào* (Radix Paeoniae), *shú dì huáng* (Radix Rehmanniae Praeparata) and *dān shēn* (Radix et Rhizoma Salviae Miltiorrhizae). *Dān shēn* (Radix et Rhizoma Salviae Miltiorrhizae) is first prescribed in a small dose of 6g, and gradually raised to 12g.[2]

3) Li Weihong employed the method of tonifying the kidney and regulating menstruation to treat habitual miscarriage:

The artificial regulation of the menstrual cycle using Chinese medicinals is created on the basis of Chinese medical theory—"the kidney stores essence", "the kidney dominates reproduction", the waxing and waning of the sea of blood and reproduction is dependent upon the balance of kidney qi, *tiān guǐ*, the penetrating and conception vessels, and the uterus — as well as the application of related theories in modern medicine. The method involves prescribing medicinals according to the changes of kidney qi and of qi and blood during the different phases of the menstrual cycle, integrated with the different developmental stages of the ovarian follicle, and tonifying the kidney as the foundation of treatment.

Integrative research has shown that Chinese medicinals for tonifying the kidney has similar functions as endocrine hormones, but do not replace their actions, which may be the significance of using Chinese medicine to tonify the kidney. Tonification of the kidney has a bidirectional regulative effect on the function of pituitary-gonadal axis, and can improve the regulatory function of the hypothalamus-pituitary-ovary axis.

Select *Tao Hong Si Wu Tang* 桃红四物汤 during menstruation to remove old blood and engender new blood, thus unblocking the flow of menstrual blood; new blood can be produced once old blood has been dispelled. After menstruation, prescribe *Gui Shen Wan* 归肾丸 to enrich the kidney and nourish blood. The formula's primary function is to nourish the liver and kidney with *shú dì huáng* (Radix Rehmanniae Praeparata), *shān yào* (Rhizoma Dioscoreae), *shān zhū yú* (Fructus Corni) and *xù duàn* (Radix Dipsaci). During mid-cycle, prescribe medicinals that tonify the kidney, assist yang, invigorate blood and transform stasis to promote ovulation.

Use *Gui Shen Wan* 归肾丸 to nourish kidney yin. Add *xù duàn* (Radix Dipsaci), *tù sī zǐ* (Semen Cuscutae) and *lù jiǎo* (Cornu Cervi) to tonify kidney yang; use *dāng guī* (Radix Angelicae Sinensis), *chì sháo* (Radix Paeoniae Rubra) and *wǔ líng zhī* (Faeces Togopteri) to invigorate blood and transform stasis to promote ovulation (this method is also referred to as facilitating the transformation of yin into yang).

Select *Shou Tai Wan* 寿胎丸 to tonify both yin and yang equally and regulate both qi and blood, which helps the body to prepare for conception. [3]

4) Tian Bingzhao points out that one must tranquilize the heart in order to calm the fetus:

The heart stores the spirit and dominates the physiological activities of the body and the mental activities of the conscious mind. Various symptoms of threatened miscarriage can be exacerbated by an unpeaceful mind, mental stress, fear, worry, a spirit that has no residence, and severe anxiety. The securing of the fetus is the "storing" function of the kidney, which is also regulated by the heart spirit; when the spirit is bright, the kidney's function of stabilizing the fetus is normal. Therefore, it is necessary to calm the heart in order to pacify the fetus; when the heart is still and the kidney is solid, there is an abundance of essence, the uterus is able to store, and the fetus is secure. Add *huáng lián* (Rhizoma Coptidis), *lián zǐ xīn* (Plumula Nelumbinis) and *suān zǎo rén* (Semen Ziziphi Spinosae) to the prescription. Advise the patient to listen to gentle relaxing music to soothe her mind. In addition, spiritual counseling is important for the healing process and is therefore highly recommended.

5) Tonifying the kidney and nurturing the spleen is the first important step in calming the fetus:

He Tonglu advocates the adoption of this method to prevent miscarriage. He repeated the wisdom the ancients: "the kidney stores essence, governs reproduction, and is known as the root of congenital constitution", "the uterine vessels are connected to the kidney", "the spleen is the root of acquired constitution and the source of qi and blood production", and "the fetal stalk is connected to the spleen, which hangs like a bell on a beam; if the pole is wobbly, the beam will be unstable." The spleen is the source of qi and blood production and transformation; if qi is sufficient, the fetus can be fastened; if blood is abundant, the fetus can be pacified. Restless fetus, threatened miscarriage with vaginal bleeding and recurrent miscarriage can be caused by deficient spleen qi which is unable to hold and contain things in their rightful positions. [5]

(2) Specific Formulas

a) *Zi Shen Yu Tai Wan* 滋肾育胎丸:

Contains *rén shēn* (Radix et Rhizoma Ginseng), *bái zhú* (Rhizoma Atractylodis Macrocephalae), *tù sī zǐ* (Semen Cuscutae), *sāng jì shēng* (Herba Taxilli), *xù duàn* (Radix Dipsaci) and *ē jiāo* (Colla Corii Asini). It was used to treat 221 cases of early threatened miscarriage and 10 cases of late threatened miscarriage with a total effectiveness rate of 91.89%. [6]

b) *Zhu Huang Bao Tai Wan* 助黄保胎丸:

Contains *dǎng shēn* (Radix Codonopsis), *huáng qí* (Radix Astragali), *bái zhú* (Rhizoma Atractylodis Macrocephalae), *bái sháo* (Radix Paeoniae Alba), *tù sī zǐ* (Semen Cuscutae), *dù zhòng* (Cortex Eucommiae) and *huáng qín* (Radix Scutellariae). It was used to treat 115 cases of threatened miscarriage (68 cases with primary luteal phase defect, 65 cases with primary endometriosis, 50 cases with a history of miscarriage). 108 cases (93.3%) achieved full recovery from the illness; 7 (6.1%) cases had no effect. [7]

c) *Shou Tai An Zi Tang* 寿胎安子汤:

Contains *chǎo xù duàn* (Radix Dipsaci, stir-fried) 12g, *sāng jì shēng* (Herba Taxilli) 10g, *tù sī zǐ* (Semen Cuscutae) 10g, *zhù má gēn* (Radix Boehmeriae Ramie) 30g, *huái shān yào* (Rhizoma Dioscoreae Oppositae) 15g, *chǎo huáng qín* (Radix Scutellariae, stir-fried) 10g, *hàn lián cǎo* (Herba Ecliptae) 10g and *tài zǐ shēn* (Radix Pseudostellariae) 15g. It was used to treat 80 cases threatened miscarriage with the following results: 66 cases fully recovered from the illness, 3 cases showed improvement, and 11 cases showed no effect. [8]

d) Modified *Shi Xiao San* 失笑散:

Includes *Shi Xiao San* (wrapped), *chǎo chuān xiōng* (Rhizoma Chuanxiong) 10g, *mǔ dān pí* (Cortex Moutan) 10g, *zhì dà huáng* (Radix et Rhizoma Rhei, processed) 10g, *chǎo dāng guī* (Radix Angelicae Sinensis, stir-fried) 15g, *chǎo lián fáng* (Receptaculum Nelumbinis, stir-fried) 15g, *zhì mò yào* (Myrrha, processed) 6g, *táo rén* (Semen Persicae) 6g, *mǎ chǐ xiàn* (Herba Portulacae) 24g and *yì mǔ cǎo* (Herba Leonuri) 24g. This formula was used to treat 24 cases of incomplete miscarriage with the following results: a cure in 17 cases, improvement in 4 cases, and no effect in 3 cases. [9]

e) *Gu Tai San* 固胎散:

Contains *shú dì huáng* (Radix Rehmanniae Praeparata) 6g, *shān zhū yú*

(Fructus Corni) 6g, *huái shān yào* (Rhizoma Dioscoreae Oppositae) 6g, *chǎo bái zhú* (Rhizoma Atractylodis Macrocephalae, stir-fried) 6g, *dǎng shēn* (Radix Codonopsis) 9g, *bái sháo* (Radix Paeoniae Alba) 7.5g, *chǎo dù zhòng* (Cortex Eucommiae) 7.5g, *gǒu qǐ zǐ* (Fructus Lycii) 7.5g, *huáng qín* (Radix Scutellariae) 4.5g, *yán hú suǒ* (Rhizoma Corydalis) 6g, *chǎo biǎn dòu* (Semen Dolichoris Lablab, stir-fried) 7.5g, *qiàn cǎo tàn* (Radix et Rhizoma Rubiae, carbonized) 6g, *jīng jiè suì tàn* (Spica Schizonepetae Carbonisata) 6g and *gān cǎo* (Radix et Rhizoma Glycyrrhizae) 3g. It was used in the treatment of 76 cases of restless fetus with the following outcome: a cure in 70 cases, and no effect in 6 cases. The effectiveness rate was 92.1%.[10]

f) *Bao Tai Fang* 保胎方:

Contains *tù sī zǐ* (Semen Cuscutae) 15g, *xù duàn* (Radix Dipsaci) 15g, *sāng jì shēng* (Herba Taxilli) 15g and *ē jiāo* (Colla Corii Asini) 10g. The formula was modified to treat 47 cases of spontaneous abortion of unknown cause. The results were: 38 (80.8%) cases had a full-term delivery. The formula was thought to have a relationship with cellular immunity and humoral immunity, and can enhance the functions of gonads and endocrine system. [11]

g) Modified *Sheng Hua Tang* 生化汤:

Contains *dāng guī* (Radix Angelicae Sinensis) 15g, *chuān xiōng* (Rhizoma Chuanxiong) 9g, *táo rén* (Semen Persicae) 9g, *zhì gān cǎo* (Radix et Rhizoma Glycyrrhizae Praeparata cum Melle) 3g, *wēi jiāng* (Zingiber Officinale Rosc.) 1.5g, *yì mǔ cǎo* (Herba Leonuri) 15g, *jīn yín huā* (Flos Lonicerae Japonicae) 15g, *lián qiào* (Fructus Forsythiae) 15g and *hóng huā* (Flos Carthami) 6g. This formula was used to treat 84 cases of incomplete miscarriage with the following results: full recovery in 73 cases (87%) after one course of treatment, a full recovery in 8 cases (9.5%) after two courses of treatment, and no effect in 3 cases (3.5%). These 3 cases were later revealed to be ectopic pregnancies by transabdominal examination.[12]

h) Modified *Shou Tai Wan* 寿胎丸:

Contains *tù sī zǐ* (Semen Cuscutae) 10g, *xù duàn* (Radix Dipsaci) 10g, *ē jiāo* (Colla Corii Asini) [to be decocted first] 10g, *dǎng shēn* (Radix Codonopsis) 10g, *chǎo huái shān yào* (Radix Dioscoreae Oppositae, stir-fried) 10g, *bái sháo* (Radix Paeoniae Alba) 10g, *huáng qín* (Radix Scutellariae) 10g and *sāng jì shēng* (Herba Taxilli) 25g. The formula was modified and used to treat 110 cases of threatened miscarriage. The results were: improvement in 106 cases (96.36%). Clinical trials showed that the formula can inhibit uterine smooth muscle activity and enhance the luteotrophic function of the pituitary-ovary axis. Every single medicinal in the formula was shown to possess hormone-like functions.[13]

i) Modified *Bao Tai Yin* 保胎饮:

Contains *tù sī zǐ* (Semen Cuscutae), *chuān duàn* (Radix Dipsaci), *dù zhòng* (Cortex Eucommiae), *dǎng shēn* (Radix Codonopsis) and *bái sháo* (Radix Paeoniae Alba). It was used to treat 36 cases of miscarriage according to pattern differentiation and treatment. The total effectiveness rate was 94.4%. The modified *Bao Tai Yin* has the effect of tonifying the kidney, fortifying the spleen, benefiting qi, nourishing blood, and stabilizing, controlling and calming the fetus. [14]

j) Self-composed *Bao Tai Yin* 保胎饮:

Contains *bái zhú* (Rhizoma Atractylodis Macrocephalae), *shā rén* (Fructus Amomi), *shú dì huáng* (Radix Rehmanniae Praeparata), *chuān duàn* (Radix Dipsaci), *tù sī zǐ* (Semen Cuscutae), *sāng jì shēng* (Herba Taxilli) and *dù zhòng* (Cortex Eucommiae). The formula was modified according to pattern differentiation and was used to treat 86 cases of threatened miscarriage. The effectiveness rate was 90%. The formula has the effect of harmonizing qi and blood to pacify the fetus.[15]

k) Modified *Bu Shen Yi Kang Tang* 补肾抑抗汤:

Contains *tù sī zǐ* (Semen Cuscutae), *shú dì huáng* (Radix Rehmanniae Praeparata), *chuān duàn* (Radix Dipsaci), *gǒu qǐ zǐ* (Fructus Lycii), *lù jiǎo jiāo* (Colla Cornus Cervi), *dāng guī* (Radix Angelicae Sinensis), *bái sháo* (Radix Paeoniae Alba), *dān shēn* (Radix et Rhizoma Salviae Miltiorrhizae), *fú líng* (Poria) and *gān cǎo* (Radix et Rhizoma Glycyrrhizae). This formula was modified to treat 36 cases of positive ACA after repeated miscarriage. The results were the following: 35 cases became negative. The effectiveness rate was 96%. The formula has the effect of tonifying the kidney, nourishing blood, inhibiting antibodies, and eliminating ACA antibodies. [16]

l) Modified *An Tai Fang* 安胎方 :

Contains *dǎng shēn* (Radix Codonopsis), *huáng qí* (Radix Astragali), *bái zhú* (Rhizoma Atractylodis Macrocephalae), *shā rén* (Fructus Amomi), *tù sī zǐ* (Semen Cuscutae), *shú dì huáng* (Radix Rehmanniae Praeparata), *bái sháo* (Radix Paeoniae Alba), *xù duàn* (Radix Dipsaci), *sāng jì shēng* (Herba Taxilli) and *gān cǎo* (Radix et Rhizoma Glycyrrhizae). The formula was used to treat 26 cases of habitual miscarriage. 6 cases had premature delivery, 4 cases had a C-section delivery, and 16 had a smooth full term delivery. [17]

m) Modified *Gu Chong An Tai Yin* 固冲安胎饮 :

Contains *tù sī zǐ* (Semen Cuscutae), *xù duàn* (Radix Dipsaci), *sāng jì shēng* (Herba Taxilli), *ē jiāo* (Colla Corii Asini), *huáng qí* (Radix Astragali), *bái sháo* (Radix Paeoniae Alba), *guī jiǎ* (Carapax et Plastrum Testudinis) and *chǎo dù zhòng* (Cortex Eucommiae, stir-fried). The treatment of 60 cases of threatened miscarriage using this formula resulted in: a cure in 38 cases, excellent improvement in 10 cases, moderate improvement in 5 cases, and no effect in 7 cases. The total effectiveness rate was 83.3%. The formula was shown to inhibit uterine contraction, enhance the luteotrophic function of the pituitary-ovary axis, possess estrogen-like qualities and promote the development of the embryo. [18]

n) Modified *Bu Zhong Yi Qi Tang* 补中益气汤 :

Contains *huáng qí* (Radix Astragali), *rén shēn* (Radix et Rhizoma

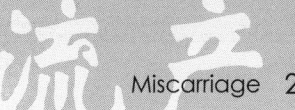

Ginseng), *bái zhú* (Rhizoma Atractylodis Macrocephalae), *dāng guī* (Radix Angelicae Sinensis), *chén pí* (Pericarpium Citri Reticulatae), *shēng má* (Rhizoma Cimicifugae), *chái hú* (Radix Bupleuri), *zhì gān cǎo* (Radix et Rhizoma Glycyrrhizae Praeparata cum Melle), *huái huā* (Flos Sophorae), *dì yú* (Radix Sanguisorbae) and *cè bǎi tàn* (Cacumen Platycladi, carbonized). The formula was used to treat 68 cases of threatened miscarriage, of which 56 cases fully recovered from the illness, 10 cases showed improvement, and 2 cases had no effect. The total effectiveness rate was 97.06%. [19]

o) *Tiao Mian No. 1* 调免I号:

Contains *nǚ zhēn zǐ* (Fructus Ligustri Lucidi), *shēng dì huáng* (Radix Rehmanniae Recens), *shān zhū yú* (Fructus Corni), *zhī mǔ* (Rhizoma Anemarrhenae), *huáng bǎi* (Cortex Phellodendri Chinensis), *dān shēn* (Radix et Rhizoma Salviae Miltiorrhizae) and *táo rén* (Semen Persicae). It was used in the treatment of 42 cases of recurrent spontaneous abortion with testing indexes AcAb, EmAb, AsAb and zPAb. The results were: 9 cases became negative in the first course of treatment, 25 cases became negative in the second course of treatment, and 6 cases became negative in the third course of treatment. The effectiveness rate was 80.9% after two courses of treatment, and 95.2% after three courses of treatment. The formula had the effect of regulating the body's immunological function. [20]

p) Modified *Yan Xue Bu Shen Gu Tai Tang* 养血补肾固胎汤:

Contains *tù sī zǐ* (Semen Cuscutae) 10-15g, *zhù má gēn* (Radix Boehmeriae Ramie) 10-15g, *chuān xù duàn* (Radix Dipsaci) 12g, *sāng jì shēng* (Herba Taxilli) 12g, *shān zhū yú* (Fructus Corni) 10g, *gǒu qǐ zǐ* (Fructus Lycii) 10g, *chǎo bái zhú* (Rhizoma Atractylodis Macrocephalae, stir-fried) 10g, *chǎo bái sháo* (Radix Paeoniae Alba, stir-fried) 15g, *shā rén* (Fructus Amomi) 6g, *huáng qín* (Radix Scutellariae) 6g and *zhì huáng qí* (Radix Astragali Praeparata cum Melle) 10-20g. It was used to treat 88 cases, of which 75 cases fully recovered from illness. There was no recovery in

13 cases. The recovery rate was 85.2%. This formula tonifies kidney qi, transforms and transports spleen qi, and eliminates fetal heat to enable it to be nourished and stabilized. [21]

(3) Acupuncture and Moxibustion

Acupuncture and moxibustion is less commonly selected to treat miscarriage, but if used properly, it can also play an important role in treatment. Yu Rongcai used warming needle acupuncture bilaterally on DU 20, ST 36, SJ 5, LR 2, SP 6, SP 10 and RN 4. Result after treating 41 cases of habitual miscarriage: 75.5% effectiveness rate.[22]

Zhou Liming needled LI 4 with drainage and SP 6 with supplementation to tonify blood and drain qi. The gathering of blood and qi has the effect of stabilizing the fetus.[23]

It has been clinically proven by Fufu Hongzhi that needling BL 67, SP 6 and KI 1 can not only inhibit uterine contraction, but also significantly increase uterine blood flow. The treatment is both effective and safe. [24]

(4) Additional Treatment Modalities
a) External Application of Medicinals:

Ingredients: *Ē jiāo* (Colla Corii Asini) 10g and *ài yè* (Folium Artemisiae Argyi) 10g. Decoct *ē jiāo* first. Dry *ài yè* over fire and grind it into a powder. Mix *ē jiāo* and *ài yè* and together and stir them into a paste. Apply this medicinal paste on the patient's RN 8 (shén quē). Cover with a gauze, use adhesive tape to keep it in place, and heat it with a hot pack over the umbilicus. This procedure is done 1 to 2 times a day to warm the channels, nourish blood and calm the fetus. It is suitable for threatened miscarriage, restless fetus and habitual miscarriage of qi and blood deficiency.[25]

Ingredients: *Dù zhòng* (Cortex Eucommiae) and *bǔ gǔ zhī* (Fructus Psoraleae) of equal quantity. Grind the medicinals into a fine powder and store the powder in a bottle. Take an appropriate amount and stir it in water to form a paste. Apply this medicinal paste on the umbilicus, and cover it with a gauze. Keep it in place with adhesive tape. This remedy primarily treats habitual miscarriage of the kidney deficiency type. [25]

Ingredients: *Dù zhòng* (Cortex Eucommiae) 18g, *bǔ gǔ zhī* (Fructus Psoraleae) 20g, *ē jiāo* (Colla Corii Asini) 50g, *ài yè* (Folium Artemisiae Argyi) 15g and *zhù má gēn* (Radix Boehmeriae Ramie) 30g. First, heat *ē jiāo* (Colla Corii Asini) in a pot until it melts, then grind the other medicinals into fine powder and add them to the melted *ē jiāo* (Colla Corii Asini). Stir well to form a paste. Apply an appropriate amount of this medicinal paste on the patient's BL 67 and RN 8, affixing it with a cloth (or gauze) and adhesive tape. This remedy is suitable for various patterns of threatened miscarriage.[26]

Ingredients: *Hán shuǐ shí* (Calcitum) 120g (60g is raw, and 60g is calcined red) is ground into fine powder and mixed thoroughly with 15g of *zhū shā* (Cinnabaris) until the color is peach red. Use only 0.9g of this powder at a time, stirring it in cold water to make a thin paste. Place a piece of paper on the patient's umbilicus first, and then pour the medicinal paste onto the paper. The formula has the effects of invigorating blood, transforming stasis and expelling the fetus. It is appropriate for treating retention of dead fetus. [25]

b) Tui Na

The patient lies down in supine position, and uses both palms to massage the abdomen clockwise for 5 to 10 minutes. The main location is the lower abdomen, and the acupoints emphasized are RN 12, ST 25, RN 6, RN 4, RN3, ST 29, ST 30, and zǐ gōng. Press and knead each acupoint for 1 minute, and push along the conception vessel from the pubic symphysis to the umbilicus with the thenar eminence. This protocol is repeated 7-9 times to treat threatened miscarriage.

When patient is in prone position, apply rolling and rotation at the lumbosacral region for 5-7 minutes. Press and knead BL 17, BL 20, BL 21,

BL 18, BL 24, BL 23 and DU 4 for half a minute on each point. Knead *bā liáo* (BL 31-34) for 2 minutes on each point, then apply horizontal scrubbing. Stop scrubbing when the skin is hot and slightly red. Finally, knead DU 20, ST 36, SP 6, SP 10 and PC 6 for 1 minute on each point. This protocol treats threatened miscarriage. [25]

2. Experimental Studies

Research on the pathogenesis and treatment of miscarriage has gradually shifted from clinical research to experimental research, which provides powerful evidence of the efficacy of Chinese medical treatment, as well as create new treatment approaches for miscarriage. Research on the pharmacodynamics of single herbs is comparatively less, and those conducted on herbal formulas can be seen below:

(1) Research on the Efficacy of Herbal Prescriptions

a. *Yun Kang Kou Fu Ye* 孕康口服液 relaxes uterine smooth muscle and reduces uterine sensibility: Wang Qinmao developed *Yun Kang Kou Fu Ye*, which was based on the empirical formula of the late physician Yang Xinwu (*Wu You Bao Tai Fang* 无癇保胎方), to treat threatened miscarriage. The oral solution contains *gǒu jǐ* (Rhizoma Cibotii), *huáng qí* (Radix Astragali), *huái Shān yào* (Radix Dioscoreae Oppositae), *tù sī zǐ* (Semen Cuscutae), *sāng jì shēng* (Herba Taxilli), *dāng guī* (Radix Angelicae Sinensis), *xù duàn* (Radix Dipsaci), *dù zhòng* (Cortex Eucommiae), *dǎng shēn* (Radix Codonopsis), *bái sháo* (Radix Paeoniae Alba) and *bǔ gǔ zhī* (Fructus Psoraleae). Experiments show that it has a similar effect as progesterone, and relaxes uterine contraction in rats and mice. also In addition, it can antagonize the excitatory effects of oxytocin and acetylcholine on the uterus.[27]

b. *Zhu Yun No. I* (助孕Ⅰ号) and *Zhu Yun No. II* (助孕Ⅱ)号 can strengthen immunity in patients who have immune-response spontaneous abortions or immune infertilities. Luo Songping designed *Zhu Yun No. I* to enrich the kidney. It is composed of *tù sī zǐ* (Semen Cuscutae), *nǚ zhēn zǐ* (Fructus Ligustri Lucidi), *jīn yīng zǐ* (Fructus Rosae Laevigatae), *gān cǎo* (Radix et Rhizoma Glycyrrhizae), *dāng guī* (Radix Angelicae Sinensis), *táo rén* (Semen Persicae), *shú dì huáng* (Radix Rehmanniae Praeparata) and other medicinals. *Zhu Yun No. II* was designed to warm the kidney and invigorate blood, and contains *tù sī zǐ* (Semen Cuscutae), *yín yáng huò* (Herba Epimedii), *dǎng shēn* (Radix Codonopsis), *jīn yīng zǐ* (Fructus Rosae Laevigatae), *chì sháo* (Radix Paeoniae Rubra), *dān shēn* (Radix et Rhizoma Salviae Miltiorrhizae), *gān cǎo* (Radix et Rhizoma Glycyrrhizae) and other herbs. Human semen was used as an antigen to test the effect of *Zhu Yun No. I* and *Zhu Yun No. II* on ASAb. The serum ASAb test showed that all are positive before the experiment. After the experiment, there was no antibody titer larger than 1:80 in the group that used *Zhu Yun No. I*. 5.3% of the *Zhu Yun No.II* group and 90% of the control group had antibody titers larger than 1:80. The difference between the groups was significant. Endocrine hormone testing showed that the level of estradiol in male rats were raised significantly ($P<0.05$) after using *Zhu Yun No.I*, but there was no change in testosterone level. Clinical trials prove that *Zhu Yun No.I* and *Zhu Yun No.II* have a positive effect on eliminating ASAb. [28]

    c. *Yun Tai Jian Bao Chong Ji* 孕胎健宝冲剂 has the effect of inhibiting uterine smooth muscle in rats. Gao Pengxiang designed *Yun Tai Jian Bao Chong Ji* which is composed of 17 Chinese medicinals, such as *rén shēn* (Radix et Rhizoma Ginseng), *cì wǔ jiā* (Radix et Rhizoma seu Caulis Acanthopanacis Senticosi) and other medicinals. Experiments proved that this formula antagonizes the effect of oxytocin, which in turn causes miscarriage in rats (without causing any malformations), and has no effect on the development of pregnant rats and their ovaries. The experiments ex vivo prove that *the dissolved medicine of Yun Tai Jian*

Bao has an inhibitory effect of varying intensity on the uterine smooth muscle of pregnant and non-pregnant rats, and antagonizes the severe contraction of uterine smooth muscle caused by oxytocin.[29]

d. *Qu Mo Tang* 去膜汤 shortens the duration of uterine bleeding after miscarriage. Zhang Tingting self-composed the formula , *Qu Mo Tang* which consists of *chuān xiōng* (Rhizoma Chuanxiong), *yì mǔ cǎo* (Herba Leonuri), *pú huáng* (Pollen Typhae) and other other medicinals. It has been shown that the formula can shorten the duration of uterine bleeding after miscarriage, reduce the quantity of bleeding, and enhance the intrauterine pressure of rabbits in utero, as well as the frequency of uterine contraction. The mechanism of this formula is eliminating stasis and stopping bleeding by contracting the uterine muscles and uterine vessels.[30]

e. *Tai Er An Chong Ji* 胎儿安冲剂 shortens bleeding and clotting time in mice. Cui Xiaoping added *wǔ líng zhī* (Faeces Togopteri), *pú huáng* (Pollen Typhae), *dān shēn* (Radix et Rhizoma Salviae Miltiorrhizae), *shā rén* (Fructus Amomi), *zǐ sū gěng* (Caulis Perillae) to *Shou Tai Wan*. Lab experiments have shown that this combination is effective in shortening the bleeding and clotting times in mice.[31]

REFERENCES

[1] Dong Kewei, Ma Lin, Na Sumei. Analysis of Chen Shiduo's Syndrome Differentiation and Treatment of Restless Fetus (Chen Shiduo Bian Zhi Tai Dong Bu An Jing Yang Tan Xi) 陈士铎辨治胎动不安经验探析. *Beijing Journal of Chinese Medicine (Beijing Zhong Yi)* 北京中医. 1997, 16(6): 5-6.

[2] Zhang Meifeng. Calming the Fetus Safely by Invigorating Blood and Eliminating Masses: Inspiration from Zhongjing's Gui Zhi Fu Ling Wan Treatment Method (Huo Xue Xiao Zheng An Tai Wu Yun: Zhongjing Gui Zhi Fu Ling Wan Fa De Qi Di) 活血消癥安胎无殒: 仲景桂枝茯苓丸法的启迪. *Shanghai Journal of Chinese Medicine and Medicinals (Shanghai Zhong Yi Yao Za Zhi)* 上海中医药杂志. 1998, (7): 27-28.

[3] Huang Jianping, Li Weihong. The Treatment of 68 Cases of Habitual Miscarriage by Tonifying the Kidney and Regulating Menstruation (Bu Shen Tiao Zhou Fa Zhi Liao Xi Guan Xing Liu Chan 68 Li) 补肾调周法治疗习惯性流产68例. *Guanxi Journal of Chinese Medicine and Medicinals (Guangxi Zhong Yi Yao)* 广西中医药. 2005, 28 (6): 15-16.

[4] Tian Bingzhao. Understanding the Treatment of Threatened Miscarriage (Xian Zhao Liu Chan Zheng Zhi Ti Hui) 先兆流产证治体会. *Hebei Journal of Chinese Medicine (Hebei Zhong Yi)* 河北中医. 2006, 28(1): 42-43.

[5] Xia Yu. He Tonglu's Brief Introduction to the Clinical Prevention of Miscarriage (He Tonglu Lao Zhongyi Ling Zheng Fu Ke Bao Tai Zheng Zhi Te Se Jian Jie) 何同录老中医临证妇科保胎证治特色简介. *Shanxi Journal of Chinese Medicine (Shanxi Zhong Yi)* 陕西中医. 2002, 23(5): 430-431.

[6] Chen Qian, Zhao Ruilin, Zou Qi. Observation of the Curative Effect of *Zi Shen Yu Tai Wan* on 231 Cases of Miscarriage (Zi Shen Yu Tai Wan Zhi Liao Xian Zhao Liu Chan 231 Li Liao Xiao Guan Cha) 滋肾育胎丸治疗先兆流产231例疗效观察. *Guangdong Journal of Pharmacology (Guangdong Yao Xue)* 广东药学. 2003, 13 (3): 44-45.

[7] Cheng Hang, Li Xiangyun. The Treatment of 115 Cases of Threatened Miscarriage with *Zhu Huang Bao Tai Fang* (Zhu Huang Bao Tai Fang Zhi Liao Xian Zhao Liu Chan 115 Li) 助黄保胎方治疗先兆流产115例. *Shanxi Journal of Chinese Medicine (Shanxi Zhong Yi)* 陕西中医. 1998, 19 (6): 241-242.

[8] Lu Qibing, Ren Qingling. The Treatment of 80 Cases of Threatened Miscarriage with *Shou Tai An Zi Tang* (Shou Tai An Zi Tang Zhi Liao Xian Zhao Liu Chan 80 Li) 寿胎安子丸治疗先兆流产80例. *The Correspondence Course of Chinese Medicine (Zhong Yi Han Shou Tong Xun)* 中医函授通迅. 1996, 15 (6): 35-36.

[9] Fu Ping. The Treatment of 24 Cases of Incomplete Miscarriage with Modified *Shi Xiao San* (Jia Wei Shi Xiao San Zhi Liao Bu Quan Liu Chan 24 Li) 加味失笑散治疗不全流产24例. *Zhejiang Journal of Chinese Medicine (Zhejiang Zhong Yi)* 浙江中医杂志. 1995, 30 (5): 205.

[10] Cong Hua, Wang Xiuqin, Yang Tao. The Treatment of Restless Fetus of the

Spleen and Kidney Deficiency Pattern with *Gu Tai San* (Gu Tai San Zhi Liao Pi Shen Xu Xing Tai Dong Bu An) 固胎散治疗脾肾虚型胎动不安. *Shandong Journal of Chinese Medicine (Shandong Zhou Yi Za Zhi)* 山东中医杂志. 1998, 17 (11): 491.

[11] Cui Shuhui, Xu Zhongqin. The Treatment of 47 Cases of Spontaneous Abortion of Unknown Causes with *Bao Tai Fang* (Bao Tai Fang Zhi Liao Yuan Yin Bu Ming Zi Ran Liu Chan 47 Li) 保胎方治疗原因不明自然流产47例. *Shanxi Journal of Chinese Medicine (Shanxi Zhong Yi)* 陕西中医. 1998, 19(6): 242.

[12] Gu Ping. The Clinical Observation of Modified *Sheng Hua Tang* in the Treatment of 84 Cases of Incomplete Miscarriage (Sheng Hua Tang Jia Wei Zhi Liao Bu Quan Liu Chan 84 Li Lin Chuang Guan Cha) 生化汤加味治疗不全流产84例临床观察. *Journal of Guiyang College of Chinese Medicine (Guiyang Zhong Yi Xue Yuan Xue Bao)* 贵阳中医学院学报. 1996, 18(3): 57.

[13] Zeng Jingen. The Treatment of 57 Cases of Threatened Miscarriage with Modified *Shou Tai Wan* (Shou Tai Wan Jia Wei Zhi Liao Xian Zhao Liu Chan 57 Li) 寿胎丸加味治疗先兆流产57例. *Practical Journal of Chinese Medicine and Medicinals (Shi Yong Zhong Yi Za Zhi)* 实用中医药杂志. 2001, 17(11): 20.

[14] Li Licai. The Treatment of 36 Cases of Threatened Miscarriage with Modified *Bao Tai Yin* (Bao Tai Yin Jia Jian Zhi Liao Xian Zhao Liu Chan 36 Li) 保胎饮加减治疗先兆流产36例. *Shanxi Journal of Chinese Medicine (Shanxi Zhong Yi)* 陕西中医. 2003, 24 (5): 397-397.

[15] Shi Shuqin, Sun Shouxin. The Treatment of 86 Cases of Threatened Miscarriage with *Bao Tai Yin* (Bao Tai Yin Zhi Liao Xian Zhao Liu Chan 86 Li) 保胎饮治疗先兆流产86例. *Shanxi Journal of Chinese Medicine (Shanxi Zhong Yi)* 陕西中医. 2002, 23 (5). 392-392.

[16] Yuan Huixia. The Clinical Research of *Bu Shen Yi Kang Tang* in the Treatment of 36 Cases of Positive Cardiolipin Antibody After Repeated Miscarriage (Bu Shen Yi Kang Tang Zhi Liao Fan Fu Liu Chan Hou Kang Xin Lin Zhi Kang Ti Yang Xing 36 Li Lin Chuang Yan Jiu) 补肾抑抗汤治疗反复流产后抗心磷脂抗体阳性36例临床研究. *Journal of Shanxi College of Chinese Medicine (Shanxi Zhong Yi Xue Yuan Xue Bao)* 陕西中医学院学报. 2005, 28(6): 28-29.

[17] Kang Yihua, Liu Fang. The Treatment of Habitual Miscarriage with *An Tai Fang* (An Tai Fang Zhi Liao Xi Guan Xing Liu Chan) 安胎方治疗习惯性流产. *Shandong Journal of Chinese Medicine (Shandong Zhong Yi Za Zhi)* 山东中医杂志. 2005, 24 (12): 754.

[18] Chen Lixing, Lin Xiaohua, Wu Xiaoke. The Treatment of 60 Cases of Threatened Miscarriage with *Gu Chong An Tai Yin* (Gu Chong An Tai Yin Zhi Liao Xian Zhao Liu Chan 60 Li) 固冲安胎饮治疗先兆流产60例. *Jilin Journal of Chinese Medicine and Medicinals (Jilin Zhong Yi Yao)* 吉林中医药. 2005, 25 (12): 15.

[19] Ding Anhua, Xu Meijie, Yu Meihong. The Treatment of 68 Cases of Threatened Miscarriage with *Bu Zhong Yi Qi Tang* (Bu Zhong Yi Qi Tang Zhi Liao Xian Zhao Liu Chan 68 Li) 补中益气汤治疗先兆流产68例. *The Forum of Chinese Medicine* (Guo Yi Lun Tan) 国医论坛. 2005, 20 (5): 28.

[20] Chen Ruiyu, Liu Rui, Yan Lefa. The Clinical Research of *Tiao Mian* No. 1 in the Treatment of Recurrent Spontaneous Abortions of Increasing Dysimmunity (Tiao Mian Yi Hao Zhi Liao Mian Yi Yi Chang Zeng Gao Xing Fan Fu Zi Ran Liu Chan Lin Chuang Yan Jiu 调免I号治疗免疫异常增高型反复自然流产临床研究. *Shandong Journal of Chinese Medicine (Shandong Zhou Yi Za Zhi)* 山东中医杂志. 2005, 24 (15): 717-718.

[21] Zhu Huiping. The Observation of the Treatment 88 Cases of Habitual Miscarriage with *Yang Xue Bu Shen Gu Tai Tang* (Yang Xue Bu Shen Gu Tai Tang Zhi Liao Xi Guan Xing Liu Chan 88 Li Guan Cha) 养血补肾固胎汤治疗习惯性流产88例观察. *Practical Journal of Chinese Medicine and Medicinals (Shi Yong Zhong Yi Za Zhi)* 实用中医药杂志. 2005, 21 (10): 593.

[22] Yu Rong. Warming Needle in the Treatment of 41 Cases of Habitual Miscarriage (Wen Zhen Zhi Liao Xi Guan Xing Liu Chan 41 Li) 温针治疗习惯性流产41例. *Shanxi Journal of Chinese Medicine (Shanxi Zhong Yi)* 陕西中医. 1993, 14 (6): 273.

[23] Zhou Liming. The Application of Needling LI 4 and SP 6 to Unblock the Channels and Calm the Fetus (Zhen Ci He Gu, San Yi Jiao Zai Tong Jing An Tai Fang Mian De Ying Yong) 针刺合谷，三阴交在通经安胎方面的应用. *Chinese Acupuncture and Moxibustion (Zhong Guo Zhen Jiu)* 中国针灸. 1995, 15 (5): 45-46.

[24] Lu Jing. The Effectiveness of Acupuncture and Moxibustion for Patients of Threatened Miscarriage (Zhen Jiu Dui Xian Zhao Liu Chan Huang Zhe De You Xiao Xing) 针灸对先兆流产患者的有效性. *Foreign Medicine. Manual of Chinese Medicine and Chinese Medicinals (Guo Wai Yi Xue. Zhong Yi Zhong Yao Fen Ce)* 国外医学.中医中药分册. 1994, 16 (3): 53.

[25] Liu Minru. *Traditional Medicine of the World: Gynecology (Shi Jie Chuan Tong Yi Xue Fu Ke Xue)* 世界传统医学妇科学. Beijing: Beijing Science Press, 1999. 287-301.

[26] Song Qiang, Yang Baimei. The Treatment of 50 Cases of Threatened Miscarriage with *Bu Du An Tai Gao* (Bu Du An Tai Gao Zhi Liao Xian Zhao Liu Chan 50 Li) 补杜安胎膏治疗先兆流产50例. *Shanxi Journal of Chinese Medicine (Shanxi Zhong Yi)* 山西中医. 2002, 18 (3): 46.

[27] Wang Qinmao, Yang Yaofang, Yao Daoyun. The Experimental Research of Preventing Miscarriage with *Yun Kang Kou Fu Ye* (Yu Kang Kou Fu Ye Bao Tai Zuo Yong De Shi Yan Yan Jiu) 孕康口服液保胎作用的实验研究. *Journal of Integrative Medicine (Zhong Xi Yi Jie He Za Zhi)* 中西医结合杂志. 1994, (7): 418.

[28] The Clinical Research of Immune-Response Spontaneous Abortion and Immune Infertility (Mian Yi Xing Zi Ran Liu Chan Yu Mian Yi Xing Bu Yun De Lin Chuang Yu Shi Yan Yan Jiu) 免疫性自然流产与免疫性不孕的临床与实验研究. *Journal of Chinese Medicine (Zhong Yi Za Zhi)* 中医杂志. 1997, 38 (6): 351-354.

[29] Cui Manhua, Gao Pengwu, Gao Pengxiang. The Experimental Research of *Yun Tai Jian Bao Chong Ji* (Yun Tai Jian Bao Chong Ji De Shi Yan Yan Jiu) 孕胎健宝冲剂的实验研究. *Journal of Chinese Medicine and Medicinals (Zhong Guo Yi Yao Xue Bao)* 中国医药学报. 1997, 12 (3): 56.

[30] Dai Deying, Wu Dunxu, Zhang Tingting. The Clinical Research of *Zhong Yao Qu Mo Tang* in the Treatment of 214 Cases of Bleeding After Drug-Induced Abortions (Zhong Yao Qu Mo Tang Zhi Liao Yao Wu Liu Chan Hou Chu Xue 214 Li Lin Chuang Yu Shi Yan Yan Jiu) 中药祛膜汤治疗药物流产后出血214例临床与实验研究. *Journal of Integrative Medicine (Zhong Xi Yi Jie He Za Zhi)* 中西医结合杂志. 1997, 17 (9): 534-536.

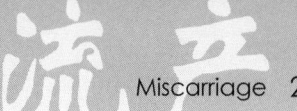

[31] Cui Xiaoping. The Experimental Research of the Hemostatic Effect of *Tai Er An Chong Ji* on Threatened Miscarriage (Tai Er An Chong Ji Zhi Liao Xian Zhao Liu Chan De Zhi Xue Zuo Yong Shi Yan Yan Jiu) 胎儿安冲剂治疗先兆流产的止血作用实验研究. *Journal of Shanxi College of Chinese Medicine (Shanxi Zhong Yi Xue Yuan Xue Bao)* 陕西中医学院学报. 2003, 26 (3): 38-40.

Index by Disease Names and Symptoms

Index by Chinese Medicinals and Formulas

General Index

G

H

I

S